MAYO CLINIC

Guide to Raising a

Healthy Child

MAYO CLINIC

Medical Editor
Angela C. Mattke, M.D.

Editorial Director
Paula M. Marlow Limbeck

Senior Editor
Karen R. Wallevand

Managing Editor
Rachel A. Haring Bartony

Senior Product Manager
Christopher C. Frye

Illustration, Photography and Production
Jeanna L. Duerscherl, Joseph M. Kane, Joanna R. King, Michael A. King, Brenda S. Lindsay, Kent McDaniel, Matthew C. Meyer, Caitlin J. Mock, James (Jim) E. Rownd, Gunnar T. Soroos, Malgorzata (Gosha) B. Weivoda, Aimee L. Wood

Editorial Research Librarians
Abbie Y. Brown, Eddy S. Morrow Jr., Erika A. Riggin, Katie J. Warner

Copy Editors
Miranda M. Attlesey, Alison K. Baker, Nancy J. Jacoby, Julie M. Maas

Indexer
Steve Rath

Contributors
Devon O. Aganga, M.D.; Jyoti Bhagia, M.D.; Bridget K. Biggs, Ph.D., L.P.; Patricia M. Collins; Kari A. Cornell; Caroline J. Davidge-Pitts, M.B., B.Ch.; Dawn Marie R. Davis, M.D.; Jessica M. Davis, M.D.; Daniel R. Hilliker, Ph.D., L.P.; Flora R. Howie, M.D.; Robert M. Jacobson, M.D.; Alexandra C. Kirsch, Ph.D.; Kelsey M. Klaas, M.D.; Suresh Kotagal, M.D.; Seema Kumar, M.D.; Heather L. LaBruna; Jocelyn R. Lebow, Ph.D., L.P.; Jarrod M. Leffler, Ph.D., L.P.; Mark S. Mannenbach, M.D.; Sarah R. McCarthy, Ph.D., M.P.H., L.P.; Mark W. Olsen, M.D.; David B. Soma, M.D.; Tori L. Utley; Allison C. Van Dusen; Brett C. Vermilyea; Laura H. Waxman; Jennifer (Jen) A. Welper; Stephen P. Whiteside, Ph.D., L.P.; Paul E. Youssef, D.O.; Michael J. Zaccariello, Ph.D., L.P.; Katherine A. Zeratsky, RDN, LD

Published by Mayo Clinic

© 2019 Mayo Foundation for Medical Education and Research (MFMER)

For bulk sales to employers, member groups and health-related companies, contact Mayo Clinic, 200 First St. SW, Rochester, MN 55905, call 800-430-9699, or send an email to SpecialSalesMayoBooks@mayo.edu.

Library of Congress Control Number: 2018911443

ISBN 978-1-893005-48-8

Printed in the United States of America

Introduction

Raising a child is an adventure with a lot of rewards and many unknowns. Fortunately, there are plenty of opportunities to provide your child with balanced, healthy life choices, and to build a strong foundation that allows your child to weather life's inevitable ups and downs.

How you teach your child at an early age to face challenges and setbacks will prepare him or her to face bigger challenges in middle school, high school and beyond. Don't worry too much if your family encounters struggles ahead. Parenting in any shape or form is rarely an easy task, but a commitment to a loving and nurturing relationship with a child has profound and lifelong rewards.

We understand that every family is different in its makeup and how it functions to raise a healthy child. When we use the word *parent*, it means any loving and supportive person devoted to raising a child. We hope that no matter what your parenting situation, you'll find the information in this book helpful and meaningful.

This book is the work of many individuals with a special interest or expertise in childhood development. A special thanks to all of those who helped make it possible.

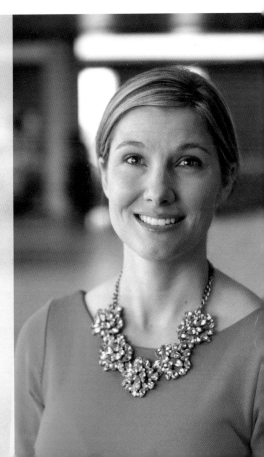

Angela C. Mattke, M.D., is a pediatrician in the Division of Community Pediatric and Adolescent Medicine at Mayo Clinic Children's Center in Rochester, Minn. In her daily work, she most enjoys seeing her patients smile and helping families who are struggling with health challenges. Dr. Mattke has a special interest in using social media to connect with patients and families and hosts a Facebook Live show with Mayo Clinic called #AsktheMayoMom. She lives in Rochester, Minn., with her husband and two sons.

How to use this book

To help you easily find what you're looking for, *Mayo Clinic Guide to Raising a Healthy Child* is divided into the following seven sections.

Part 1: Growth and development

Here you'll discover what to expect as your child moves through the preschool years all the way to getting ready for middle school. Check developmental milestones, read the latest recommendations on technology use, get a preview of puberty and much more.

Part 2: Health and wellness

Part 2 covers key elements to keeping your child healthy and safe. Get the latest information on child care, vaccines, dental health and sleep. You can also find out what to do in common first-aid and emergency scenarios.

Part 3: Fitness and nutrition

These are big topics in raising a child. In this section, you'll find trusted and up-to-date information on fitness and sports recommendations, commonsense guidelines for feeding your family a balanced diet, and proven strategies for preventing and treating childhood obesity and maintaining a healthy body image.

Part 4: Emotions and behaviors

Part 4 gives you step-by-step instructions for helping your child develop positive behaviors, cultivate resilience and foster friendships. Also learn what you can do to help your child cope with tough times and how to address common childhood mental health concerns.

Part 5: Common illnesses and concerns

Here you'll find helpful tips and remedies for managing conditions that commonly affect children, such as allergies, colds, stomachaches and others.

Part 6: Complex needs

Some children need more care than others, whether it be medical, behavioral or school-related. Part 6 addresses some chronic conditions that occur during the preschool and school-age years, as well as tips for parenting a child with complex needs.

Part 7: Being a family

Families come in all shapes and sizes. But there are some fundamental principles that every successful family adheres to as they live and learn together. Here's what you need to know.

Contents

PART 1

Growth and development

CHAPTER 1

Welcome to the preschool and school-age years

You've made it through the all-consuming baby and toddler years with your child. It's been quite a ride — exhilarating, exhausting and everything in between. You've poured your heart and soul into this little being, who has required so much of your time and energy but has given you so much in return. You've delighted in all the ways he or she has grown and changed. With each passing day, you've learned a little more about who your child is.

Throughout it all, your routines and parenting strategies have no doubt evolved to match your changing son or daughter. Adapting to these changes, you've realized, is a big part of being a parent.

Now you're embarking on a new phase: the preschool years. This period is sometimes called the wonder years. No longer in need of constant supervision, your child has become an explorer, filled with wonder and curiosity. Boundaries are being tested and the world beyond the family is opening up. Your little one is making friends and connecting with teachers or other adults. He or she is becoming much more talkative, expressing likes and dislikes — often loudly and clearly! You've noticed that your child's increasing ability to cooperate with daily tasks goes hand in hand with a desire for more independence. These changes can be both exciting and challenging.

Maybe you're already beyond the preschool years. In middle childhood, days spent at home or in a child care setting give way to hours immersed in school life, sports, and extracurricular and social activities. Your son or daughter will continue to undergo enormous changes in all areas of development — from growing physically and emotionally to making amazingly logical arguments about allowances and cellphone privileges. You'll celebrate the pleasures of this newfound

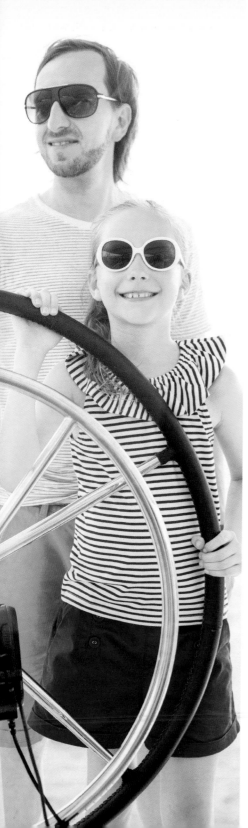

confidence and independence right along with your child and offer guidance during times of struggle. As your child's ability to reason, communicate and manage his or her feelings increases, you'll marvel at the way your baby is growing up into his or her own person.

Through all these stages, you'll continue to experience glorious and not-so-glorious moments with your child. Like everything else in life, parenting has its ups and downs. One minute you're loving the sounds of laughter and joyful noise filling the house. The next minute you're tearing your hair out because all you want is some peace and quiet. Some days you feel as if you know what you're doing, and other days — maybe most — you feel as if you're winging it. That's completely normal and to be expected. After all, parenting is the ultimate learn-as-you-go job.

BEING A GOOD PARENT

With a couple of years of parenting under your belt, you know a lot more than you did when you first held your newborn baby. Even so, every day seems to bring more to learn. You're still trying to figure out the best way to do this parenting job. This book was written to help you along the way. But don't let the desire to be a good parent turn into pressure to be the "perfect" parent.

Just as there are no perfect children, there are no perfect parents. Even parents who seem to have it all together bungle things or lose their patience sometimes. Messing up is a normal — even healthy — part of parenting. It's how we learn and improve. You won't "ruin" your child if you make a mistake (and be prepared to make plenty of them). Your child is tougher, wiser and more resilient than you think.

Instead of expecting to do everything right all the time, focus on being a committed parent. Set yourself reasonably high standards but recognize that you'll sometimes fall short. What matters is how you view those inevitable blunders and misguided parenting attempts — that you see yourself as being in this for the long haul and know that one mistake isn't the end of the world. Rather than beating yourself up or dwelling endlessly on every mishap, look at failures as opportunities to try a new approach. Use your missteps as a chance to reflect on your parenting style and assess how it's matching up with your child. Forgive yourself for not getting it right the first time, and strive to do better next time. What your child will notice is that you care and are trying.

By cutting yourself some slack, you'll be able to relax and enjoy parenting a lot more. And that will free you up to be more loving and empathetic toward your child. What's more, you'll be modeling a healthy approach to life's challenges by letting your child see that you're willing to learn from your experiences. If you and your child can face the struggles ahead together, you'll also learn to be a family together — people who can lean on each other no matter what happens.

As you step forward on this wonderful parenting journey, here are a few key points to keep in mind:

Trust your instincts You know more than you think you do. Have confidence in your ability to figure things out, even if it takes some trial and error. On the flip side, remember that even the most seasoned parents sometimes find themselves at a complete loss. It's OK to seek advice from friends, family and medical professionals. If you get unsolicited advice, take the advice that "fits" with your parenting values and feel free to forget the rest.

Make time to reflect Life as a parent can be downright hectic, and you may feel as if you barely have time to breathe. Sometimes it's enough just to get through the day and collapse into your bed at night. But if possible, try to carve out some time alone or with your partner now and then to look at the big picture. What parenting strategies are working? What might need to be tweaked or reinvented? What used to work when your child was a preschooler but isn't working so well now that he or she is a kindergartner? Asking yourself these kinds of questions will help keep you in tune with your child and the kind of parenting required at the present moment.

Appreciate your child As chaotic as life may seem with a child, these are precious years. Give yourself permission to step back and enjoy your son or daughter. Make room for one-on-one time, when you can really be present. Pay attention to your child and try to see things from his or her point of view. Take joy in the little things. For all the challenges that come with raising a child, parenting also brings an incredible richness to daily living.

Take care of yourself Taking good care of your child involves taking good care of yourself. The better you feel, the better able you'll be to care for and enjoy your son or daughter. Give yourself permission to take breaks from the responsibilities of parenting. Make time to do things you enjoy. Nurture your interests, friendships and relationships. Your child may be the center of your universe, but

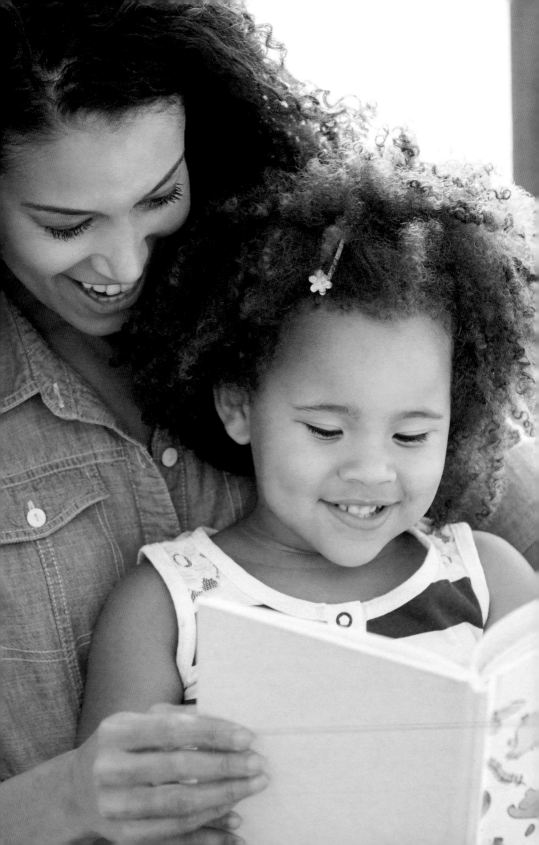

it's important to find fulfillment in other ways, too. This is another way of modeling mental and emotional well-being for your child.

Keep a sense of humor Everyone has bad days — parents and children. Sometimes things might get so frustrating that the only way out is to laugh it off and start over. Seeing the humor in a situation can lighten your mood, give you a clearer perspective and help you stay balanced. It can also help teach your child resilience and how to take a positive approach toward life's challenges. Using humor with your child can be a powerful tool in your parenting toolkit.

THIS BOOK

As you maneuver the ins and outs of parenting, a little guidance and reassurance can be of great help. *Mayo Clinic Guide to Raising a Healthy Child* is designed to help you find answers to common questions during your child's preschool and middle years. The book is also intended to provide you with reassurance that you're doing well and that the emotions and concerns you may be experiencing are the same as those of many other parents.

Dig in with whatever approach works best for you. You can turn the page and begin reading, or you can selectively choose those chapters or sections that are most important to you right now. Keep the book handy so that you can return to it when a concern arises or to prepare yourself for what may be in store in the years ahead. Remember that parenting is an adventure; enjoy the journey!

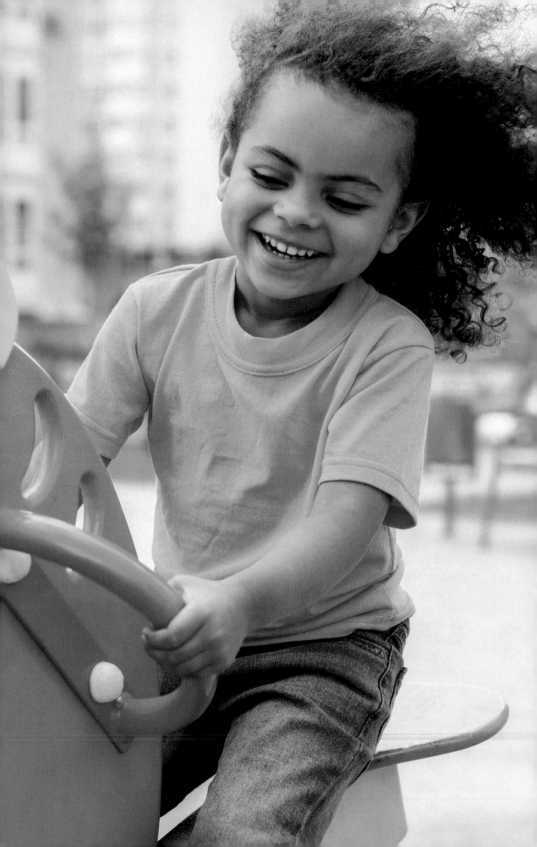

CHAPTER 2

Preschool years

The preschool years are an active time for parents. Preschoolers are full of energy and enthusiasm. Their zest for life is contagious but also sometimes exhausting. Their physical abilities and curiosity are on the upswing, yet they still need close supervision while they learn the rules of safety. Limits will need to be set and will no doubt be challenged by your child, sometimes loudly!

As preschoolers grow in confidence and improve how they communicate, they bring a whole new dimension to family life. It's exciting to watch your child grow and reach new heights. From toilet training to getting ready to enter school, there are lots of important lessons to learn between the ages of 3 and 5.

DEVELOPMENTAL MILESTONES

As children grow, they're constantly developing new skills. Things most kids can do by a certain age are called developmental milestones.

When exactly these occur varies from child to child, as each child follows his or her own growth curve and pattern of development. But checking that milestones are progressing and occur within a certain age range helps monitor development and provides early clues about any potential delays.

Tracking milestones is an important part of your child's annual checkup. Your child's medical provider may have you fill out a questionnaire that assesses your child's developmental stage and then compare that information with data from other children of the same age.

Developmental milestones are often split up into the following categories:
▶ Physical development and movement
▶ Language and speech development
▶ Social and emotional development

◗ Mental development

In this chapter you'll learn about typical preschooler milestones. If you have questions about how your child is developing at any time, don't hesitate to ask your child's medical provider.

PHYSICAL DEVELOPMENT AND MOVEMENT

Your child is becoming stronger and more agile with each passing day. In fact, you may find your child easily running ahead of you in the park, effortlessly tackling a flight of stairs, or pumping his or her legs on the swing like it's second nature.

This is also a time when your child's abilities are ahead of his or her decision-making skills, so you'll need to help your child learn to stay within safe limits and keep an eye out for potential hazards (see Chapter 10).

Height and weight gain Compared with the first couple of years of life, growth during the preschool years slows down considerably. Typical gains during this time are about 4 to 5 pounds and 2 to 3 inches in height a year. Your child's abdominal area may be starting to slim down and his or her legs are getting longer. Some children add inches to their height faster than they add pounds and may take on a thinner appearance. Most children eventually fill out as their bodies develop more muscle.

The preschool years are also a time when even good eaters can get picky about their food. This is part of growing up and becoming more independent. Eating can also be erratic, with your child refusing to eat dinner one day and devouring everything the next.

In most cases, children manage to get ample nutrition during the course of a week. Offering a variety of nutritious foods at mealtimes and letting your child decide how much he or she wants to eat is often one of the best ways to handle picky eaters. If you feel like your child may not be getting proper nutrition, talk with your child's medical provider.

Gross motor development At this age, your child is probably performing some pretty complicated moves using his or her large muscles — throwing a ball, riding a bike or climbing a tree.

How well a child does with these large-muscle tasks varies from child to child during this time. As long as your child seems to be improving his or her skills, there's typically no cause for worry. However, if you're concerned about delays, reach out to your child's medical provider.

Walking with the knees turned slightly inward (knock-kneed) and having mild flat feet — where arches in the feet are less pronounced — aren't uncommon in this age group and usually don't require treatment.

Fine motor development Increased development in brain and muscle coordination allows your preschooler to use his or her hands and fingers as much more precise tools than in the toddler years.

Preschoolers are learning to manipulate forks and spoons to feed themselves, and manage buttons and zippers to get themselves dressed.

The objects in your child's drawings are becoming more recognizable, and you may be flattered to see you're often a subject of these pictures. Children tend to depict in their drawings and paintings those things that are important to them.

DEVELOPMENTAL SKILLS BY AGE

By a certain age, most children can do certain things.

	Physical	Language	Social	Mental
Age 3	• Walk up and down stairs, alternating feet • Climb, run and pedal a tricycle • String small beads together • Cut awkwardly with scissors from side to side	• Speak 250 to 500 words or more • Speak in three- and four-word sentences • State first name • Speak clearly enough for strangers to understand about 75 percent of the time	• Take turns • Express affection openly • Easily separate from parents • Understand routine (may get upset with major changes)	• Turn book pages one at a time • Copy a circle • Do puzzles with three or four pieces
Age 4	• Hop or stand on one foot for two seconds • Catch a bounced ball most of the time • Use scissors with supervision	• Answer simple questions • Use sentences with four or more words • Speak clearly all of the time • Use words for feelings	• Cooperate with other children • Talk about likes and dislikes • Become more creative with make-believe play	• Print some capital letters • Draw a person with two to four body parts • Understand the idea of counting • Start to understand time
Age 5	• Stand on one foot for at least 10 seconds • Hop, skip, swing and do somersaults • Use the toilet independently	• Understand rhyming • Use sentences that give multiple details • Use the future tense • State full name	• Want to be like his or her friends • Follow rules and instructions • Be aware of gender • Like to sing, act and dance	• Know about common items, such as food and money • Count 10 or more objects • Copy a triangle and other geometric patterns

Vision Though eyesight can vary, by the age of 4 many children have developed 20/20 vision. However, eye problems may develop in childhood and it's important to address them promptly to help your child see better and prevent complications.

Have your child's vision checked by an ophthalmologist, optometrist, pediatrician or other trained eye specialist at least once between ages 3 and 5.

Your child's eye doctor can check for and treat common childhood eye conditions, such as crossed eyes (strabismus) and decreases in vision (amblyopia). These involve problems with the muscles of the eye and coordination between eye and brain activity.

Treatment can help correct the problem and improve your child's vision; it may include the use of eyeglasses, eyedrops or an eye patch.

Dental At this point, all of your child's baby teeth should be in place. Encourage twice daily brushing with fluoride toothpaste as well as daily flossing, and visit your child's dentist regularly for dental checkups and cleaning. Taking care of your child's teeth now can help prevent painful and costly dental problems in the future (see Chapter 7).

Sleep By this age, many children can sleep for 11 to 13 hours at night. By age 4, many children stop taking naps. Even when this is the case, though, plan for a quiet period of rest at a regular time each day. This helps prevent your child from becoming too excited or tired.

Keep a regular bedtime routine for your child. Bedtime may come earlier when naps are stopped. Encourage your child to fall asleep in his or her own bed and sleep there through the night (see Chapter 8).

LANGUAGE AND SPEECH

It's amazing to think how far your child has come in a few short years, from the babbling of babyhood to the expanding vocabulary of preschool.

This period marks the most rapid growth in terms of language development. By now, your child may know close to 2,000 words and his or her sentences are more complex.

As a general rule, your child's sentences typically will include words for each year of his or her age — for example, four-word sentences for a 4-year-old.

He or she will begin understanding concepts such as "bigger" and "smaller," follow more-involved instructions, name colors, and learn to count to 10 by age 5. Children at this age also begin using the past and future tense.

Evolving language in a young child is an important development. It provides him or her with the tools to communicate without having to act out emotions.

If your child seems to have a language delay, make sure to discuss it with your child's medical provider to rule out an underlying disorder.

Parents may become concerned if they notice their preschooler is stuttering. Rest assured: It's not uncommon for children to stutter at this age — for example, pausing while speaking or stumbling a bit on the beginning sounds of words. This may occur more often when your child is excited or feeling stressed — sometimes it's hard to get those words out fast enough!

However, if your child's stuttering is severe, occurs frequently or causes you concern, don't hesitate to talk to your child's medical provider. The provider may recommend evaluation by a speech pathologist. Speech therapy may be helpful for some children.

DEVELOPMENTAL DELAYS

The term *developmental delay* is used when a child doesn't gain skills following typical pediatric milestones. Delays can affect multiple areas, including physical abilities, socialization, and language and speech skills.

Because every child develops at his or her own pace, it can be difficult to tell whether a child is just following his or her own path or whether a developmental delay is present. Talk to your child's medical provider. If there is a developmental delay, getting your child the proper interventions and therapy early on can help manage, improve or resolve the delays by the time he or she starts school. Your child's provider can offer guidance in obtaining any needed interventions.

If at any point in your child's development, your child seems to lose skills that he or she once had, consult with your child's medical provider.

Potential signs of a developmental delay

Age 3	Age 4	Age 5
• Falls down a lot or has trouble with stairs • Drools or has very unclear speech • Can't work door handles or simple toys, such as pegboards or simple puzzles • Doesn't speak in sentences • Doesn't understand simple instructions • Doesn't play pretend or make-believe • Doesn't want to play with other children or with toys • Doesn't make eye contact	• Can't jump in place • Has trouble scribbling • Shows no interest in interactive games or make-believe • Ignores other children or doesn't respond to people outside the family • Resists dressing, sleeping and using the toilet • Can't retell a favorite story • Doesn't follow three-part commands • Doesn't understand "same" and "different" • Doesn't use "me" and "you" correctly • Speaks unclearly	• Doesn't show a wide range of emotions • Shows extreme behavior (unusually fearful, aggressive, shy or sad) • Unusually withdrawn and not active • Easily distracted, has trouble focusing on one activity for more than five minutes • Doesn't respond to people, or responds only superficially • Can't tell what's real and what's make-believe • Doesn't play a variety of games and activities • Can't give first and last names • Doesn't use plurals or past tense properly • Doesn't talk about daily activities or experiences • Doesn't draw pictures • Can't brush teeth, wash and dry hands, or get undressed without help

Source: Centers for Disease Control and Prevention

LIGHT THE SPARK

Positive habits that will help encourage your child's development in the preschool years include:

1. *Responsibility.* Let your child help you with simple chores, such as setting the table or putting clothes away.
2. *Sharing.* Take turns turning the pages of a book at bedtime or playing favorite characters during games of make-believe.
3. *Socialization.* Set up play dates with children who are about the same age as your child. Community recreation classes and sport leagues are great ways to meet children who share similar interests with your child.
4. *Independence.* Offer your child choices — for example, let him or her pick out an outfit to wear or what he or she would like for snack time.
5. *Listening and following directions.* Add multiple steps to your requests, such as "Please hang up your coat on the coat rack, wash your hands, and then help me set the table for dinner."
6. *Quiet time.* Have your child engage in a quiet activity for a short amount of time, and then gradually increase the time spent doing a low-key activity.
7. *Reading and language.* Avoid baby talk. Ask questions, encourage your child to participate in conversations and read to your child every night. Make frequent trips to your local library or bookstore. Read road signs and menus together and listen to audiobooks or kid-friendly podcasts on car rides. Practice sounding out letters. Teach your child the alphabet song and sing along, too!
8. *Writing.* Have your child practice holding a pencil or crayon correctly. Make practice fun by offering connect-the-dots puzzles or mazes. Supervise activities such as sorting coins or stringing beads to help improve grasp.
9. *Mathematics.* Practice counting to 100. Make learning shapes fun by identifying circles, triangles, squares and other shapes as you go for a walk or on your next car ride.
10. *General knowledge.* Plan trips to museums, zoos and child-friendly live theater.

SOCIAL AND EMOTIONAL DEVELOPMENT

The preschool years are a time of greater exploration and interaction with other children. Your child's sharing skills have likely improved and he or she is eager to make friends — and please them. Children this age are also getting better at handling their emotions, making tantrums a little less frequent. These are all developments that help smooth the transition to kindergarten.

Play When your child was younger, he or she likely engaged in "parallel play," which is playing alongside other children rather than playing with them. Now that your child is older, he or she is likely to play more cooperatively with friends and invent games with his or her own rules. Don't be surprised to see one "leader" in

THE IMPORTANCE OF UNSTRUCTURED PLAY

To you, it looks like a simple game of make-believe — story hour for an imaginary classroom full of students or the wrangling of a menagerie of stuffed animals as head zookeeper. In reality, your child is developing a wealth of skills. Everyone's favorite neighbor, Mr. Rogers from the beloved PBS television show *Mister Rogers' Neighborhood* summed it up best when he said, "Play is often talked about as if it were a relief from serious learning. But for children, play *is* serious learning."

In simple terms, unstructured play is an activity that is decided upon by your child and is guided only by his or her imagination and decisions — though you may supervise for safety's sake. This includes playing with dolls, stacking blocks, running, jumping, dancing and playing on playground equipment.

Play has been shown to help further cognitive, physical, social and emotional development in children. It can help children fine-tune decision-making skills, acquire new interests and allow them to move at their own pace. Academically, such play has been shown to improve the skills needed to interact with peers and solve problems. Play also gives you bonding time with your child, which is connected to increased confidence and resilience.

Unfortunately, playtime can sometimes get cut out of a child's schedule as he or she becomes more interested in watching television or playing video games. However, television and video games are considered "passive" — meaning they require little to no imagination — so it's important to make sure your child isn't losing playtime to them.

You'll also want to consider how many community and school activities your child participates in. Participating in a lot of activities can sometimes lead to "over-scheduling," which leaves little downtime for children to engage in free play and has been associated with increased anxiety and stress in children.

these play sessions. This is a common time for dominant children to start to lead other children around, which children generally don't seem to mind.

Your child's play may involve some familiar moves, including pretending to talk on a cellphone or make dinner. However, you'll also notice your child's imagination taking flight during this stage. Play is becoming more complex, such as landing a spaceship on Mars, turning into a superhero who saves the world from dinosaurs or becoming a famous ice cream inventor. Your child may turn to imaginary friends or use stuffed animals to act out his or her fantasies.

It's also common for children to tell over-the-top stories at this age. They're still learning to distinguish between what's real and what's make-believe. By age 5, though, most children can tell the difference.

Budding empathy helps preschoolers relate to others and begin to see things from another's point of view. Often, kids this age will show unprompted affection toward friends and feel bad if someone else gets hurt.

Behavior Preschoolers are famous for testing their limits and that of their parents. This early resistance can try a parent's patience, but it's also an integral part of a child's social and emotional development.

This is a time where your child is discovering two important things: (1) that he or she still has some physical limitations, which can be a frustrating barrier to what he or she wants to do, and (2) that you don't allow him or her to do certain things, which is how he or she learns about boundaries.

While preschoolers should be allowed to explore the world around them, they need clear and consistent rules to keep them safe. That's why it's important to keep enforcing rules, or you may find yourself being tested often.

Temper tantrums may still occur at this age, though they're likely to be less frequent than during the toddler years. If your child is having lengthy tantrums or having them several times a day, talk to your child's medical provider about it. The provider may offer some tips or strategies that can help and can check for any underlying issues that might be contributing to your child's mood and behavior.

Children at this age also want to please their parents. Your child wants to be like you and will mimic the things you do and say. Consider this when you talk about yourself and interact with your child and others. Early examples of positive behavior will help your child learn about healthy social interactions.

At the same time, because of a growing appreciation for rules and certain ways of doing things, children may get upset with major changes in routines. It's important to keep a consistent schedule for your child. If big changes are coming up, try to prepare your child ahead of time.

Sexuality It's normal for preschoolers to be curious about sex. Masturbation is common, as children often discover during this time that touching their own genitals brings pleasurable feelings. Sometimes children may touch their genitals in public. If this happens, try to distract your child or pull him or her aside and give a gentle reminder about the importance of privacy. By age 4 or 5, children generally understand that they should masturbate only when they're alone. As a parent, avoid overreacting to a child's masturbation.

The preschool years are also the time when your child may develop greater

TOILET TRAINING

Did you envision your 4-year-old child completely toilet trained at this point? If you find that your child is still having accidents, you probably now realize how individual this milestone is for children. As tempting as it may be to compare your child's progress with that of another child of the same age, try not to. Toilet training is often a marathon, not a sprint.

It's not uncommon for preschool-age children who stay dry during the day to have occasional nighttime accidents. As a rule, girls tend to toilet train faster than boys, and successful nighttime toilet training takes longer than daytime toilet training. If your child is still having accidents, avoid disciplining your child. Instead, assure him or her that having accidents happens and that he or she will eventually master this task as he or she grows. While you wait for this transition to happen, you can make your life easier by investing in products such as nighttime trainers and waterproof mattress covers. Keep spare clothing and sheets easily accessible, in case of an accident.

If your child seems to be having a particularly difficult time with toilet training or if it's become a power struggle between the two of you, consider backing off. Respond gently to accidents but make an effort to transfer full responsibility for toileting to your child. Once your child realizes it's up to him or her to use the toilet when the urge arises, he or she is more likely to do it independently. You can also offer incentives, such as a treat or screen time, along with plenty of praise for every time your child uses the toilet independently. Reward freely at first to increase your child's motivation.

If your child was previously dry and is now having accidents again, talk with his or her medical provider. A common cause of daytime accidents is chronic constipation. The muscles that control bowel movements also have an effect on urination. Treating the constipation will help resolve urinary leakage (see page 325).

feelings of modesty about his or her body, going from changing clothes in the middle of the living room to changing in his or her bedroom, behind closed doors.

For many parents, discussing sex begins with teaching your child about genitalia, and the correct names for them. Discussions about sex should be open and honest, but in simple terms that a child this age can understand.

Though popular culture has depicted "the sex talk" as one monumental — and sometimes awkward — conversation, living with a curious child will likely mean it will be many conversations over the years. Part of being a parent is having awkward moments and conversation. Don't let it stop you. While sex may be uncomfortable or awkward to discuss in the beginning, know that you'll likely get a lot more practice as time goes on.

Parents also worry about the danger of sexual abuse in a young child. If your child seems overly preoccupied with things of a sexual nature or seems to know more about sex than expected for his or her age, be alert to the possibility of inappropriate exposure to sexual matters or abuse. Talk to your child about the importance of privacy and that no one has the right to touch his or her genitalia. Reiterate that if someone does try to do so, your child should tell you right away (see page 150).

MENTAL DEVELOPMENT

Preschoolers' minds are buzzing with activity: solving puzzles, telling stories, creating art and just being curious. During this time you can expect your child to work his or her way up to counting to 10 and beyond, begin printing numbers and letters, and play age-appropriate board or card games. These new skills will serve him or her well as school approaches.

Off to preschool If you're getting ready to send your child to preschool, you may wonder how it will go. As your child's first teacher, you showed him or her everything from how to use a fork at dinner to how to pedal a tricycle.

So it's natural to be a little nervous or anxious about handing over the reins to someone else. If your child has spent his or her time mostly at home up till now, you may also worry about how he or she will adjust to a new setting.

Preschools offer a variety of teaching styles and settings. You can look for one that best suits your child.

Traditional preschool classrooms These tend to be teacher-led classrooms, meaning children learn in a more structured environment using curriculum developed by the teacher. The curriculum is often centered around the idea that children learn through play.

Alternative teaching styles These may focus on child-centered curriculum and let the students' interests be the guide for daily learning, rather than relying on set topics.

The child-led method is another approach, which is focused on each child's learning experience and gives children individual control over what developmentally appropriate activities they will do. Examples of alternative styles include Montessori method, Waldorf, Reggio Emilia, HighScope and Bank Street.

Faith-based settings Preschools may be faith-based, such as those located in houses of worship or sponsored by a parish or faith community. They may reflect a religion's particular beliefs.

IS YOUR CHILD READY FOR KINDERGARTEN?

As a child's fifth birthday approaches, parents often start to wonder — is he or she ready to enter school?

Knowing the alphabet and how to count can be helpful but being developmentally ready is just as important, if not more so. Your child may be ready for kindergarten when he or she displays these abilities:

▶ Listening and taking turns while talking or asking questions
▶ Following set rules
▶ Cleaning up when asked
▶ Focusing on an activity
▶ Doing basic tasks independently, such as using the toilet and washing hands
▶ Asking for help when needed

Cooperatives Some preschools may be cooperative, which requires parents to help run the school, such as helping to clean the school on certain days, organize events or fundraising.

State and federal programs Other programs, such as universal pre-K or Head Start, are public programs offered free of charge in some communities.

When selecting a preschool, you might look for one that offers educational activities that help prepare your child for kindergarten. Ideally, preschool teachers encourage expanded thinking and language skills by frequently engaging your child in conversation, asking your child questions that can't be answered with a simple yes or no, and using new words to help broaden his or her vocabulary.

To help further reading skills, teachers may read a story and then discuss story elements and what messages they convey. Look for writing, science, math and art components in your child's curriculum. The program should also offer feedback on your child's progress and allow you to meet with teachers. Consider your child's personality and how he or she seems to learn best.

Kindergarten readiness In most school districts, children must be age 5 by a certain date to enroll in the upcoming academic year. However, a child's readiness to start school goes beyond a numeric age.

The yardstick for determining if a child is ready has shifted away from focusing on academic preparedness — for example, knowing the alphabet and being able to count to 10 — to incorporating a range of factors. These include physical health, social and emotional development, learning style, language development, and mental development. Your child's school may perform a screening prior to the start of kindergarten to evaluate these areas.

Having difficulties in some of these areas doesn't necessarily mean your child shouldn't start school on time. School

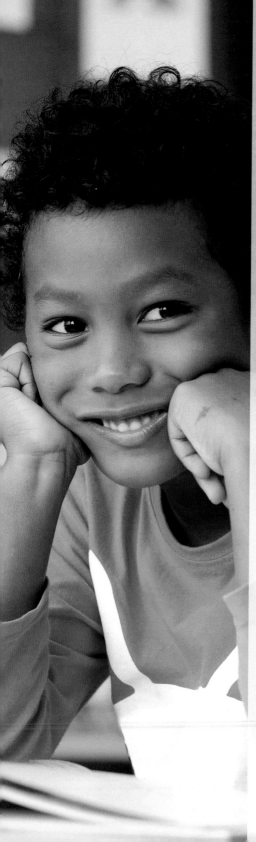

staff can help you determine when would be best for your child to start.

In case of a developmental delay or a chronic medical condition, work closely with the school district to ensure your child receives any special services he or she may need to succeed at school. For children ages 3 and up, this typically involves an evaluation by psychologists and educators, who will determine if your child qualifies for special education services (see page 463).

For some parents, concerns about their child not being ready may lead them to consider delaying kindergarten until the following year, particularly if the child's birthday is near the school district's cut-off date. This is a decision best made after careful consideration of the pros and cons and with input from the child's medical provider and teachers.

Technology At this age, you're still the biggest influence on your child. But slowly, elements such as TV and the internet are shaping how your child sees and responds to the world — even in the preschool years.

Time spent on tech devices, commonly known as screen time, has the potential to be both intellectually stimulating and intellectually stifling. But there are ways you can manage how much it influences your preschooler's development.

The American Academy of Pediatrics (AAP) recommends no more than one hour of screen time daily for preschoolers. This includes television, tablets, smartphones, video games and computers.

The reasons for this don't differ greatly from the reasons to limit screen time as your child gets older: Too much screen time can be disruptive to sleep and cut into bonding time with your child. Excessive screen time has also been associated

FIRST-DAY JITTERS

Starting preschool or kindergarten can be a nerve-wracking time for your child. But you can prepare him or her for this milestone:

▶ Have your child pick out fun school supplies, such as a backpack in his or her favorite color or a superhero-themed pencil box.

▶ Reassure your child that many children will be in the same position and also be scared on the first day. Ask your child if there's something particular about the first day of school that he or she is worried about, so that you can better address it. If your child is nervous, send him or her with a favorite object, such as a book or blanket, to offer comfort.

▶ Take advantage of any early tours. Many school districts offer an opportunity for incoming kindergarteners to visit their classroom and drop off supplies before the first day of school, when things are less chaotic. You and your child may also have an opportunity to meet the teacher.

▶ Highlight all the fun things that your child will get to do in the coming year, such as reading stories, attending class parties and going on field trips.

▶ Adjust your child's sleep schedule about a week ahead of the start of school, so tiredness doesn't make anxiety worse.

▶ Have your child spend time with adult relatives or friends if he or she isn't used to being separated from you. Set a specific time for your return to show your child that you will come back.

with problems such as lack of physical activity and difficulty paying attention.

Some parents feel pressure to introduce technology early. Given how media savvy the world has become, it's understandable that parents may feel that their child should learn how to navigate technology at a young age. But since most technology today is user-friendly and easy to learn, don't feel that you have to introduce your child to gadgets early. Your child will learn quickly when the time is right.

To help curtail the overuse of technology, consider establishing screen-free zones, such as the bedroom, and screen-free times, such as mealtime, playtime and bedtime.

If you need help formulating a media plan, visit the AAP's website for parents, HealthyChildren.org, and search for its media plan tool.

Consider these recommendations for use of specific devices, within appropriate time limits:

Television There's nothing wrong with television in moderation. However, it's a good idea to limit your child's viewing schedule to shows that offer high-quality programming. Learning is enhanced when your child has an emotional investment in a show and its characters. A show such as *Sesame Street,* for example, can be enjoyable and educational for your child.

Avoid shows with violent content and advertising, which children can have a hard time processing. Ensure your child is watching appropriate content by watching with him or her. This will also give you the opportunity to look for teachable moments and discuss what your child watches — for example, what lessons the main character learned. When your child isn't watching, turn off the television to eliminate unnecessary background noise.

Computer games and apps Not all games and apps are created equal. Many that are billed as educational have limited or no evidence of being effective. They often aren't designed to allow parents to play with their children, which can aid learning. They also don't always cover skills needed for school preparedness, such as creative thinking, which is better learned through free play. If your child does use apps, monitor his or her activity and take the app for a test drive yourself to ensure it's appropriate for your child's age.

Smartphones At this stage in your child's life, your child's smartphone use probably consists of using your phone to play games and look at photos or videos. It's up to you whether to allow your child a little time on your phone, but avoid using it to calm your child. Consider placing all of the apps your child is permitted to use on one screen or in one folder, to avoid access to apps that are meant for adults or older children.

Ebooks Depending on the ebook, there may be multiple distracting features, such as pop-ups or sound effects, which can take away from the learning experience. If you plan on purchasing ebooks or borrowing them from the library, try to go with the simplest format, and read them with your child. Interact as you would with a printed book. Shared reading time has been shown to enhance learning.

For any internet-enabled device you let your child use, make sure to implement basic safety rules. For example, a computer, smartphone or tablet should be kept in a highly visible area of your home, so that you can monitor your child's activity.

Have your child guide you through the games or other activities he or she likes to engage in. You may want to limit activity to only certain educational sites or block permission for certain functions, such as sending pictures or emailing.

Finally, one of the most important things you can do as a parent is to set a good example. Though there may be times when you need to use your phone or computer for extended periods because of work, try to limit that time so your child doesn't think screen time is a replacement for face-to-face time.

THE BIG PICTURE

The preschool years mark a wonder-filled time for parents and children. It can also be a fast-paced period as you and your child learn to face new challenges and adapt to new rules. But the more work you put in early on, the easier things tend to be later.

Sometimes, parents worry that their child may be missing a particular milestone or that their child's skills aren't progressing as expected.

Follow the schedule your child's medical provider suggests for well-child exams. These regular checkups focus on your child's growth and development. Talk with your child's provider about any concerns you may have. This can help alleviate fears and answer your questions.

Don't forget to look at your child as the unique individual he or she is. Enjoy your child's budding personality during this time. Give your child your time, attention and unconditional love.

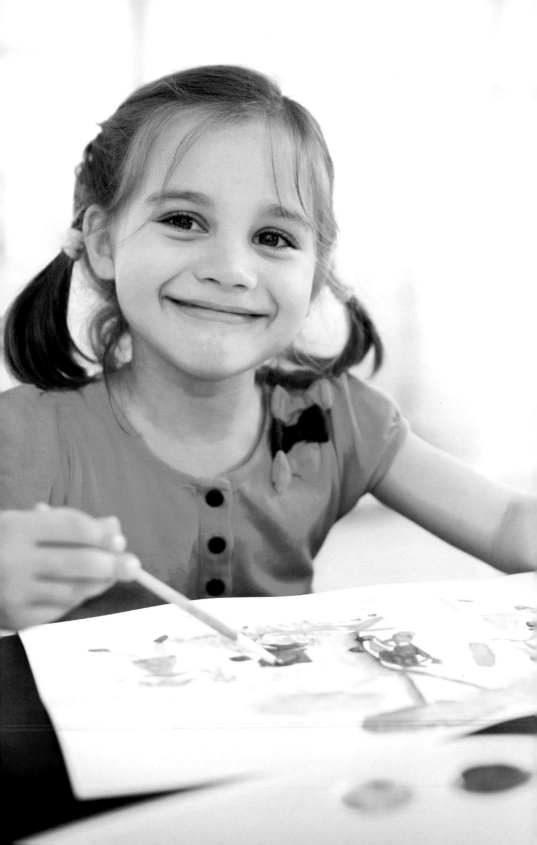

CHAPTER 3

Early elementary school years

"Look what I can do!" is a phrase you'll hear often during the early years of middle childhood. So many interesting and fun skills to learn! Children at this age can't wait to show you what they've accomplished and for you to celebrate their successes with them.

This is also a time when children start to establish the necessary life skills that will help them interact with the world as adults. As your child takes on and masters new challenges, you'll notice some major themes emerging, including budding independence and self-confidence, formation of deeper friendships, learning to try new things, and figuring out how to cope with failure.

Children this age are starting to formulate their own ideas and plans and put them into action. They're also improving in their ability to control their emotions and talk about what's bothering them.

At the same time, school is becoming a major component of your child's life. Your own relationship with your child will begin to change as classmates, teachers, coaches and others come into the picture. Your child will gradually rely on you less, but don't think of this blossoming independence as growing away from you. Think of it as your relationship evolving. You'll still be providing plenty of guidance and supervision as your child grows and matures.

PHYSICAL DEVELOPMENT AND MOVEMENT

Between the ages of 6 and 8, children continue to grow at a steady rate, even though there's plenty of variation between kids. Some children develop more slowly than others, while others develop faster. Both are OK. Vision and dental concerns may become apparent at this age, but treatment options are widely available.

As your child grows into middle childhood, here are some changes you can expect.

Height and weight gain Fairly slow and steady growth will be punctuated with growth spurts. Overall, kids grow about 2½ inches in height and gain 6 to 7 pounds in weight a year during middle childhood.

Keep in mind that physical growth and development varies from child to child based on many factors, including genetics. As long as your child is eating a balanced diet, getting plenty of exercise, and tracking along his or her own growth curve, there's generally no cause for concern about differences between children.

If you're worried that your child isn't growing or developing as expected, don't hesitate to bring it up with your child's medical provider.

Gross motor development Your child is getting stronger and more coordinated, which means he or she may be able to pull off some more-complex motions, such as mastering new dance moves or finally getting that basketball in the hoop. Your child may also be able to confidently climb a tree, catch a ball with two hands, swim or ice skate. He or she may begin to favor particular sports, especially ones he or she feels confident in.

Examples of gross motor skills at this age include:
▶ Running
▶ Galloping
▶ Hopping
▶ Skipping
▶ Kicking
▶ Climbing
▶ Throwing
▶ Catching

As with other age groups, there will be a wide variation in exactly when and how well a child can do a certain task. However, if you have any concerns, don't hesitate to reach out to your child's medical provider to address them.

Sometimes, these differences can leave your child feeling bad about himself or herself. For example, if he or she isn't as skilled as classmates in gym class or if learning to ride a bike is more difficult than your child thought it would be.

This can be tough. Support your child through the frustration. Encourage your child to keep practicing and also to discover his or her own unique strengths.

As your child learns from these experiences, it will become easier for your son or daughter to handle disappointment and move on. It will also help your child become more resilient when facing adversity (see Chapter 17).

The middle childhood years also mark a period when some children become less active. A more sedentary lifestyle can lead to health concerns down the road, such as obesity and diabetes.

At a time when children are becoming increasingly aware of their appearance and conscious of their body image, it's important to keep encouraging physical activity and healthy-eating habits as a family.

If you're concerned about your child's weight, talk with his or her medical provider. The provider can look at your child's growth charts and body mass index measurements to get a clearer picture of your child's weight and growth patterns. Part 3 of this book has more-detailed information on fitness and nutrition, as well as on preventing obesity and eating disorders.

Fine motor development As your child's fine motor skills are developing, he or she likely won't need your help as much to complete tasks. Examples of things your child may be able to do now include:
▶ Getting dressed
▶ Brushing hair and teeth
▶ Tying shoe laces

- Drawing more-detailed pictures
- Grasping a pencil correctly and writing neatly

Vision Visual skills such as the ability to focus or track moving objects are continuing to develop and improve.

At the same time, vision problems may become more apparent during these years, especially once kids start school and are assigned seats in the classroom.

If you notice that your child persistently squints, sits close to the television or complains of not being able to read the board at school, it may be that your child is having difficulty seeing properly.

Vision problems may include:

Nearsightedness (myopia) Nearsightedness is when you can't see things far away very well. It usually occurs when the eyeball is longer than normal or the

CAUSE FOR CONCERN

No two children act exactly the same. But certain behaviors, such as those listed here, may raise red flags. If these behaviors persist for more than two or three weeks, seek the help of your child's medical provider or a child psychologist.

Emotional concerns
- Frequently sad, worried or afraid
- Overly worried about trying and failing or making mistakes
- Excessively clingy or has difficulty falling asleep alone

Behavioral concerns
- Regresses to younger behaviors
- Avoids family activities or interacting with family members
- Loses interest in activities that used to be favorites
- Acts on impulse or appears out of control; takes unsafe risks
- Has difficulty dealing with emotions, such as anger
- Is preoccupied with violence, fire, or cruelty to animals or siblings

Peer concerns
- Is uncooperative with other children
- Bullies other children
- Doesn't have friends or mentions losing friendships
- Is easily hurt by peers

Cognitive concerns
- Doesn't express own ideas or interests
- Has problems communicating

School concerns
- Intense dislike of school
- Difficulty focusing or staying on task compared with peers
- Disruptive behavior in the classroom
- Strong avoidance of homework

Physical concerns
- Can't physically keep up with peers
- Has bedwetting or stool accidents
- Has a negative body image
- Sleeps too much or too little
- Reports ongoing complaints of stomachache or headache
- Experiences weight loss or excessive gain
- Misses school repeatedly due to illness

cornea is curved too steeply. Instead of being focused precisely on the retina, light is focused in front of the retina. The result is that things look blurry from a distance.

Farsightedness (hyperopia) Farsightedness means that objects or letters look blurry close-up. This occurs when the eyeball is shorter than normal or the cornea is curved too little. The effect is the opposite of nearsightedness.

Astigmatism This common problem occurs when the cornea or lens is curved more steeply in one direction than in another. Astigmatism can make things seem a bit blurry all of the time.

An optometrist or ophthalmologist can perform a complete eye exam and provide prescription eyeglasses if needed. Contact lenses are often reserved for when children are older and can assume greater responsibility for care and use of the lenses. Mild astigmatism doesn't always need correction.

In general, children need to be screened for eye disease and have their vision tested by a pediatrician, an ophthalmologist, an optometrist or another trained screener before first grade and every two years during school years, at well-child visits, or through school and public screenings.

Dental Starting at around 6 years old, your child will begin to lose baby teeth, which are replaced by permanent teeth. The average child loses about four baby teeth a year.

Around this age, your child's dentist also may be able to tell you the likelihood of your child needing braces based on problems with your child's tooth alignment, tooth spacing or bite. If there are any concerns, the dentist will refer your child to an orthodontist for a consultation (see page 108).

Have your child brush twice a day with a pea-sized amount of fluoride toothpaste. Avoid sugary drinks and foods, which can damage teeth. Ask your child's dentist whether your child might benefit from a fluoride rinse (see Chapter 7).

LANGUAGE AND SPEECH

By middle childhood, children are improving their reading and writing, and can speak in words and sentences that are easily understood.

Your child is also starting to learn that to communicate and cooperate with others more effectively, it helps to take turns when speaking, stay on topic and follow instructions.

Vocabulary is also growing. By 8 years old, most children know about 20,000 words and learn an average of 20 new ones each day.

SOCIAL AND EMOTIONAL DEVELOPMENT

Children at this age are developing a stronger sense of what is right or wrong. If you start hearing the expression "That's not fair!" more frequently, don't be surprised. Your child may get upset when someone or something goes against what he or she views as "just."

As your child gets older, you can help him or her realize that there are many different viewpoints and that the world isn't so black and white. At the same time, your child's ability to feel compassion and sympathy toward others is expanding.

7 TIPS FOR HANDLING SIBLING FIGHTS

If you have more than one child, you've witnessed your fair share of sibling bickering. This is a healthy part of childhood. Typically, children who are close in age show the most rivalry. Help your children learn to handle their own conflicts in these ways:

1. Try to stay out of minor quarrels.
2. If your children come to you with a problem, encourage them to solve the disagreement peacefully on their own.
3. Intervene if a fight escalates. Don't allow hitting, breaking things or name-calling, for example.
4. If you need to get involved, try to remain fair and neutral. Avoid comparing your children.
5. Give each child a chance to freely express his or her point of view without interruption.
6. Encourage empathy toward one another by asking your children to look at the dispute from different viewpoints.
7. Encourage your children to strive for a compromise.

Your child is also learning that hard work can yield rewards — a good grade on a project that took a lot of time and effort. He or she is also realizing that not every endeavor will be successful — diligently practicing soccer skills doesn't mean always being able to score a goal. Learning that not every attempt will end in success is a difficult but important life lesson. Offer your child support and encouragement to keep trying and not take these disappointments to heart.

Play Most likely, your child will gravitate toward playmates who are the same sex and who enjoy playing the same games. He or she also is learning that people are complex. For example, a person can be your friend and play with you but can disappoint you sometimes. Chapter 18 has more on childhood friendships.

While fantasy play dominated the preschool years, children in the school-age years start gravitating toward games where there are rules and the ultimate goal is "to win." Continue to encourage your child to engage in free play. Unstructured playtime can help boost young brains (see page 29).

Behavior As they get older, children start to care more about what their peers think. In an attempt to fit in, your child may start to do or say things that he or she knows are wrong, including things that are potentially dangerous.

Now is also a common time for children to test boundaries by lying, cheating or stealing. Talk to your child about peer relationships and friendships, and how he or she can still fit in with peers without engaging in unacceptable or dangerous behavior. Avoid harsh punishments that don't fit the crime. See Chapter 16 for more on encouraging positive behavior.

Dealing with prejudice Children notice differences among people at an early age, even as early as 6 months old. By the time they're preschoolers, children already start to internalize stereotypes, biases and prejudices that they notice in those around them and what they see and hear in the media.

You can teach your child to respect and appreciate human differences. Talking about differences doesn't increase prejudice. It's important that your child receive simple, matter-of-fact answers to questions about differences in characteristics such as ethnicity, race, social class, religion, ability, gender identity or sexual orientation.

Parents often find they need to confront their own biases before teaching their children how to handle the stereotypes and prejudiced viewpoints their children may encounter.

It may help to think about the worldviews and "filters" you've acquired over time. Are they accurate and reflective of current realities? Are they kind and compassionate? Kids quickly become aware of attitudes and unspoken rules. Examine your actions and the messages you're sending to your child.

To counteract stereotypes and biases your child may be exposed to:

▶ *Set a good example.* The way you treat people who differ from you will create a foundation for your child's behavior. Show your child what it's like to treat all people with respect and courtesy, even when it involves personal discomfort or standing out from the crowd.

▶ *Discuss prejudice.* If your child displays intolerant behavior, talk to him or her about it. Ask why your child acts or feels that way. An honest discussion will help you and your child identify and correct developing biases.

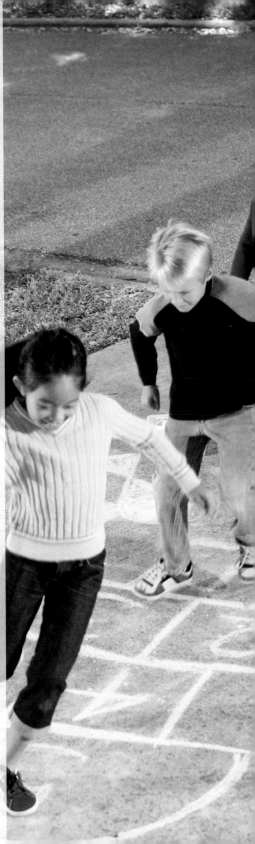

When you see an example of prejudice or a stereotype in a movie or in a magazine, point it out to your child. Explore how stereotypes project an oversimplified view of individuals who, in fact, can be very complex.

▶ *Expose your child to diversity.* Encourage your child to interact and form friendships with children from all backgrounds. One of the best ways to learn about other people is to be friends with them. Read books and watch movies about other cultures. Help your child understand that the world is a big and interesting place.

▶ *Talk about your family heritage.* Help your child understand the diversity in his or her own background. Share any family history of immigration.

▶ *Get active.* Be a voice against prejudice in your community.

An atmosphere of prejudice can deeply affect children, creating social and emotional tension and causing anxiety and hostility.

Being rejected or harassed because of personal characteristics can cause emotional and sometimes physical harm. It can make a child feel unworthy. This can lead to social withdrawal, anxiety, depression and lower academic performance.

If your child experiences bias or prejudice, allow your child to express his or her feelings, which may include anger, fear or sadness. Provide emotional support and look for ways to bolster your child's self-confidence. Talk with your child about the best way to respond.

Sexuality Interest in sex gradually increases as children get older. Though children often still think of the opposite sex as icky, children this age are becoming increasingly interested in how boys and girls differ. Masturbation is common. It's important for children not to be shamed or punished for their inquisitive nature or actions.

Your child may start approaching you more often to answer his or her questions about sex. It may feel awkward talking with your child about sex, but strive to be open and honest in your discussions, and let your child know that you'll always be there to talk. By doing so, you show your child that it's OK for him or her to come to you with questions or concerns — an important step in protecting your child from sexual abuse.

Accurate and open communication also increases the odds that your child will understand your values and make appropriate choices about sex later on. Here are some tips for talking with your child about sex:

▶ Let your child set the pace with questions. Or if necessary, ask your child if he or she has any questions.

▶ Answer questions in terms your child can easily understand.

▶ Teach your child the correct terms for body parts and sexual activity. This gives your child the vocabulary to ask questions and express concerns.

▶ Look for everyday opportunities to bring up sex, sexuality and relationship issues in an age-appropriate manner.

▶ As your child matures and asks more-detailed questions, provide more-detailed answers.

MENTAL DEVELOPMENT

Your child's mind is developing rapidly during middle childhood. Awareness of the future and the concept of time is improving. Children may enjoy planning out the days and weeks ahead. They may start thinking about what they want to be when they grow up.

GENDER IDENTITY

By middle childhood, most children have developed curiosity about their gender identity, which may be expressed through clothing, behavior, interactions with others and how a child speaks about self-identity.

While gender identity is often the same as the sex your child was born as (sex assigned at birth), this is not always the case. When a child identifies as something other than the sex assigned at birth, this is referred to as "gender nonconforming." Some children will not identify with either gender, and some may identify with the opposite gender. Still others may feel like they fall somewhere in between genders. Distress that may accompany the mismatch between sex assigned at birth and gender identity is called gender dysphoria. However, cross-gender behaviors are common in children and may not be associated with dysphoria or persist into adulthood.

Children who are gender nonconforming may be at risk of stigma, prejudice and discrimination, particularly at school. It's natural as a parent to want to protect your child. Some parents may try to encourage a child to adopt more-traditional gender-related behaviors or write the child's behavior off as a phase. However, children who are gender nonconforming have better health outcomes when they're affirmed and supported. The most important thing a parent can do for the child is to provide a safe home where the child receives unconditional love and acceptance.

If you have any questions about your child's gender identity, speak to your child's medical provider, who can provide resources for you. This may include a referral to a specialist with experience in gender-related concerns.

You may also notice that your child is becoming better at problem-solving. As their brains mature, children at this age are able to contemplate decisions and devote longer periods of time to tasks. These are important milestones for being able to learn in school.

School success Being involved in your child's education is an important way to help increase your child's academic success, especially during these early years. Transitioning between grades can be difficult for children, as learning environments become more structured and class work becomes more challenging.

The first few years of elementary school are focused on reading, writing and basic math. By the third grade, the amount of schoolwork increases, and children are required to focus on increasingly complex tasks for at least 45 minutes.

Reading moves from recognizing words on sight to reading comprehension and working to understand the content. Writing progresses from spelling words correctly or writing neatly to creating sentences that convey a theme or idea.

If you notice your child is struggling, reach out to your child's teacher to share and confirm your child's difficulties. The teacher may have some strategies to help your child. Touch base with teachers frequently to gain observations about your child's learning. A note of encouragement from you, tucked inside a lunchbox or book bag, can give your child an emotional boost during the day.

Establishing routines in these areas can help your child stay organized and on track:

▶ *Homework.* Set aside a specific time each day for your child to do homework or study or review topics he or she learned that week. Avoid having your child do homework right before bedtime, which can encourage procrastination and detract from your child's sleep schedule. Help your child create a calendar with all of his or her assignments. This will help your child plan ahead and avoid missing deadlines for homework.

▶ *Sleep schedule.* Enforce a consistent wake-up time and bedtime to ensure your child gets enough sleep each night. Not getting enough rest can negatively impact school performance and behavior (see Chapter 8).

▶ *Reading.* Spend time each night reading with your child.

Learning disorders Learning disorders affect a child's ability to complete a task or use certain skills, particularly in school, and make it difficult to read, write or do simple math.

Unfortunately, children can go a long time before they're diagnosed with a learning disorder. This can impact academic success and affect a child's self-esteem and motivation.

Signs of a potential learning disorder include:

▶ Problems recognizing and writing letters of the alphabet
▶ Persistent letter confusion
▶ Trouble understanding letter sounds
▶ Limited ability to recognize words on sight
▶ Difficulty with basic reading and writing tasks
▶ Poor handwriting, even with effort
▶ Extremely tight pencil grip
▶ Difficulty with timed tasks
▶ Difficulty learning basic math facts or multiple-step arithmetic
▶ Problems understanding directions, and resultant behavior issues
▶ Poor performance in some academic areas compared with others
▶ Problems interacting with peers
▶ Persistent reluctance to go to school

If you think your child may have a learning disorder, talk to your child's medical provider and teacher. Early diag-

THE IMPORTANCE OF THE ARTS

The National Endowment for the Arts published a review of almost 20 studies, looking at how the arts impacted social-emotional development. The studies looked at children who participated in activities such as music, dance, theater, drawing and painting. These children were found to have strong social-emotional skills, such as helping, sharing, empathizing and regulating their emotions. It's believed that the arts can help foster connections to people and allow children to express feelings and emotions.

nosis and intervention can help your child cope with these obstacles and establish a more secure academic foundation (see Chapter 22).

The gifted child Children may be considered "gifted" in any number of areas, including academics, music, the arts and sports. While there's no one recognized standard for what makes a child "gifted," intelligence and skills beyond the child's years are one hallmark. IQ scores are sometimes used to identify varying degrees of academic "giftedness." However, these scores aren't always accurate, as factors such as language barriers, attention or behavioral challenges, and poor test-taking skills can affect the results.

It might be tempting to think parents of gifted children have an easier time raising their children because of their children's talents. However, these children may have their own challenges.

Children who are considered gifted or advanced for their age may have problems fitting in with peers because their social skills don't always match that of their peers. They may have behavioral problems that stem from the frustration of being bored in the classroom.

Gifted children can also struggle with learning disorders and other conditions that can hinder their progress in school, such as attention-deficit/hyperactivity disorder (ADHD), autism spectrum disorder, anxiety and depression.

To help your child develop his or her gifts, find a program that aligns with your child's abilities and is challenging enough to keep him or her engaged but not so challenging as to lead to discouragement.

Usually, a combination of methods is needed to get the best educational experience. This might include supplemental measures such as accelerated or enrichment classes, or more-comprehensive

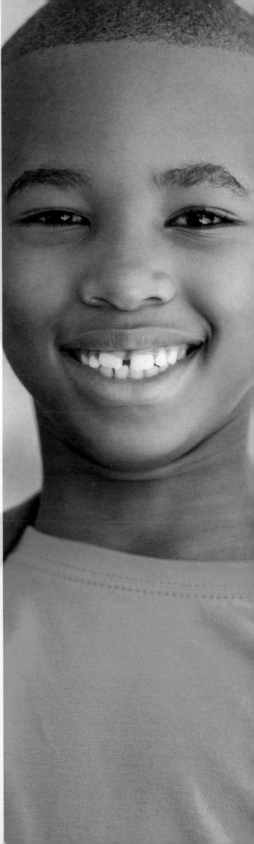

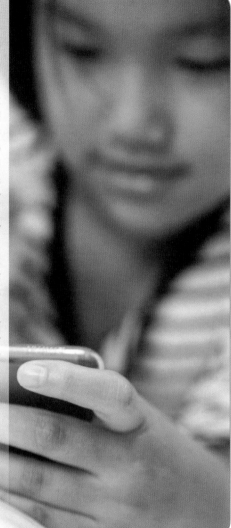

SHOULD I GET MY CHILD A CELLPHONE?

Some parents wonder when is a good time for children to get their own phones. Cellphones are a convenient way to keep in touch with your child and can be very helpful in an emergency. However, having a smart phone also exposes a child to risks associated with internet and social media use. In addition, scrolling through apps may replace other more healthy activities, such as playing outside with friends or studying.

Among experts, there's no clear-cut consensus on this issue. You know your child best. Consider your child's maturity and responsibility before making a purchase. You might consider purchasing a phone that allows for phone calls and texting but has very few "bells and whistles," such as internet access.

solutions such as classrooms or schools that cater to those children with similar advanced intelligence or skills.

Technology Used appropriately, technology can have benefits for children at this age. The internet can offer children new or differing ideas and knowledge. Email or messenger tools can provide children with the opportunity to connect and collaborate with classmates on homework and school projects.

Social media can provide resources to children and their families who are looking for support networks within a certain school or neighborhood, or for a certain health condition. Online groups can also provide inclusion and understanding to children who identify as lesbian, gay, bisexual or transgender, and their parents.

On the other end of the spectrum, excessive screen time at this age has been linked to lack of physical activity and sleep disturbances, and later on, depression and other mental health concerns. The internet can also contain misinformation and inappropriate content for children, as well as present privacy issues.

Currently, the American Academy of Pediatrics (AAP) recommends two hours or less of screen time daily for this age group — including computers, cellphones, television and tablets.

Consider these tips for guiding your child's media use, based on AAP recommendations:

▶ Be clear with your child about what types of media he or she is permitted to use.

▶ Set limits on duration of media use.

▶ Monitor the content your child is being exposed to.

▶ Use parental control tools to limit your child's exposure to inappropriate material.

▶ Teach your child about online responsibility and safety, such as treating others with respect, avoiding cyberbullying, staying away from online solicitation, and avoiding communication that compromises personal privacy and safety.

▶ Develop a network of trusted adults, such as grandparents or other relatives, with whom your child can interact online.

▶ Discourage use of entertainment media during homework.

▶ Set aside screen-free times, such as during meals, so you can interact as a family.

▶ Make sure that screen time doesn't interfere with your child's sleep and physical activity.

▶ Shut off screens one hour before bedtime to allow time to "unplug."

▶ Don't allow electronic devices in the bedroom during sleep hours.

To set clear and consistent rules on screen time, consider developing and following a family media use plan that outlines times and places for media use.

ENJOY THESE YEARS

As your child grows, learns and discovers, each day will bring a new layer of identity and potential. Enjoy your child during this time, and know that your support, guidance and unconditional love play a big part in this amazing transformation.

Be a good example for your child. He or she watches what you do. Model the behaviors and beliefs you hope to see in your child. This helps your child understand what you value. And don't forget to incorporate some fun along the way.

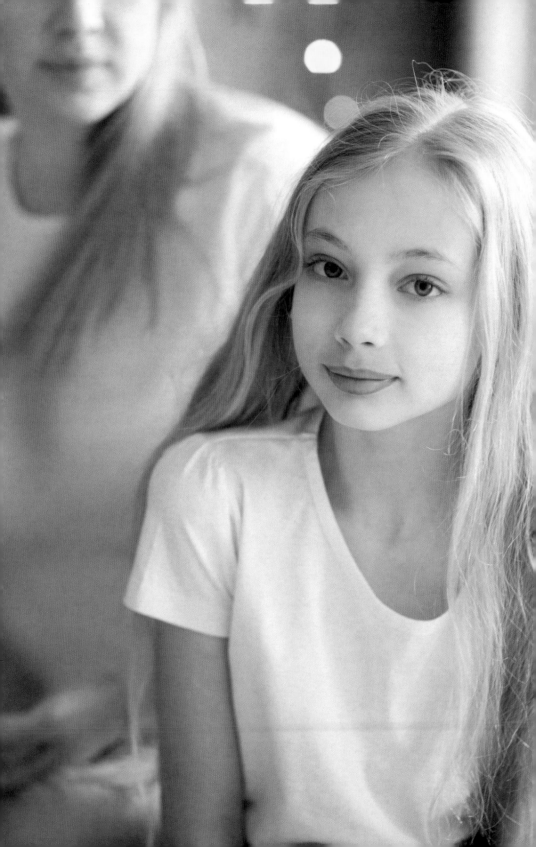

CHAPTER 4

Late elementary school years

Children in middle childhood are fun to be around. On one hand, they're becoming more independent and don't require the labor-intensive attention of the earlier years. On the other hand, they still like to spend time with their parents, telling silly stories and sharing the latest knowledge they've acquired.

Children now begin to develop a more complex sense of who they are and what their abilities are. They also begin to develop a sense of their place in the world, and they start to learn how to cope with the ups and downs of life.

At this age, your child will likely spend much of each day with teachers, care providers, coaches and friends. But the time you spend with your child during middle childhood is just as important to his or her development as it was during younger years. He or she will still need you for unconditional love and support. Your child may not always come right out and ask for help — some topics, such as puberty, can be embarrassing to bring up — but stay close and available.

Don't be surprised if you find yourself getting into some thought-provoking conversations with your child. He or she has a mind that's developing in wonderful ways, including an increased ability to reason, understand cause and effect, work through hypotheticals, and discuss more-abstract ideas.

Physically, there's a lot of variance among children this age. As your child's self-concept takes shape, so, too, does the urge to compare himself or herself to peers. It's helpful to remind your child that people come in all shapes and sizes.

PHYSICAL DEVELOPMENT AND MOVEMENT

Your child's body will be undergoing some major changes during the approach to puberty, thanks to the production of the hormones estrogen and testosterone. These changes can leave children feeling a bit unsure or uncomfortable with their

CAN A CHILD'S ADULT HEIGHT BE PREDICTED?

There's no proven way to predict a child's adult height. However, several formulas can provide a reasonable guess for a child's growth. Here's a popular example:

▶ Add the mother's height and the father's height in either inches or centimeters.
▶ Add 5 inches (13 centimeters) for boys or subtract 5 inches (13 centimeters) for girls.
▶ Divide by two.

A child's height is largely controlled by genetics. Also, children grow at different rates. Some children begin their growth phases early, while others are late bloomers.

If you're concerned about your child's growth, talk to his or her medical provider. Having the provider plot your child's growth on a standardized growth chart can determine if your child is following his or her curve, as well as help predict adult height.

bodies. It's important to discuss with your child the physical and even emotional changes that can accompany puberty, ideally before they occur, so that your child is prepared for them.

Height and weight gain Growth remains fairly steady — about 6 to 7 pounds of weight gain and 2½ inches of height increase per year.

But this is also a time of growth spurts, with girls typically experiencing them at earlier ages than boys. During a growth spurt, a child can grow up to 4 to 5 inches. These growth spurts usually will correspond with periods of increased appetite and a greater need for sleep.

Because puberty-related changes to the body can result in weight gain that's concentrated in areas such as the belly, children may be tempted to diet or restrict eating.

Continue to promote healthy, flexible eating habits and plenty of physical activity. For more on helping your child maintain a healthy body image and healthy eating habits, see Chapter 14.

Gross motor development Running, jumping and skipping are likely second nature at this stage. Now that body control has greatly improved, your child is focusing more on becoming stronger and faster. He or she is fine-tuning motor skills that allow for more-coordinated movement and perhaps competing in favorite sports, such as passing a soccer ball to a teammate, walking a balance beam or dribbling a basketball.

Fine motor development Improved handwriting and drawing skills are evidence of your child's fine motor development. Your child may also display greater ability in using tools and cooking utensils, and manipulating small objects.

A preference for using the right hand or left hand, which begins to emerge in the preschool years and gradually becomes more evident, is typically set by this point.

Vision If your child wears glasses, you may notice his or her vision worsening. Visit regularly with your child's eye doctor.

CAUSE FOR CONCERN

It's not uncommon during this time to have concerns about your child's emotions and behavior. Most school-age kids feel down or act out from time to time. But if your child displays persistent negative emotions or behaviors, for several weeks, speak with his or her medical provider. Addressing concerns and identifying underlying causes at an early stage can help your child get the assistance he or she needs. Part 4 of this book has more information on childhood emotions and behaviors. Chapter 14 has guidance on body image concerns.

Emotional concerns

▶ Is sad or depressed most days
▶ Is overly anxious, nervous or worried
▶ Has extreme mood swings
▶ Loses interest in activities he or she once enjoyed
▶ Is easily discouraged by failures
▶ Talks about hurting or killing himself or herself

Physical concerns

▶ Lacks signs of growth or other physical changes
▶ Has gained more weight than expected at this age and is sedentary
▶ Shows poor appetite

Body image concerns

▶ Closely monitors food intake or counts calories
▶ Is afraid of gaining weight
▶ Binge-eats
▶ Is preoccupied with exercising

Behavioral concerns

▶ Is disrespectful or defiant; argues often
▶ Withdraws from family and friends
▶ Is overly dependent
▶ Engages in risky or potentially harmful behaviors
▶ Frequently gives in to peer pressure
▶ Has violent outbursts
▶ Bullies or harms others
▶ Has been bullied or harmed
▶ Shows signs of abusing drugs or alcohol

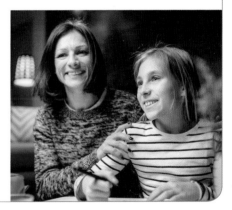

Blurry vision when looking at objects far away, called nearsightedness or myopia, typically develops during the early elementary school years and may worsen throughout the teen years. It may rapidly worsen around the ages of 11 to 13. By the late teens, vision usually stabilizes.

Dental With adult teeth coming in at a rate of approximately four per year, you can expect your child to have about eight permanent incisors — the teeth that neighbor the front teeth — and four permanent molars — the larger teeth toward the back of the mouth. Around age

11, you will see emerging premolars — the smaller teeth that are in front of the larger molars (see Chapter 7).

SEXUAL DEVELOPMENT

The first stages of puberty generally begin anywhere between ages 8 to 13 in girls and ages 9 to 14 in boys. The onset of puberty provides a good opportunity to talk with your child about sexual development, whether or not you've already done so.

You can help prepare your child for the cascade of changes that his or her body will go through during the next few years. The goal is for your child to welcome these changes without shame or anxiety that they're occurring too quickly or too slowly.

Don't worry if your child's puberty starts a little earlier or later than that of his or her peers. This is rarely a medical problem. However, your child may feel awkward and self-conscious about diverging from the average schedule.

Be sensitive to your child's feelings. Reassure your child that he or she is fine. It may help to stress that every child, including your child and each of his or her peers, is traveling along the same road toward adulthood and that everyone takes a different amount of time to arrive.

Girls and puberty Though age can vary, it's typically around 9 or 10 that girls begin to experience the first signs of puberty. Multiple factors, such as race and weight, can affect timing. Signs and symptoms include:

Breast buds These feel like small, firm lumps beneath the nipples that may feel tender or sore. It can be easy to mistake this for a cyst or other abnormal growth, but rest assured it's normal.

Pubic hair In many girls, the second sign of approaching puberty is the development of pubic hair, which typically comes in as thin, sparse hairs. As time goes on, these will begin to grow darker and coarser in texture.

Body shape Girls tend to add fat around their stomach area in preparation for redistribution to hips and breasts. Unless the weight gain is excessive, there is typically no cause for concern. However, some girls may be upset to see their body take on a more rounded appearance. Reassure your daughter that this is normal and discourage the temptation to diet.

Menstruation Girls typically get their periods about two to two and a half years after the development of breast buds, so now is the perfect time to prepare her for this milestone.

Be open and honest in discussions you have with your child about menstruation, and be available for any questions.

Boys and puberty As with girls, when boys start puberty varies, but it's often around age 10 or 11. At this time, most boys are starting to undergo significant physical changes.

Testes enlargement At the beginning stages of puberty, the testicles and scrotum almost double in size. Skin on the scrotum undergoes several changes in appearance, including darkening and the development of hair follicles, which appear as small bumps. One testicle may hang lower than the other.

Eventually, the penis grows longer, then wider. There may be pimple-like

PREPPING FOR PERIODS

Menstruation can be a bit mysterious and scary for girls. They may be afraid of suddenly getting their period at school and of being unprepared, or worry that menstruation is painful. Some may think that getting their period means they won't be able to do the things they used to do, such as swimming.

An open discussion about menstruation ahead of time can soothe these fears. Ovulation is a tricky topic for a child to understand, so you may want to show your daughter a diagram of the female reproductive system to help you explain why and how it happens. Here's an example of how to describe menstruation in a kid-friendly way:

"Your ovaries are two small, grape-sized organs filled with hundreds of thousands of tiny eggs. Around puberty, your ovaries begin to release eggs. Once this begins, if you have sex and one of your eggs is fertilized, you could become pregnant. If the egg isn't fertilized, the egg and the lining of your uterus are eliminated (shed) through your vagina. This may look like a lot of blood, but it's not really that much. When this happens, it's called having your period (menstrual cycle). You wear a pad in your underwear or a tampon to absorb the fluid and change the pad or tampon every few hours.

"Each period typically lasts two to eight days. It's very common for your first few periods to be irregular and unpredictable. Keep track on a calendar when your periods begin. Over the next two or three years, your periods will become more predictable and you'll probably start to see a pattern, so you'll know approximately when to expect the next one. On average, periods occur every 28 days, or once a month. But everyone is different. Most girls get their periods about 21 to 35 days apart."

You might also discuss that periods can be uncomfortable and that many girls have premenstrual symptoms (often called "PMS") in the days before a period begins. Common symptoms include cramps, headaches, bloating, feeling tired, mood swings and breast tenderness. Over-the-counter medications such as ibuprofen can help with pain relief.

With discussions about menstruation starting before her period begins, your daughter may be curious about when she'll actually get hers. While girls tend to get their first periods around the same time as their mothers did, there's no way to know for sure, so it's good to be prepared. Show your child how to use a sanitary pad and have her carry one in her backpack, just in case. While you child may choose to use tampons later on, it's a good idea to have her start off with pads, which are generally easier to use.

WHEN PUBERTY COMES EARLY

The term *precocious puberty* is used to define puberty signs and symptoms that come before age 8 in girls and before age 9 in boys. For girls, this might mean breast growth before age 8. For boys, it may mean enlarged testicles and penis before age 9. Both girls and boys may develop pubic or underarm hair, rapid growth, acne and adult body odor at this early age.

In many cases, the cause of precocious puberty isn't known and is attributed to a puberty process that just starts too soon. In other cases, an underlying medical disorder, genetics, or exposure to external sources of estrogen or testosterone, such as creams and ointments, may be to blame. Potential complications include shorter height and self-esteem issues.

Children displaying early signs of puberty should be evaluated by their medical provider. The provider will perform tests to determine what may be causing precocious puberty. Depending on the trigger, treatments such as medications to delay further puberty-related development until the proper age or addressing underlying medical conditions may be recommended.

---

growths close to the head of the penis — these normal growths are called papules and don't require treatment.

This is a time when boys may compare their genitalia to their peers. If your child is concerned about differences, you might point out to your child that penis size and appearance vary greatly among children, and that this is rarely a reason to worry.

Pubic hair Your son may notice a few soft hairs appear around the base of his penis, which will eventually turn thicker and curlier. Later on, the pubic hair will spread up in a thin line to the bellybutton.

Body shape As puberty sets in, some boys look to be all arms and legs. Others might be shorter than most girls for a while. In general, boys' bodies will even out during growth spurts, when height increases and the trunk of the body grows and catches up. As puberty progresses, fat is replaced by muscle.

Ejaculation and erections Though your son likely knows by now that touching his penis can bring about good feelings, this is around the time when children become sexually mature enough to orgasm and ejaculate.

Ejaculation may happen as a child masturbates or involuntarily while he sleeps (wet dream). Your child may be confused and embarrassed when he wakes up with the bed wet. Assure your son that this happens to all boys and that these involuntary occurrences will gradually stop.

Though erections are typically associated with sexual arousal, a boy's penis can become hard for no identifiable reason during puberty. There's not much a boy can do about them, except take some comfort in the fact that these occurrences will decrease in frequency as time goes on.

Voice Toward the end of middle childhood, you may notice your child's voice occasionally cracking. This is temporary and a normal part of puberty related to the growing voice box (larynx) and changing vocal cords.

Breasts Though breast growth is something more commonly associated with girls, it does occur in boys, as well. Your son may complain about sensitivity or discomfort in the nipple area. This is normal.

In some boys, breast growth may be more extensive, a condition called gynecomastia. This condition usually disappears in a year or two. However, it's a good idea to check with your child's medical provider to ensure it's not the result of an underlying condition, medication or overexposure to products containing ingredients that mimic estrogen, the hormone that most strongly influences female sexual development.

LANGUAGE AND SPEECH

By the time a child is in fourth and fifth grade, language gains many more uses. You may notice your child's increasingly

6 WAYS TO BOOST YOUR CHILD'S SELF-CONFIDENCE

1. Set aside time to hang out and talk — whether it be about friends, accomplishments or setbacks.
2. Be involved in your child's school. Maintain regular contact with your child's teachers and attend school events.
3. Encourage your child to be a "joiner," participating in school and community groups.
4. Talk about not giving in to peer pressure. Support at home and a healthy sense of self-worth can help your child handle social demands appropriately.
5. Do things together as a family.
6. Show affection and offer praise regularly.

sophisticated use of words to joke, argue and ask questions. Your child's quick wit or dry humor may catch you by surprise. You may also find that the two of you are able to hold some pretty in-depth conversations.

Slang, as well as swear words, may make their way into conversation. The latter may prompt reminders from you about what's appropriate language in your family and what's not.

This is also the time when children are getting better at understanding figurative language, such as, "It's hotter than the sun out there!" The way they talk and write sentences also is becoming more sophisticated. In fact, older children may be writing their own stories.

In late elementary years, children can typically:

▶ Translate ideas into words
▶ Learn new words by looking at the context of a sentence
▶ Better organize thoughts and information in speech and writing
▶ Write stories that include a beginning, middle and an end
▶ Conduct research to write on a specific topic

▶ Read between the lines or understand what an author means, even if the idea isn't explicitly stated
▶ Read developmentally appropriate books without many mistakes, moving from simple chapter books to more-complex stories.

SOCIAL AND EMOTIONAL DEVELOPMENT

The world is starting to develop more layers in your child's eyes. He or she is realizing that people have different points of view, and that he or she may not always agree with them. These later elementary school years also mark a time when your child can become more easily upset by criticism. As a parent, you can model constructive criticism by focusing on actions and behaviors rather than the individual.

Your child's interest in social activities is increasing at this age, and deeper bonds are formed with friends. With it, the pressure to act like peers or look like them becomes more common. Children can sometimes see their self-esteem suffer as a consequence. Support your child through the ups and downs of friendships, while continuing to reinforce your family's values (see Chapter 18).

Behavior At this age, children are capable of greater responsibility, such as doing chores around the house or helping parents by keeping an eye on a younger sibling. Greater awareness of factors such as picking up trash in the park may stem from children's growing sense of "the bigger picture," or how behavior can impact not just themselves but the people — and sometimes the world — around them.

At the same time, children this age will continue to test their parents and the rules. As your child strives for independence, he or she may act moody or rude. You may find your child doing things you don't approve of or that may be risky. Though your child likely understands that what he or she is doing is unacceptable, it's important to clarify your expectations and follow through with appropriate consequences (see Chapter 17).

Sparks of romance Children at this age may develop their first crush. It's also not uncommon for children this age to develop platonic crushes on peers of the same sex. These early crushes are generally temporary but may provide an opportunity to discuss why people fall in love and what elements are important in a healthy romantic relationship.

MENTAL DEVELOPMENT

In the late elementary years, school is geared toward challenging a child's critical thinking and problem-solving skills. Though your child may complain about

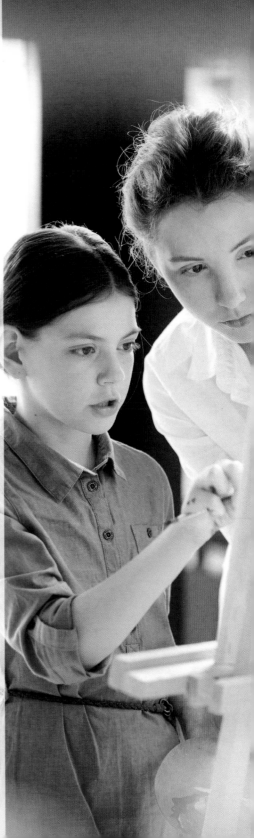

homework assignments, these after-school tasks can help him or her learn to work more independently.

Children at this age also like to be involved in family decision-making and planning, and enjoy knowing what's ahead. A shared family schedule or calendar can help family members stay up-to-date and connected.

Preparing for middle school Depending on how your local school district divides up grades, your child may be preparing to head off to middle school or junior high school soon. Starting middle school can be a scary time for a child as he or she may be confronted with several major changes all at once.

For some kids, going to middle school means there's a new building to navigate and there may be new classmates to meet. It may also mean your child will once again be the youngest in the school, and he or she may have to follow a schedule and move to different class-rooms throughout the day. Grades take on a more important role in your child's academic career.

If you ask children starting middle school what worries them the most, they may tell you about not being able to open a locker or getting lost trying to find a classroom. They may have heard stories about how mean eighth-graders are or the mountains of homework middle school teachers give out.

As a parent, you play a central role in helping to soothe your child's fears. To get your child ready:

Prep together mentally Focus on the fun things he or she will get to do, but also listen to your child's concerns and fears and address them. For example, if your child is worried about getting lost in the new school, reassure him or her that many other classmates will be in the same position, and that there will be plenty of staff to help new students find their way around.

Take advantage of orientation This is usually a time when elementary students entering middle school and their parents can learn more about the school and activities offered, meet staff, and take a tour of the school. There may be "ice-breaker" events to get children acquainted with middle school, such as picnics or ice cream socials, during the summer before school starts.

Get involved with the school Attend school meetings and keep in touch with your child's teacher. Consider volunteering with organizations such as your school's parent and teacher association (PTA). Find ways to have a say in what fun activities are available at your child's school.

Get help when needed The transition from elementary school to middle school isn't always smooth. Coupled with major changes associated with puberty, this can be a tough time.

If your child is showing signs of struggling — feeling persistently sad or anxious, experiencing changes in appetite or sleep patterns, or losing interest in friends and activities over a period of weeks — consider talking to someone. Your child's care provider, a guidance counselor or other mental health professional can provide you and your child with mental health strategies that can help both now and later in life.

Technology Technology is becoming increasingly important in your child's life. Schools use computers and tablets to help supplement classroom instruction.

ORGANIZATION AND TIME MANAGEMENT

As your child moves on to more-advanced grades — and multiple assignments and teachers become the norm — he or she may need to become more organized and better able to manage time constraints. To help keep your child on track:

▶ *Keep a planner.* A calendar, whether on paper or online, can be helpful to children learning to keep track of tasks and assignments.

▶ *Try a checklist.* Have your child compile a list of things he or she needs to get done for the day or week, whether it's schoolwork or chores. It can be gratifying for children to check off completed tasks and see how much they've accomplished.

▶ *Break up assignments.* Show your child how doing work in smaller chunks over a longer period can be more manageable. For example, instead of writing a book report over the weekend, set aside a week ahead of time to write a section each day.

▶ *Help your child navigate online calendars and assignments.* Many schools have websites that contain important information such as schedules and assignments. In addition, schools often require children to submit their homework online. Some elementary schools may even assign student tablets or laptops, although this is more common in middle and high school. Sit down with your child and familiarize yourselves with these online tools so that you both know what's expected. Teachers generally fill parents in on websites to be used, as well as usernames and passwords, but seek clarification if you need it.

▶ *Schedule a weekly backpack clean-out.* At the end of each week, remove papers and other items from the backpack and have your child decide what needs to be kept and what can be thrown out.

LEARNING GAMES

Looking for educational games that will keep your child engaged and learning? The National Education Association recommends browsing the websites of the following organizations:

▶ History: America's Story from America's Library
▶ Reading: Kidsreads
▶ Math: Math Playground
▶ Multiple topics: Fact Monster, PBS Kids
▶ Science and nature: WebRangers, Smithsonian Learning Lab

On the home front, some children have their own computers or cellphones, and may regularly surf the web and use social media on their own.

Many parents are concerned that children today are becoming addicted to digital media, worried about what seems like a constant stream of texting and scrolling through smartphones. While further research is needed to determine if true addiction to digital media exists in children, too much screen time can cause other problems.

For example, evidence suggests that constantly being "connected" may negatively impact a child's ability to sleep well, pay attention and learn. It may also increase a child's risk of obesity and depression. In addition, there's always a risk of your child being exposed to inappropriate content.

As with most things in life, context and balance are key. A child who spends longer periods on his or her computer composing music or writing stories isn't necessarily a cause for concern. A child who uses technology to the exclusion of physical activity or hanging out with friends may need greater screen limits. Continue to implement clear and consistent guidelines about how, when and where your child can use electronic devices and access the internet. As part of these rules:

▶ Encourage digital media and technology for specific uses, such as school projects or other activities, such as coding or learning about world events.

▶ Help your child learn the ins and outs and proper use of digital media by going online with him or her.

▶ Keep computers, tablets and other devices in a central location where you can easily monitor your child's internet activity.

▶ Reinforce rules about online safety, such as not sharing personal information and avoiding online friendships with people your child doesn't know in real life. Importantly, teach your child about online predators and make sure your child knows to never agree to meet an online friend in person without the presence of a trusted adult.

▶ If your child engages in social media, make sure he or she understands the need to treat other kids online respectfully, in the same way as in real life. Encourage your child to let you know about any kind of cyberbullying or online harassment that occurs. Let your child know that you will work with him or her to solve any problems that come up.

▶ Stress the importance of "face time" with family, friends and peers, and that virtual communication and social media don't replace personal interactions.

▶ Stick to screen-free times, such as during meals, and zones, such as bedrooms during sleep hours.

For your part, remember that parents have a great influence on a child's behavior. Model the kind of technology and social media use that you would like to see in your child.

GROW TOGETHER

There will be many more changes and obstacles in the years to come. But with continuing love and guidance from you, your child can keep growing into a healthy, well-adjusted young person.

You'll find, too, that your own parenting skills will expand and be refined as you gain experience and remain open to adjustments.

As you guide your child toward adolescence, this is an important time to help your child develop a sense of self-confidence, responsibility and empathy for others. Help your child develop a sense of right and wrong.

Engage with your child's school to keep up with your child's academic efforts and to address any issues that may arise. Peer pressure and bullying become more common as kids get older. Talk to your child about challenges that may come up.

Continue to set boundaries and guidelines. Set them for mealtime, bedtime, and daily household chores. Set them for screen time, family time, and anything else you feel strongly about.

Enjoy your child's company. Allow your relationship to evolve and bloom as your journey together progresses.

PART 2

Health and wellness

CHAPTER 5

Partnering with primary medical care

An important role as a parent is keeping your growing son or daughter as strong and healthy as possible. As a parent, you do a lot of the heavy lifting in this area — you provide nutritious meals, allow plenty of time for play and activity, wipe runny noses, encourage budding social connections, and keep bedtime on time. An important ally in this job — and one you should take full advantage of — is your child's primary medical provider.

Over the course of their lives, children may see a range of medical professionals for needs such as routine well-child checkups, vaccinations and emergency visits, as well as more specialized care for complex medical conditions. Making sure that all of these needs are being met is a primary medical provider — typically a pediatrician, family doctor, physician assistant or nurse practitioner.

It's comforting to have a central go-to person who knows your child's complete health history, who carefully follows your child's growth and development, and who can alert you to any po-

tential problems. Having a primary medical provider also gives you a ready point of contact when your child gets sick and can help minimize time spent in urgent care or the emergency room. Furthermore, the provider's office can act as a central location for your child's medical records.

In addition, the medical provider isn't there solely for your child. He or she is a valuable reference for you, too, providing guidance, advice and support for navigating the sometimes difficult terrain of parenting.

FINDING A MEDICAL PROVIDER

In many families, children continue to be seen by the same medical provider who took care of them when they were babies. This makes for a smooth transition into the preschool and school-age years.

But what if you need to find another provider? Maybe your family has recently

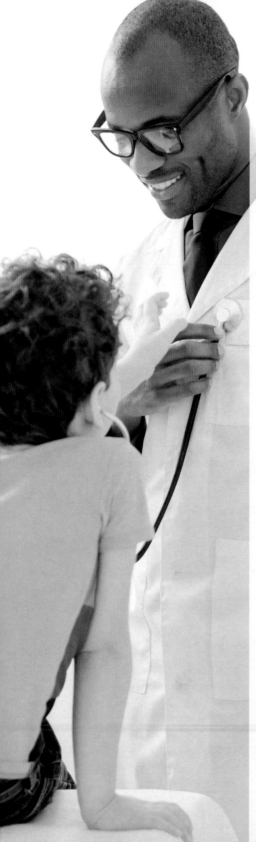

moved or your current provider for your child is retiring. Or perhaps you've yet to find a provider for your child.

In any case, it's natural to feel overwhelmed by starting a new search. Being prepared can help smooth the process. In the long run, finding a quality medical provider for your child can be well worth it in terms of time, money and stress.

The first step in the process is to think about what kind of medical provider you're looking for. Asking for provider recommendations from friends, relatives and co-workers with children, or another doctor such as your OB-GYN or other provider, is a great way to get some names and help compile a list.

Weighing your options When it comes to choosing a medical provider for your child, you have some options. Several types of medical professionals are trained to provide care to children, including:

Pediatricians A pediatrician is a doctor who specializes in caring for children from infancy through adolescence. After medical school, pediatricians complete a three-year residency program. During this time, they perform supervised care in places such as hospitals, subspecialty care and pediatricians' offices. This hands-on training gives them the knowledge to treat a wide variety of childhood illnesses.

After a pediatric residency, doctors are eligible to take a written exam, given by the American Board of Pediatrics. Passing this exam means a pediatrician is "board certified" and a fellow of the American Academy of Pediatrics — denoted by the letters "FAAP" that you might see after his or her name.

Some pediatricians choose to continue their education for an additional three or more years and train in a subspecialty such as heart care (cardiology) or the care of premature newborns (neonatology).

Many parents appreciate that pediatricians are experts in caring for both children with complex medical needs as well as healthy children, and that they can answer most questions that come up.

Once your child is older — typically between the ages of 18 and 21 — he or she will transition to a medical provider for adults, such as an internal medicine doctor (internist) or a family doctor.

Family doctors These are doctors who can provide care to all members of your family. Training in many different areas of medicine allows them to provide care to your child through adulthood and to treat most common problems, such as a cold or sore throat, and chronic illnesses, such as diabetes or high blood pressure. If he or she provides care to your entire family, this provider will have the advantage of being familiar with your family's medical history, as well.

Similar to pediatricians, family doctors complete a three-year residency after graduating from medical school and are eligible to become board certified in family medicine. During the course of this training, family doctors learn to care for young patients, though they don't focus on this area of medicine to the extent a pediatrician does.

If you're interested in having your child seen by your family doctor, ask if he or she is seeing children.

Midlevel providers Midlevel providers include nurse practitioners and physician assistants. Nurse practitioners are registered nurses who have advanced education — such as a master's or doctorate degree in nursing — and additional training in a specific area of medicine, such as pediatrics or family health.

After completion of nursing school, nurse practitioners go through a formal education program in their chosen specialty area. Pediatric nurse practitioners see children of all ages, from infants to teens, while family nurse practitioners see children and adults. These providers may work on their own or closely with or under the supervision of one or more doctors, depending on what state you live in.

Physician assistants are medical professionals who are trained and licensed to diagnose illness, develop and manage treatment plans, and prescribe medications. A physician assistant generally works with or under the supervision of a doctor, depending on state guidelines, and may serve as your primary medical provider. Physician assistants work in all areas of medicine, including pediatrics and family medicine.

Factors to consider Before selecting a medical provider, think about what makes a good fit for you and your child. Information such as office hours and educational background can often be found on the provider's website or other online profile. In addition, the following questions are worth considering as you do your research:

What are your needs? Though all of the medical providers mentioned earlier are trained to care for your child, certain aspects of training may be more important to you than others. For instance, does the provider you're considering have plenty of experience with children? Does he or she list areas of expertise that you consider key to providing care to your child — for example, treating children with asthma or diabetes? Or maybe you're looking for someone with expertise in behavioral health.

WHEN YOUR CHILD'S NEEDS ARE MORE COMPLEX

If your child has a chronic health condition or complex health care needs, visits to your child's medical provider are often more frequent and you may have additional appointments with other specialists.

For example, a child with asthma may see several medical providers in addition to his or her primary medical provider. These providers might include a respiratory specialist, an allergist, or an ear, nose and throat doctor. For a child with autism, a social worker, a mental health specialist, a developmental pediatrician, occupational and physical therapists, and speech and language therapists may be part of the team. Coordinating all of this care can be a full-time job. And, in fact, it is.

Many medical practices are aware of the burden that care coordination places on families. As a solution, a growing number of medical providers are offering the services of a care coordinator. A medical practice or health care organization that offers care coordination is sometimes referred to as a medical home. This means that it serves as a home base for most or all of your child's health care needs.

After your child receives a diagnosis, a care coordinator facilitates communication between you, your child's primary medical provider and appropriate specialists. Parents play an active role in care coordination, and their feedback is a critical component when creating a treatment plan.

The care coordinator uses input from your family, your primary medical provider and other specialists to help set up a treatment plan for your child. In addition, the care coordinator helps your child get access to services and resources in the community and at school. A care coordinator also serves as a gatekeeper of your child's medical records, providing a central access point where all past test results and other health information can be stored.

Finding a practice that offers care coordination may be worth consideration if your child requires more complex care involving one or more specialists. Some research has shown that such coordinated care may result in advantages, such as fewer emergency room visits and school absences, and lower out-of-pocket expenses for families.

In some cases, care coordination may not be available. Whether you ultimately find a medical home or not, you might find it useful to keep an up-to-date written record of your child's medical history that's quickly and easily accessible. This could be an app, an online document, or a notebook or planner.

The important thing is to detail information such as vaccinations, hospitalizations, sick plans, allergies, medications, appointments, insurance and pharmacy information, and anything else that will help coordinate treatment. You can bring the information with you to your child's medical appointments or on vacation, in case of an emergency.

The National Center for Medical Home Implementation has a wide range of printable pages and other resources to help you get your recordkeeping started. Go to the center's website and visit the section for families and caregivers.

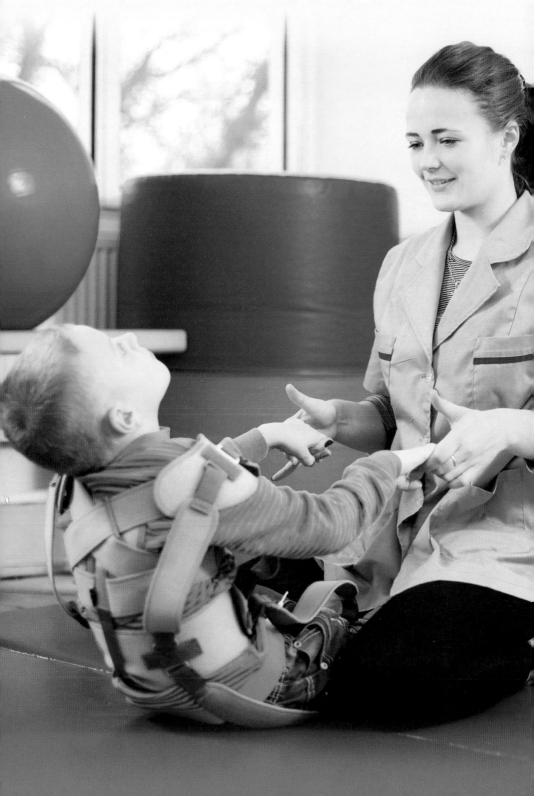

Does the provider accept your insurance? Even if the provider is listed in your benefits book or on your health insurance company's website as being in the company's network, it's always a good idea to double-check with the provider's office.

Where is the office located? Travel time can be an important factor. Having to drive a long distance for your child's yearly visit may not be that big of a deal, but it can quickly become inconvenient when you have a sick child to transport. And during cold and flu season, those trips can be frequent.

Are appointments convenient? It's not always easy to squeeze an appointment into the typical 9-to-5 schedule. You may find it more convenient if your child's provider offers evening hours or weekend appointments.

Will you always see the same provider? It's becoming more common these days for medical providers to be part of a larger group consisting of multiple medical professionals, including doctors and nurse practitioners. If it's important to you that your child see a specific provider in the group, double-check that you'll be able to request that provider for appointments.

Is the provider easily reached? Think about the type of communication you're looking for between you and your child's medical provider. What if you have questions or concerns after hours? Will the provider offer guidelines on what illnesses or other concerns warrant an office visit, and which ones can be handled over the phone?

You may prefer to contact the provider directly by email, or through a messaging service via an online patient portal.

Medical providers typically have an answering service for relaying after-hours messages, and some offices may offer a nurse line, where you can call in with your questions.

Where does the provider have hospital privileges? If you favor a specific hospital, you'll want to make sure that the medical provider you're considering has privileges to see your child at that facility, in the event your child needs care there.

How do you handle referrals? Ask the medical provider about his or her referral process for specialists. Some providers may be limited to referring your child to someone who is practicing in the same health care network or at certain medical institutions.

Taking these questions into consideration can help you narrow down your choices for medical providers. After you've narrowed down the candidates, call the provider's office and verify that he or she is accepting new patients and that the office accepts your insurance.

WHAT TO EXPECT AT A WELL-CHILD VISIT

After age 2, most children move to a yearly exam schedule with their medical provider. The benefits of these regular visits are numerous:

- They allow your child's provider to follow up on your child's development.
- Visits keep your child up to date on vaccinations.
- They provide an opportunity to screen for any abnormalities, which may have better outcomes if caught early.
- They allow the provider to monitor ongoing concerns.

Since a well-child visit is just that — a checkup with a child who's not sick or in for another reason — it's often pretty low-key and may offer an opportunity for you, your child and the medical provider to get to know each other in a more relaxed setting. Typically, a well-child visit involves a brief physical exam, vaccinations if needed and the rest of the time spent in conversation. Depending on the age of your child, the provider may ask you most of the questions, or ask your child to answer them. As your child gets older, it can be helpful to let your son or daughter develop his or her own relationship with the provider.

Here are the areas you can likely expect to cover at a well-child visit.

Physical exam This includes taking your child's blood pressure, checking his or her height and weight, listening to the heart and lungs, feeling the belly area, and testing reflexes. The provider also checks eyes, ears and mouth, spine alignment, genitalia, walking pattern (gait), and any other physical aspect you might have concerns about.

Growth Growth charts usually are a standard feature of a well-child visit. These detailed charts plot your child's height and weight measurements over time in order to show your child's rate of growth (growth curve).

In general, your child's medical provider will be more attentive to your child's pattern of growth over time, rather than to specific one-time measurements. Typically what you'll see is a smooth curve that arcs upward as the years go by. Regularly reviewing your child's growth chart also can alert you and the provider to unexpected delays in growth or changes in weight that may suggest the need for additional monitoring.

The rapid pace of growth in the infant and toddler years slows down a bit as your child reaches the preschool and school-age years. You'll often hear growth measurements expressed as percentiles — for example, 50th percentile for height and 20th percentile for weight. These numbers represent a comparison of your child with children who are of the same age and sex.

If you have a son who is in the 20th percentile for weight, for example, that means 20 percent of boys the same age weigh less than your son and 80 percent of boys the same age weigh more.

To hear that 80 percent of children weigh more than your child may sound concerning, but it's important to put these numbers in context. Each child is unique. The most important thing is that your child is following his or her own growth curve. See growth charts on pages 74 and 76.

Development Your child's medical provider will likely check to see if your child is reaching appropriate developmental milestones based on his or her age.

If your child is younger, that might mean your medical provider will ask you to fill out a standardized developmental questionnaire. This screening tool reviews many areas of your child's development including fine motor, gross motor, communication, emotional development, and self-help skills.

For example, the questionnaire may ask if your child's vocabulary has expanded to contain a certain number of words, or whether he or she is able to follow a number of commands or draw specific shapes.

The medical provider may ask your child to perform specific actions to test motor skills, such as being able to hop on one foot. If some milestones aren't being

2 to 20 years: Girls
Stature-for-age and Weight-for-age percentiles

NAME _____

RECORD # _____

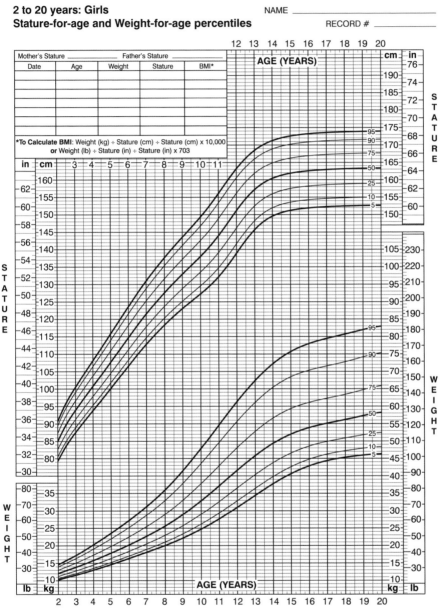

SOURCE: Centers for Disease Control and Prevention

2 to 20 years: Girls
Body mass index-for-age percentiles

NAME _____

RECORD # _____

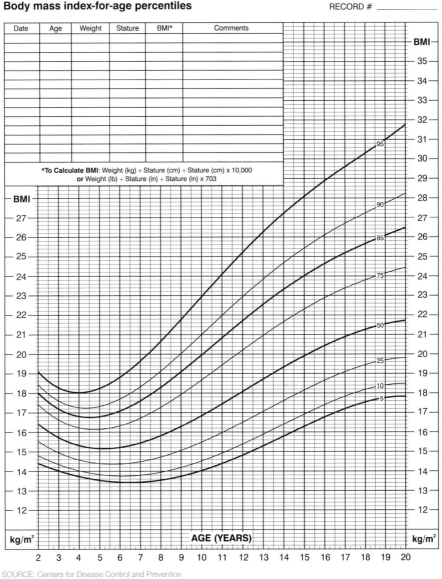

Date	Age	Weight	Stature	BMI*	Comments

*To Calculate BMI: Weight (kg) ÷ Stature (cm) ÷ Stature (cm) x 10,000
or Weight (lb) ÷ Stature (in) ÷ Stature (in) x 703

AGE (YEARS)

SOURCE: Centers for Disease Control and Prevention

2 to 20 years: Boys
Stature-for-age and Weight-for-age percentiles

NAME _____

RECORD # _____

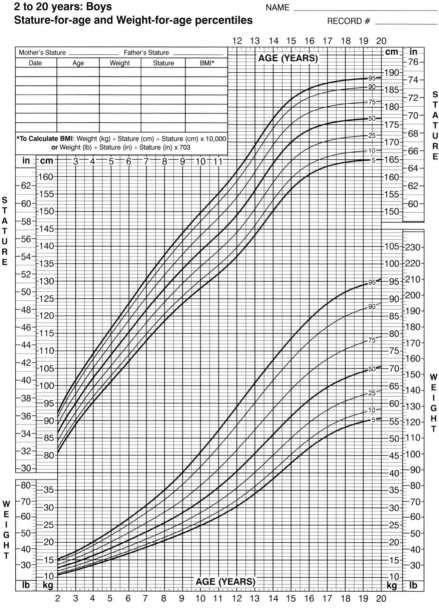

*To Calculate BMI: Weight (kg) ÷ Stature (cm) ÷ Stature (cm) x 10,000
or Weight (lb) ÷ Stature (in) ÷ Stature (in) x 703

SOURCE: Centers for Disease Control and Prevention

2 to 20 years: Boys
Body mass index-for-age percentiles

NAME _____

RECORD # _____

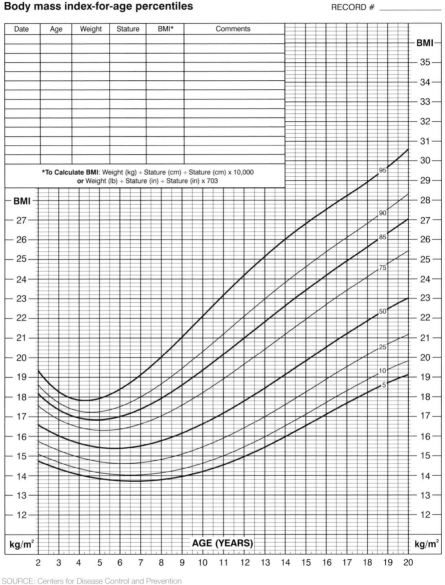

Date	Age	Weight	Stature	BMI*	Comments

*To Calculate BMI: Weight (kg) ÷ Stature (cm) ÷ Stature (cm) x 10,000
or Weight (lb) ÷ Stature (in) ÷ Stature (in) x 703

AGE (YEARS)

SOURCE: Centers for Disease Control and Prevention

WHY MEASURE MY CHILD'S BMI?

Starting at age 2, your child's medical provider may start measuring your child's body mass index (BMI). This is a screening tool based on population averages that uses weight in relation to height to estimate whether a person might be underweight, overweight or obese.

BMI for children is not expressed in the same way as it is for adults. When measuring children and young adults, BMI percentiles (also called "BMI-for-age percentiles") are preferred. Percentiles allow for more flexibility than standard BMI measurements, taking into account growth over time and the fact that children will carry varying amounts of body fat as they develop. Children who are in the fifth to 84th percentile are generally considered to be within a healthy range. A child might be considered to be underweight if he or she is in the fourth percentile or lower, and overweight if he or she placed in the 85th to 94th percentile. Children who are in the 95th percentile and above may be considered obese. See BMI charts on pages 75 and 77.

Which percentile your child's BMI falls into is only one part of the picture, though. Your child's medical provider will mostly want to see if your child is tracking consistently along his or her individual growth curve over time. The provider will also look at your family's medical history and your child's overall diet and activity levels. If your child's growth is consistent — say, your child has always tracked in the 87th percentile for BMI — there's generally no reason to worry. If there's a large change in BMI percentile over the previous year's measurements — suddenly dropping to the 50th percentile or increasing to the 98th percentile — this might be a sign of an unhealthy shift in weight.

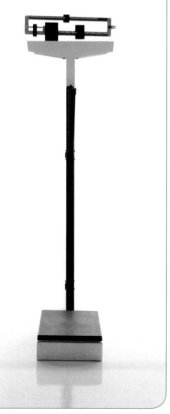

If your child's weight is a concern for you, talk to your child's medical provider. It's important to remember that BMI has limitations as a screening tool. It can't diagnose obesity, and says little on its own about an individual child's health. Not every child who tracks in a higher percentile necessarily has a health problem. Some children have larger frames than others; others have more muscle mass. Factors such as these can skew a child's BMI higher even though the child is healthy. A more important gauge may be whether your child is keeping up with his or her peers in terms of physical activity, such as on the playground or in gym class.

met, your child's provider can help you determine the next step, whether it be a wait-and-see approach or a more specialized evaluation.

With older kids, the medical provider may ask about school and extracurricular activities — how they're doing with grades, homework and standardized testing and whether they're meeting with tutors or taking remedial or advanced classes. If you or your child has concerns in this area, this is a good opportunity to let the provider know, too.

Emotional well-being Your child's medical provider will also want to know how your child is doing socially and emotionally, and how this is expressed in his or her behavior.

The medical provider may ask questions about different aspects of your child's family and social life to ensure he or she is adjusting well. The provider may ask you if there are any behavioral issues you might be concerned about, such as difficulties getting along with other children or following rules at home or school.

If your child is a preschooler, you may be asked to fill out a standardized social-emotional questionnaire to help flag any difficulties your child may be having in these areas. These questionnaires can help identify early on moods and behaviors that tend to accompany conditions such as autism, and for which early intervention is crucial.

Most of the time, though, this is an opportunity for the medical provider to reassure you that you're not alone in your concerns and that your family is, in fact, very much like other families experiencing the stressors of everyday life. He or she may be able to provide some tips or resources that can help you sustain a positive family environment.

Vaccinations Vaccines are a critical part of making sure your child stays healthy because they can greatly reduce your child's risk of getting certain diseases.

Vaccines don't end after age 2. Boosters and new vaccines are needed as your child gets older, including the annual flu vaccine.

If your child isn't up to date on his or her immunizations, it's generally not too late to catch up. Talk to your child's medical provider about getting caught up as soon as possible. See Chapter 6 for more on vaccinations.

Nutrition At each well-child visit, your child's medical provider will likely want to know about your child's eating patterns and favorite foods. He or she also may discuss whether your child is getting enough of certain nutrients, such as calcium and vitamin D. See Chapter 13 for more on nutrition.

Bowel and bladder function A well-child visit is a great opportunity to discuss bathroom issues. Younger children, particularly boys and heavy sleepers, may still wet the bed at night. This typically isn't too much of a concern for children under the age of 7.

But if your child was previously sleeping through the night without accidents and is now wetting the bed, or if your child is still having regular daytime accidents, these can sometimes be signs of an underlying problem, such as a bladder infection. Sometimes stress, perhaps due to a move to a new home or starting a new school, can lead to a relapse in bladder control.

A well-child visit is also your opportunity to address concerns about bowel function and any irregularities, such as frequent loose stool or constipation (see page 325).

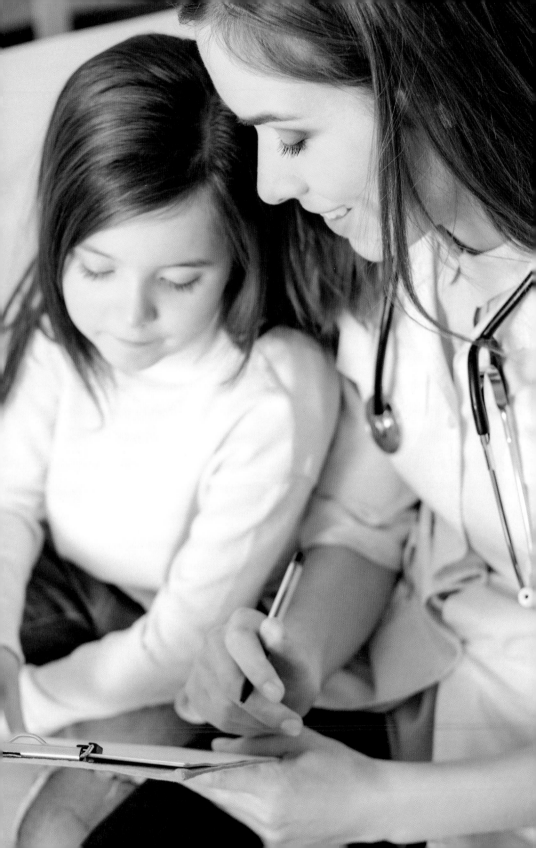

MAKING THE MOST OF YOUR VISIT

Visits with a medical provider are often fairly short and, in many medical practices, limited to a specific amount of time allotted for each type of visit.

While most medical providers do their best to cover all of your questions, you may want to consider prioritizing your concerns beforehand. This will help ensure that the most important questions you have are covered during the visit, and you get the most out of your time with the provider.

If you have multiple concerns in different areas or otherwise need a lengthier well-child visit, make sure to mention this when you schedule your appointment, so more time can be allotted.

It can help to write down questions that come up between appointments — maybe keep a running list in a notebook, smartphone or tablet — so that you remember them when it comes time for your child's next appointment. Also jot down life events that might cause stress or otherwise may affect your child's normal behavior — for example, the birth of a baby brother or sister, or the loss of a beloved grandmother.

There are digital tools available to help you plan for a visit, as well. One example you can search online for is the Child and Adolescent Health Measurement Initiative's free Well Visit Planner for children up to 6 years old.

Hearing and vision Your child's medical provider may periodically evaluate your child's hearing and vision using various methods. Hearing tests will look for signs of hearing loss, which at this age is typically the result of an infection, trauma or noise exposure. Your child's provider may check for potential eye abnormalities and assess how sharp your child's vision is (visual acuity).

Sleep Getting enough sleep is critical for healthy child development. Your child's medical provider will likely ask about your child's sleep habits, such as bedtime routines and the amount and quality of sleep your child gets. Your child's provider also can offer guidance on cementing healthy sleep habits (see Chapter 8).

Prevention and safety Your child's medical provider will discuss preventive health measures, such as regular dental exams, exercise guidelines and limiting screen time. He or she can offer tips on keeping your child safe both in and out of the home. The provider may offer guidance on how to store and administer medications, for example, and explain guidelines for use of safety devices, such as car seats and booster seats.

Remember that the relationship between your child's medical provider and your family is a partnership — one that will likely take time and effort to cultivate. But the payoff is substantial: Such a partnership will ensure that your child is getting personalized, comprehensive and effective care.

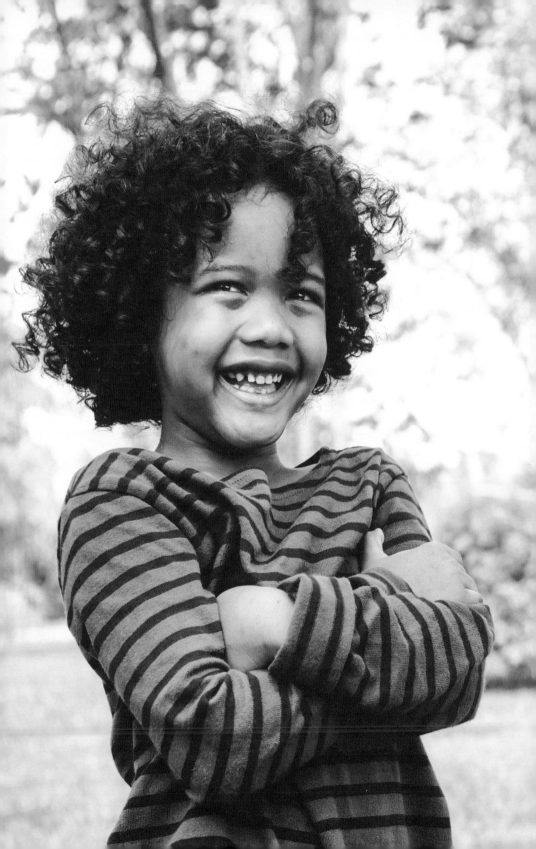

CHAPTER 6

Vaccinations

By following the recommended vaccine schedule, most children will be immunized against a wide range of diseases. During the preschool and school-age years, vaccines continue to be an important of your child's health care. Timely vaccination can help protect your entire family against diseases that only a few generations ago caused serious illness, permanent disability and death.

As parents, it's reassuring to live in an age in which medicine can provide this kind of protection to young children and to the community at large. When people become immune to a certain illness, there's less chance that they will pass that illness on to others. That makes everyone around them safer — a valuable phenomenon called herd immunity.

In this chapter you'll find what you as a parent need to know about vaccines — information on how they work, the latest on vaccine safety and what vaccines are recommended for children at what ages. You'll also find a variety of helpful tips, including how to ease the discomfort of shots, keep track of vaccine records, and meet school and travel requirements. At the end of the chapter is a breakdown of all the diseases that vaccines can prevent in preschoolers and school-age children.

HOW VACCINES WORK

Every day, everyone is exposed to a host of circulating bacteria, viruses and other germs. But most humans aren't too bothered by germs, even the disease-causing ones. This is because of the way the immune system works. When a harmful germ enters your body, your immune system mounts a defense, producing proteins called antibodies to fight off the invader. The goal of your immune system is to neutralize or destroy the foreign invader, rendering it harmless and preventing you from getting sick.

One way the body's immune system fights off sickness is through developing a specific immunity to a foreign element after being exposed to it. Once you've been infected with a certain disease-causing organism, your immune system has a tendency to "remember" that particular organism. If the germ shows up again, your immune system puts into play a complex array of defenses to prevent you from getting sick again from that type of virus or bacteria.

Another way to help the immune system prevent disease is through vaccine immunity. With this method, a person acquires immunity without having to get sick. A vaccine contains just enough of a killed or weakened form or derivative of an infectious germ to trigger your immune system into action without developing the actual disease.

When given to you before you get infected, the vaccine makes your body think that it's being invaded by a specific organism, and your immune system begins building defenses against the organism to guard against it in the future. If you're exposed to the disease after vaccination, the invading germs will meet antibodies prepared to defeat them. In addition, vaccines can be given without the risk of serious disease complications.

Sometimes it takes several doses of a vaccine for a full immune response — this is the case for many childhood vaccines. Some people fail to build immunity to the first doses of a vaccine, but they often respond to later doses.

It's important to note that the immunity provided by some vaccines, such as tetanus and pertussis, isn't lifelong. Because the immune response may decrease over time, you may need another dose of a vaccine (booster) to restore or increase your immunity. And for some diseases, the organism evolves, and a new vaccine is needed against the new form. This is the case with the annual flu (influenza) shot.

VACCINE SAFETY

If you're feeling apprehensive about giving your child vaccines, that's understandable and a common sentiment among parents.

While you know from your doctor that vaccinations are important and safe, you've also heard claims that they could be harmful. You may worry after hearing or seeing reports about a severe "reaction" that occurred shortly after a child's vaccination visit or of children who've developed a chronic condition after being vaccinated. Stories such as these frequently circulate on the internet.

Many, many studies have been done on vaccines and the conclusions are that vaccines are extremely safe. In fact, they are some of the safest and most studied medical products used today.

Before vaccines can be used, they must meet strict safety and effectiveness standards set by the Food and Drug Administration (FDA). Meeting these standards requires a lengthy development process of years of study in the laboratory, followed by three phases of clinical trials that may take seven or more years. These studies, unlike drug studies, involve tens of thousands of individuals. Only a few vaccines studied ever get licensed. Once licensed, the FDA requires ongoing safety studies for the vaccine.

Out of all the vaccines licensed by the FDA, only some of the licensed vaccines are selected for recommendation to the public. Experts in the field, supported by the Centers for Disease Control and Prevention (CDC), examine how frequently the vaccine-preventable disease occurs and how useful the licensed vaccine would be if recommended. Only vaccines that are recommended by this group are put into the routine vaccine schedule.

Once the vaccine is recommended, the FDA and the CDC continue to conduct safety studies as well as studies monitoring the vaccine's impact in preventing disease and maintaining immunity over time. Furthermore, vaccines are subject to ongoing research, review and refinement by doctors, scientists and public health officials. Those who provide vaccines — such as vaccine manufacturers, doctors, nurses and other health workers — must report any side effects they observe to the FDA and the CDC.

Millions and millions of vaccine doses are given out each year, but serious side effects are rare. Statistically speaking, your child's chances of being harmed or fatally injured by a disease are far greater than his or her chances of being harmed by the vaccine used to prevent the disease.

Vaccine additives In addition to the killed or weakened microorganisms that make up vaccines, small amounts of other substances may be added to a vaccine to prevent contamination, enhance the immune response, and stabilize the vaccine against temperature variations and other conditions. Vaccines may also contain small amounts of materials used in the manufacturing process, such as gelatin.

Some people worry that some of these additives may be harmful. But to date, there's little scientific evidence to support these concerns. Examples include:

Thimerosal Thimerosal is a preservative used for flu vaccines that are prepared in multidose vials. The thimerosal prevents the growth of bacteria and fungus when new needles are inserted into the vials for each dose. Today, most childhood vaccines come in single-dose vials that don't use thimerosal. Flu vaccine is also available in single-dose vials that don't contain thimerosal.

VACCINES AND AUTISM

Given the stories that regularly appear in the news, blogs and various media outlets, it's no wonder that parents become concerned about a possible connection between the use of vaccines and conditions such as autism. As a parent, you want to protect your children from potential harm, and rightly so.

But it's also important to get the whole story. The suggestion that vaccines might be linked to autism dates back to 1998 when a group of scientists published an article in *The Lancet,* a medical journal. The article suggested that elements in the measles, mumps and rubella (MMR) vaccine led to inflammatory bowel disease, which allowed harmful proteins to circulate through the bloodstream and damage the brain.

The study, however, was based on false information and has since been taken back by the journal. In addition, the main investigator, who eventually lost his medical license, failed to disclose that his research was being funded by a group seeking legal action against vaccine manufacturers — a serious conflict of interest.

The study had other shortcomings. It was conducted in a very small group of children — 12 in all. It's difficult to consider such a small size as representative of the larger population, and it isn't big enough to reveal reliable associations. In addition, even large studies require confirmation. Science relies on a consistent pattern of replication through multiple independent studies to confirm whether a hypothesis is true. In the case of this particular study, other researchers were unable to reproduce its results — multiple studies since including thousands of children have found no connection between the MMR vaccine and autism.

Research on autism is ongoing. For example, a 2017 study examining infant brain scans found that neurological changes related to autism may begin as early as 6 months, before the MMR vaccine is given. To date, there's no medical evidence that the MMR vaccine causes autism. Hopefully in the near future, researchers will be able to explain what causes autism and come up with effective treatments or even cures.

When ingested, the body eliminates thimerosal quickly. No evidence shows that children have been harmed by its use in vaccines.

Aluminum Aluminum gels or salts have been used in vaccines for over 70 years to help stimulate a better immune response. Federal regulations limit aluminum content in vaccines so that total exposure is substantially less than the minimal risk level established by federal agencies. Most of the aluminum is rapidly eliminated from the body after injection, and there's no evidence showing a link between any remaining aluminum and damaging side effects.

Formaldehyde This substance is used to inactivate the virus or bacterium central to a vaccine and to avoid contamination of the vaccine with other germs. Most of the formaldehyde is removed from the vaccine before it's packaged. Generally, toxic exposure to formaldehyde occurs as a result of breathing in large quantities of it, such as from paints or varnishes.

Side effects Vaccines are considered very safe. However, as with all medications, they aren't completely free of side effects.

Most side effects are minor and temporary. Your child might experience a mild fever, or soreness or swelling at the injection site. Serious reactions, such as a seizure or high fever, from a dose are rare.

The risk of a life-threatening allergic reaction (anaphylaxis) occurs on the order of 1 per million of doses. The risk of death from a vaccine is so slight that it can't be accurately determined. Still, when any serious event occurs following a vaccination, it must be reported and it receives careful scrutiny from the FDA and the CDC.

Some vaccines are blamed for chronic illnesses, such as autism or diabetes. (See opposite page for more on autism and vaccines.) Sporadic reports have, at times, suggested an association between vaccine use and such conditions. But when other researchers have tried to duplicate those results — a test of good scientific research — they haven't been able to reproduce the findings. In fact, many large studies conducted around the world have failed to find a consistent link between vaccines and these illnesses.

When to avoid vaccination There are only a few circumstances in which vaccination should be postponed or avoided. Talk to your child's medical provider if you have questions about postponing your child's vaccinations.

Vaccination may be inappropriate if your child has:

- Had a serious or life-threatening reaction to a previous dose of that vaccine.
- A known, significant allergy to a vaccine component. A history of egg allergy no longer precludes a child from receiving the flu vaccine. No special precaution needs to be taken for children who are allergic to eggs.

A serious medical condition, such as AIDS or cancer, that's compromised your child's immune system and could allow a live virus vaccine to cause additional illness.

Vaccination may need to be delayed if your child:

- Is in the early, acute stages of a moderate to severe illness
- Has recently taken immunocompromising medications for an extended period
- Received a transfusion of blood or plasma or was given blood products within the past year

Vaccination shouldn't be delayed because your child has a minor illness, such as a common cold, an ear infection or mild diarrhea. The vaccine will still be effective. It also won't make your child any sicker.

If your child lives in a household with people at risk of serious complications from vaccine-preventable diseases, such as an older grandparent or a family member with a weakened immune system, it's especially important that your child receive timely vaccinations to help protect those individuals from getting sick.

VACCINES BEFORE PRESCHOOL AND KINDERGARTEN

Individual states have their own vaccination requirements before a child can enter school. These laws typically apply not just to public schools but to private schools and child care facilities, as well. Most schools, preschools and day care centers require a certificate of immunization prior to enrollment. It's important to keep your own record of the vaccines your child has received. But your child's medical provider should be able to provide you with a record of your child's immunization.

You can find out the requirements in your state by checking with your child's medical provider, your child's school, or your state's immunization program or department of health.

The CDC doesn't set immunization requirements for schools and child care centers, but it has a lot of information on vaccines and a search tool to help you find information about your state's school vaccination requirements. Visit the CDC's website for more.

Fully immunizing your child not only helps protect the health of your child but also that of friends, classmates, teachers and others.

Gone but not gone It can be easy to take the benefits of widespread vaccination for granted. Because many vaccine-preventable diseases are now uncommon in the United States, some people feel that these diseases are gone for good. As a result, many people feel less urgency about getting themselves or their children vaccinated.

If you wonder if it's necessary to vaccinate your family and keep everyone's vaccinations up to date, the answer is yes. Many infectious diseases that have virtually disappeared in the United States can reappear quickly. The germs that cause the diseases still exist — many countries are still working to get vaccination programs in place. These germs can be easily acquired and spread by people who aren't protected by immunization.

As travelers unknowingly carry disease from one country to another, a new outbreak may be only a plane trip away. From a single entry point, an infectious disease can spread quickly among unprotected individuals. Outbreaks of mumps and measles have repeatedly occurred this way in the United States in the past few years.

FINDING IMMUNIZATION RECORDS

If you need an official copy of your child's immunization records or you just want to update your personal records, there are several options you can pursue to find the records you need:

▶ Check with your child's medical provider or your local health clinic.

▶ Check with your state's health department or the state where your child last received his or her shots. Most states have a computer-based immunization information system (IIS) that doctors and public health clinics may use to keep track of the vaccines their patients receive.

▶ Check with a child care center, school or summer camp that your child attended. You may have had to submit an immunization record along with your application or registration, and the administrators may still have a copy. However, they generally only keep such records for a year or so after your child leaves the program.

If your child's records can't be located, the assumption is that your child is vulnerable to disease and will need to receive the appropriate vaccines. Your doctor can help you figure out which ones your child needs. Blood tests may detect antibodies (immunity) to certain diseases. But it won't harm your child to be revaccinated even if he or she received the vaccine in the past.

Finding immunization records can sometimes be a concern in cases of adoption or foster care. Your adoption agency or coordinator may have access to these records. Revaccination is recommended when records can't be located, are incomplete, can't be understood, or you or your child's medical provider suspects the records are inaccurate.

IS IT OK TO DELAY OR SPREAD OUT SHOTS?

Some parents worry about their child getting too many vaccines at once. It can be tempting to delay vaccines until your child is older or until the timing seems better. But it can be a challenge to follow through on these intentions, and skipping or delaying vaccines can leave your child vulnerable to vaccine-preventable diseases that may be going around.

In addition, there's no scientific evidence that alternate vaccine schedules are as safe and effective as the regularly recommended vaccine schedule published by the CDC. In fact, alternate schedules:

▶ Delay onset of immunity
▶ Increase pain and distress for your child
▶ Make it harder to keep up with vaccine doses
▶ Complicate your child's medical record

Mayo Clinic doctors, nurses, researchers and other experts — based on the best available evidence — recommend following the vaccine schedule published by the CDC.

VACCINES BY AGE

A number of vaccines are recommended for preschoolers and school-age children, including the flu vaccine and several boosters that can help further strengthen immunity to illnesses such as diphtheria, tetanus, whooping cough (pertussis) and others.

If you've missed one or more vaccines, now is a good time to catch up. An interruption in your child's schedule doesn't mean you have to start a series over or redo any doses. But until your child receives the entire vaccine series, he or she won't have maximum possible protection against diseases.

The CDC's website has comprehensive vaccine information. But identifying which vaccines your child needs can be confusing between the charts and the footnotes. Talk with your child's medical provider to determine which vaccines your child needs and when.

3-year-olds By age 3, most children should have completed their primary vaccinations series begun at birth. If you're not up to date on vaccines, talk to your child's medical provider about catching up on any your child may have missed or following up on an incomplete series of doses. The earlier in life vaccines are given, the sooner your child is protected from certain diseases.

Also, you and your children should receive flu shots every year. Flu shots are recommended just as strongly as all other vaccines, and they prevent an illness far more common than any other vaccine-preventable infection, other than perhaps the human papillomavirus (HPV).

Flu shots typically become available in the fall and can help protect against a variety of influenza types. Flu shots are especially important for younger kids and pregnant moms, who are often more vulnerable to complications of the flu.

MINIMIZING THE DISCOMFORT OF SHOTS

Vaccines aren't completely painless, unfortunately. They do sting a bit and some kids — and even parents — have a very real fear of needles. Dismissing your child's anxiety or telling him or her that the shot won't hurt isn't necessarily true and in fact, risks undermining your child's trust in you.

Instead, answer questions honestly. Keep in mind that your child will look to you for reassurance and guidance. If you maintain a calm, comfortable, no-non-sense disposition, it's more likely that your child will take a similar approach.

You also might want to try some of these tips for minimizing your child's anxiety and discomfort:

▶ *Pack a comfort object.* A favorite stuffed animal, blanket, book or other object from home may help soothe your child during the visit.

▶ *Have a seat.* Being seated during the shot appears to be less painful than lying down. You might hold your child in your lap or sit or stand next to your child for support.

▶ *Save some for last.* If your child is receiving two or more vaccines at a visit, ask to receive the most painful vaccine last. For example, the MMRII (a vaccine against measles, mumps and rubella) is known to be slightly more painful than others. Your child's medical provider will likely do this anyway, but it doesn't hurt to ask.

▶ *Draw attention elsewhere.* For younger children, distraction in the form of con-versation, singing or drawing may help.

▶ *Give it a rub.* Some evidence suggests that rubbing the injection site just before the shot helps reduce pain. Other research hasn't found this to be true, how-ever.

▶ *Breathe.* Encouraging your child to focus on his or her breathing or taking a few deep breaths together during the injection may also help.

▶ *Ask your child's medical provider about other measures.* Some offices provide additional options such as applying a numbing spray or an anesthetic cream, or using a cooling or vibration pack in an effort to desensitize nearby nerves.

▶ *Don't get up too quickly.* Sometimes, receiving a shot can make people a little dizzy, so it might help to sit for a few minutes after the vaccine before getting up to walk.

▶ *Use pain relievers afterward.* Your child may experience mild side effects from the vaccine, such as redness, pain or swelling at the injection site. Ask your doctor what to expect. Automatically giving doses of a pain reliever after every vaccination to prevent side effects is no longer recommended. Research shows that doing so may inhibit the body's immune response to the vaccine. But if your child is irritable or in pain after vaccination, do use acetaminophen to reduce discomfort as needed. Follow the label instructions for the correct dose, or ask your child's medical provider for specific dosing instructions.

VACCINES AT A GLANCE

Blue = All children
Green = Catch-up immunization
Purple = Certain high-risk groups

Vaccine ▾ Age ▸	2-3 years	4-6 years	7-10 years	11-12 years
Influenza	Annual (1-2 doses)	Annual (1-2 doses)	Annual (1-2 doses)	Annual (1 dose)
Diphtheria, tetanus, pertussis (DTaP): < 7 yrs		DTaP 5th dose		
Tetanus, diphtheria, pertussis (Tdap): ≥ 7 yrs				Tdap
Inactivated poliovirus (IPV)		IPV 4th dose		
Measles, mumps and rubella (MMR)		MMR 2nd dose		
Varicella (VAR)		VAR 2nd dose		
Hepatitis A				
Hepatitis B				
Haemophilus influenzae type b				
Pneumococcal conjugate				
Meningococcal (MenACWY)				MenACWY 1st dose
Human papillomavirus (HPV)				HPV (2 doses)
Meningococcal B (MenB)				MenB
Pneumococcal polysaccharide (PPSV23)		PPSV23		

Source: Advisory Committee on Immunization Practices, Centers for Disease Control and Prevention, 2018

Getting flu shots for your immediate family indirectly helps protect older relatives, such as grandparents, who may be susceptible to more-severe manifestations of the flu. Reducing your own risk of getting the flu also reduces your risk of passing it on to others.

4- to 6-year-olds Sometime between the ages of 4 and 6 — usually before entering kindergarten — your child should receive a group of booster shots that will further enhance his or her immunity. These booster shots help refresh your child's immune "memory list" of potential infectious invaders. They include:

▶ Diphtheria, tetanus and whooping cough (pertussis) (DTaP)
▶ Inactivated poliovirus (IPV)
▶ Measles, mumps and rubella (MMR)
▶ Chickenpox (varicella)

It's safe and effective for your child to receive all of the booster shots at the same time. In fact, it's better to do them all at once. Separating them over several visits results in more pain from injections and leads to delayed or missed doses. Receiving multiple vaccinations at once has no harmful effect on a healthy immune system. All of the booster shots should be received before entering school for greatest effectiveness.

Don't forget about getting your annual flu shots. These can be especially helpful if your child is getting ready to enter a group setting such as preschool or kindergarten for the first time. Getting the flu shot can help reduce your child's risk of getting the flu in the face of increased exposure and minimize sick days at home. Again, flu shots are recommended just as strongly as other routine vaccines.

7- to 11-year-olds Kids between ages 7 and 11 need the annual flu vaccine to protect against seasonal influenza.

Once your child is 11, he or she will need a booster vaccine for tetanus, diphtheria and pertussis (Tdap).

Also around age 11, your child should receive a dose of the meningococcal vaccine to protect against infection by meningococcal bacteria, which can lead to severe infection of the brain and blood.

Mayo Clinic recommends that children get two doses of the human papillomavirus (HPV) vaccine starting at 9 years of age. The HPV vaccine protects against some strains of human papillomavirus infection and cancers caused by HPV. It's generally recommended at age 11 or 12, but Mayo Clinic recommends early administration to take advantage of the body's strong immune response at this age. The HPV vaccine is recommended just as strongly as any of the other vaccines.

This is also a good time to catch up on vaccinations your child may have missed. Talk to your child's medical provider about a catch-up schedule that will meet your child's needs.

VACCINE-PREVENTABLE DISEASES

Illnesses that current vaccines can help prevent in preschoolers and school-age children include:

Chickenpox Chickenpox (varicella) is a common childhood disease that causes an itchy, blistery rash and fever. For most children, it's not life-threatening, but for some it can be very serious, leading to hospitalization and even death. It can also affect adults who aren't immune.

The chickenpox virus is spread mainly by direct contact with the rash, which is the best-known sign of the disease.

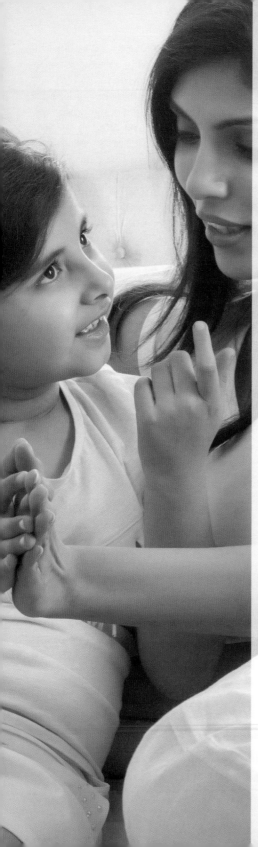

The rash begins as superficial spots on the face, chest, back and other areas of the body. The spots quickly fill with a clear fluid, rupture and turn crusty. The rash can spread over the whole body and the itching can be very uncomfortable.

Children with chickenpox generally end up missing about a week of school or child care.

Vaccine recommendation The first recommended dose of the chickenpox vaccine is given between ages 12 and 18 months. A second dose is given sometime between ages 4 and 6 years. To catch up, two doses are recommended. Talk to your child's medical provider about timing.

Diphtheria Diphtheria is a bacterial infection that spreads from person to person through airborne droplets, such as when a person coughs or sneezes. It starts with a sore throat, fever and chills. Next, it causes a thick covering (membrane) to develop in the back of the throat that makes it hard to breathe.

Diphtheria can lead to severe respiratory problems, paralysis, heart failure and death. The disease is fatal in as many as 1 out of 5 children under age 5.

Thanks to widespread use of the vaccine, reported cases in the United States have been close to zero for the last two decades.

Vaccine recommendation The diphtheria vaccine typically is given in combination with the tetanus and whooping cough (pertussis) vaccines (DTaP). A child should receive five shots in the first six years of life, starting at two months of age. Catch-up shots can be scheduled with your child's medical provider. A booster Tdap shot, which helps protect against tetanus, diphtheria and whooping cough, is recommended at age 11 or

12, and then a Td booster, for tetanus and diphtheria, every 10 years thereafter.

Flu (influenza) Influenza is a viral infection that sickens millions of people each year. It can cause serious complications in some people, especially children with a chronic illness, such as asthma or diabetes, and older adults.

Flu-related deaths are uncommon among children. Deaths typically occur because of a secondary bacterial infection, such as bacterial pneumonia, or because the flu aggravated an existing illness. But data from 2004 through 2012 show that almost half the pediatric flu-related deaths occurred in previously healthy children. In addition, most of the children who died had not received the seasonal flu vaccine.

Flu vaccines are designed to protect against strains of flu virus expected to be in circulation during the fall and winter. The vaccine is generally offered by the end of October and is available through the entire flu season. In most states, flu season runs through April or May.

Vaccine recommendation The influenza vaccine is now recommended yearly for everyone, beginning as early as age 6 months. If your child is less than 9 years old and getting the flu shot for the first time, he or she needs two doses of the vaccine the first time around. That's because children at this age don't develop an adequate antibody level the first time they get the vaccine.

Hepatitis A Hepatitis A is a highly contagious liver disease caused by the hepatitis A virus. The virus is found in an infected person's stool. It's usually spread by eating or drinking contaminated food or water or by touching contaminated objects, such as a used diaper or a doorknob.

Children under age 6 often have no symptoms of hepatitis A, but they can pass the disease to older children and adults, who can become very sick. Signs and symptoms — which may include nausea, vomiting, jaundice, fatigue and joint pain — can last up to six months. Rarely, hepatitis A can lead to liver failure and death.

Vaccine recommendation The two-dose series of hepatitis A vaccine is recommended for all children in the U.S. The first dose is generally given at 12 months and the second dose at 24 months. Catch-up vaccinations at an older age are also available.

Hepatitis B The hepatitis B virus can cause a short-term (acute) illness marked by loss of appetite, fatigue, diarrhea, vomiting, jaundice, and pain in muscles, joints and the abdomen. More commonly, it causes a silent infection that persists for decades and can lead to long-term (chronic) liver damage (cirrhosis) or liver cancer.

The virus is spread through contact with the blood or other body fluids of an infected person, whether or not the person has symptoms. This can happen by touching open sores or cuts of an infected person, sharing their toothbrushes or other personal items, having unprotected sex, sharing needles when injecting illegal drugs, or during birth, when the virus passes from an infected mother to her baby. However, over one-third of people who have hepatitis B in the U.S. don't know how they got it.

Vaccine recommendation The hepatitis B vaccine is given to children in three doses — at birth, at least one month later (ages 1 to 4 months) and then at 6 to 18 months. Catch-up doses can be given at older ages.

Haemophilus influenzae type b (Hib) Hib bacteria can spread from person to person through coughing or sneezing. When the bacteria spread to the lungs or bloodstream, the infection can cause serious and potentially fatal problems, most commonly meningitis — an infection of the membranes (meninges) surrounding the brain and spinal cord.

Most children with Hib infection need hospital care. Even with treatment, Hib-related meningitis is fatal in as many as 1 out of 20 children. And 1 out of 5 children who survive will have brain damage or hearing problems. Hib infection can also lead to severe swelling in the throat and infections of the blood, joints, skin and bones.

Vaccine recommendation The Hib conjugate vaccine is typically given to children in four doses recommended at ages 2 months, 4 months, 6 months and 12 to 15 months. Ask your child's medical provider for a personalized schedule if you need to catch up.

Children between the ages of 15 months and 5 years who haven't received any Hib vaccinations typically need one dose to catch up. Children over age 5 generally don't need a Hib vaccine unless they have a missing spleen or sickle cell disease.

Human papillomavirus (HPV) Your child may not get vaccinated against this infection until middle school, but it's worth knowing about. HPV is a common virus that has many different strains. According to the CDC, HPV infections occur in about 14 million people each year, primarily older teens and young adults.

A vaccine is available to protect against certain strains that can cause genital warts and several forms of cancer in both girls and boys. These strains of the virus are generally spread through sexual contact.

The goal of the vaccine is to protect your child long before the possibility of exposure to the virus. In addition, the HPV vaccine produces a higher immune response in preteens than older kids, which is why appropriate timing of the vaccine is important.

Vaccine recommendation The HPV vaccine is recommended for preteens, starting at age 11 or 12. Mayo Clinic recommends starting all children earlier, at age 9, for a better immune response. Those starting the series before age 15 only need two doses. Those starting at age 15 or later will need three doses. The vaccine is given as a series of shots over several months.

Measles Measles (rubeola) is caused by the most contagious human virus known. The virus is transmitted through the air in droplets, such as from a sneeze.

Signs and symptoms include rash, fever, coughing, sneezing, runny nose, eye irritation and a sore throat. Measles can sometimes lead to pneumonia, seizures, brain damage and death. It's most common in children but can affect adults.

According to the CDC, almost everyone who hasn't been vaccinated against measles will get the measles if they're exposed to the virus. In the U.S., people usually get the measles from travelers coming from other countries. This type of viral hitchhiking has led to widespread outbreaks among U.S residents who aren't fully immunized.

Vaccine recommendation Typically, two doses of the combined measles, mumps and rubella (MMR) vaccination are given, beginning at ages 12 to 15 months and then again at 4 to 6 years. But you can catch up at older ages, as well.

Meningococcal disease Meningococcal disease is caused by infection with meningococcus bacteria (*Neisseria meningitidis*). This type of bacterial infection can lead to life-threatening illnesses that affect the lining of the brain and spinal cord (meningococcal meningitis) and the blood (meningococcemia).

Meningococcal bacteria are spread by close contact with an infected person's saliva, such as by kissing, sharing food or coughing in close proximity. Because the infection can progress quickly, prompt treatment with antibiotics is imperative.

Vaccine recommendation All preteens should receive a single shot of the meningococcal conjugate vaccine at age 11 or 12, with a booster dose given later at age 16.

Mumps Mumps is caused by a virus that's transmitted through droplets of saliva or mucus, such as when an infected person coughs or sneezes. The disease causes fever, headache, fatigue and swollen, painful salivary glands. Mumps is usually a mild disease. But in some children it can lead to deafness, meningitis, and inflammation of the testicles or ovaries, with a remote possibility of sterility.

Vaccine recommendation Two doses of the combined measles, mumps and rubella (MMR) vaccine are given, usually beginning at ages 12 to 15 months and then again at 4 to 6 years. Use of this vaccine has markedly decreased the incidence of mumps in the United States. Catch-up MMR shots can be given at older ages.

Pneumococcal disease Pneumococcal disease is the leading cause of bacterial meningitis and ear infections among children younger than 5 years old. It can also cause blood infections and pneumonia.

Pneumococcal disease is caused by *Streptococcus pneumoniae* bacteria. The bacteria become airborne when a person with the infection coughs or sneezes and spread when another person inhales them. Because many strains of the bacteria have become resistant to antibiotics, the disease can be difficult to treat.

DOES MY CHILD NEED SHOTS BEFORE TRAVELING TO ANOTHER COUNTRY?

If you're planning an international trip with your child, check in with your child's medical provider — and your own — to make sure you're up to date on vaccinations. A number of vaccine-preventable diseases, such as measles, remain common in certain countries, and pre-trip vaccination may be appropriate. In addition, specific travel vaccines may be required depending on where you're going.

Make the appointment at least four to six weeks (or longer) before you leave as it may take this long to complete a vaccine series and for your body to build up immunity. For example, some countries require proof of yellow fever vaccine before allowing entry, and the certificate must be stamped at least 10 days before travel. If your medical provider doesn't stock travel vaccines, you may need to visit a travel clinic.

The Centers for Disease Control and Prevention provides specific travel vaccine recommendations based on your destination, available on its website.

Vaccine recommendation Pneumococcal conjugate vaccine (PCV) can help prevent serious forms of pneumococcal disease, such as meningitis and pneumonia. It can also prevent some ear infections. The vaccine is recommended in four doses between ages 2 and 15 months, but a catch-up dose can be given to children between ages 2 and 5 who haven't been fully immunized for their age.

Polio Polio is caused by a virus (poliovirus) that spreads through the saliva or stool of an infected person. The infection may lead to mild, flu-like symptoms. But it can also be more severe. Approximately 1 out of 200 people who become infected develop weakness and limb paralysis that can last a lifetime. Some children die because their breathing muscles become paralyzed. Even those children who recover may develop new symptoms as adults.

No polio cases have been reported in United States for over 30 years, but the disease is still common in some parts of the world. And the virus could be brought to the U.S. For that reason, getting children vaccinated against polio continues to be important.

Vaccine recommendation The vaccine, called inactivated poliovirus (IPV) vaccine, contains the chemically killed virus. IPV is given in four doses, at ages 2 months, 4 months, 6 to 18 months, and a booster shot between ages 4 and 6 years. If your child needs to catch up, talk to your doctor about a personalized schedule.

Rubella Rubella, also known as German measles, is caused by a virus that spreads through the air when people with the infection cough or sneeze. It's typically a mild infection that causes a rash and slight fever. However, a rubella infection during pregnancy may lead to a miscarriage, or the baby could be born with problems.

Vaccine recommendation Usually, two doses of the combination measles, mumps and rubella (MMR) vaccine are given, the first at ages 12 to 15 months and the second at ages 4 to 6 years. Catch-up shots can be given later, as well.

Tetanus Tetanus is a dangerous disease that causes headache, jaw cramping and painful tightening of the muscles, usually all over the body. It can be difficult to open your mouth (lockjaw) or swallow. Tetanus can also cause violent seizures, fever and rapid heart rate. It can take months to recover from tetanus, and the disease is fatal in up to 20 percent of cases.

The tetanus bacteria live in soil and manure. They enter the body through deep or dirty cuts or wounds. Tetanus isn't a contagious disease, so there's no herd immunity against it. Each person needs to be vaccinated for his or her own protection.

Vaccine recommendation The tetanus vaccine usually is given in combination with those for diphtheria and pertussis (DTaP). Vaccination typically begins at 2 months of age and is given in a series of five shots in the first six years of life. A booster shot, Tdap, against tetanus, diphtheria and pertussis, is recommended at age 11 or 12 and then a Td booster, for tetanus and diphtheria, every 10 years thereafter. Talk to your child's medical provider if you need a catch-up schedule. If your child is age 7 or older, this may involve a shot of Tdap.

Whooping cough Whooping cough (pertussis) is a disease that causes severe coughing spells and is especially dangerous for infants and toddlers. The word *pertussis* is from the Latin word for "cough." These coughing fits can last for weeks and can cause severe complica-

tions such as pneumonia, seizures, brain damage and even death. Severe whooping cough primarily occurs in children younger than 2 years.

Whooping cough spreads easily through infected droplets of saliva or mucus, often coughed into the air by an older child or adult with a mild case of the disease. Vaccines protecting against whooping cough have reduced the number of related deaths from approximately 8,000 a year to less than 20 annually. Outbreaks still occur, however, so full immunization continues to be important.

Vaccine recommendation The DTaP vaccination combines vaccines for diphtheria, tetanus and pertussis. It's given as a series of five shots typically beginning at age 2 months and continuing to between ages 4 and 6. At age 11 or 12, a booster of the vaccine, called Tdap, is recommended.

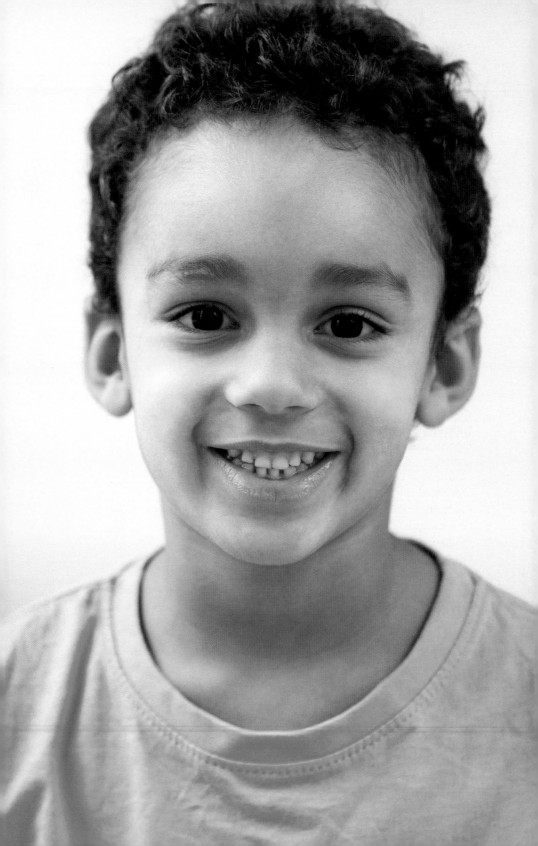

CHAPTER 7

Protecting your child's teeth

There's not much that can melt a parent's heart faster than a child's toothy — or not so toothy — grin. But keeping that charming smile healthy isn't always easy. Although children at this age are becoming increasingly independent when it comes to taking care of their own personal hygiene, getting children to brush their teeth or floss is a daily struggle many parents face. Some kids may not like the taste of toothpaste or the feeling of the toothbrush in their mouths, or they may be too engrossed in playtime to want to stop and clean their teeth. It can be exhausting, but don't give up. This is a crucial time to reinforce good brushing habits, which can prevent many dental health issues.

The American Dental Association (ADA) recommends that children begin seeing a dentist within six months of the appearance of their first tooth, or no later than their first birthday. After the first visit, most children will see the dentist every six months for teeth cleanings and to check for cavities. In many ways, it can be considered a "well-child" visit for the teeth. If your child has special needs or is more prone to cavities, your dentist may suggest more-frequent visits.

DENTAL EXAM

By now, your child may have had his or her teeth checked by a dentist at least a few times. If not, now's the time to catch up. If you're in search of a dentist, know that both pediatric dentists and many general dentists see young patients. Pediatric dentists receive at least two years of additional training beyond dental school, focusing on pediatric dental concerns, and they limit their patients to children and adolescents. A general dentist is trained to treat patients from childhood through adulthood.

During a checkup, the dentist or hygienist will assess your child's dental health and risk of cavities. A hygienist is a dental professional who assists the dentist with various tasks, including cleaning your child's teeth, taking dental X-rays and explaining strategies for maintaining good dental health.

The dentist may recommend dental X-rays for a closer look at your child's teeth to see if there are areas of decay, analyze how the teeth's roots are developing, and make sure the upper and lower jaw fit together properly. If your child has a habit that can affect teeth, such as thumb sucking, your child's dentist can evaluate whether it will impact development. As your child gets older, the dentist may discuss any need for orthodontic treatment, such as braces.

Your child's dentist will also be one of your best resources for help in fighting cavities — one of the most common dental problems in children. He or she can advise you on proper brushing and flossing techniques, apply sealants to help protect teeth from decay, and offer guidance on limiting tooth decay through diet.

FIGHTING TOOTH DECAY

During a typical dental appointment, one of the things your child's dentist or hygienist might do is inspect your child's mouth with a thin metal instrument or probe, tapping suspicious areas in search of soft spots that can indicate tooth decay is present. But what exactly causes tooth decay?

Everyone's mouth is filled with all kinds of bacteria. Like bacteria elsewhere in the body, some are beneficial, while others are harmful. Some harmful bacteria use sugar in the foods your child eats to produce acid. When sugary or starchy foods are eaten regularly, the acid produced can wear away enamel on teeth and rob them of protective minerals.

Over time, cavities can develop, and the only treatment for them is to drill out the damaged areas and replace them with a filling.

However, tooth decay is not a foregone conclusion. If caught early enough in the process, tooth damage can be stopped and even reversed. The calcium naturally present in your child's saliva, combined with good oral hygiene habits, fluoride from your child's toothpaste or water, and limits on sugary foods are the keys to stopping damage. Steps to help protect against tooth decay include:

Brushing The cornerstone of maintaining healthy teeth is brushing them. Depending on the age of your child, you may have to help with this. As a general rule, most kids need assistance with brushing until about age 8 or when they can tie their own shoes — a milestone that demonstrates they can likely also use a toothbrush effectively.

The dentist or dental hygienist can help give you and your child a tutorial on proper tooth brushing. Here are some tips: Have your child hold the brush angled at the gums, or at 45 degrees, gently moving the brush back and forth in short strokes and making sure to get at the inner surfaces and other harder-to-reach places. Encourage your child to also brush his or her tongue, which helps remove bacteria. Brushing is recommended twice daily for two minutes each time.

It's not necessary to buy the most expensive toothbrush you can find. A small, soft-bristled toothbrush that's designed to fit a child's mouth is all you need. And while there's been some debate about which is better — manual or electric toothbrushes — both have been found to do the job well when used correctly. Basically, it comes down to which type your child finds easier to use — or which one

ENCOURAGING TOOTH BRUSHING

It's common for a child, especially a young one, to put up a fight when it comes to tooth brushing. But it's also frustrating for you to try and convince an unwilling participant to keep his or her teeth clean. So what can you do about a child who hates brushing or just needs some encouragement? Try making tooth brushing a fun activity. For instance:

Take your child shopping for a new toothbrush and toothpaste Being able to pick out a kid-friendly flavor of toothpaste and a toothbrush in a favorite color or adorned with a beloved cartoon character can be a great incentive to brush. And your child will be happy to be included in the decision on what to purchase.

'Tune in' your child to tooth brushing Children can take some convincing when it comes to tooth brushing and its importance. Why not try some catchy music videos that stress the importance of brushing to young children? You can usually find these online. "Kids Just Love to Brush," a song featured on *Sesame Street* and inspired by Cyndi Lauper's "Girls Just Want To Have Fun," is an example. There are also numerous books featuring popular cartoon characters that cover how important brushing your teeth is.

Make timed tooth brushing enjoyable In a child's mind, the recommended brushing schedule of two minutes twice a day can seem like an eternity. But you can help pass the time. There are fun smartphone apps that keep track of how long your child brushes. Alternatively, you can read aloud your child's favorite book or crank up a favorite song while he or she brushes. Let your child choose the activity.

Offer rewards Create a rewards chart. For each successful brushing session, your child earns a star. If he or she gets a certain number of stars, offer a prize, such as a special trip to the library, getting an extra 30 minutes at the playground or choosing what your family has for dinner one night. Be sure to also offer your praise for a job well-done.

Make brushing part of 'family time' Brushing your teeth at the same time as your child is a great opportunity to demonstrate how to brush correctly and let your child know that even adults must brush their teeth.

Sometimes, having to offer these incentives to get your child to brush can feel time-consuming. But the good news is twofold: You probably won't have to do this for long, and you're instilling the importance of good dental hygiene at a young age — a practice that will follow your child for the rest of his or her life.

he or she is more likely to use. Whichever you decide to go with, make sure to replace the toothbrush every three to four months. When bristles become frayed or damaged, they don't clean teeth as well as they should.

Fluoride Fluoride is a naturally occurring mineral that helps strengthen teeth's enamel or repair spots on the teeth that have been damaged by acid. You can ensure your child gets the protective benefits of fluoride by using toothpaste that contains it.

Depending on the age of your child, you may need to help him or her apply the proper amount of toothpaste to the toothbrush — about the size of a pea. Supervise to make sure the toothpaste is being spit out after he or she is done brushing to avoid exposure to too much fluoride. If your child can't reliably spit out the toothpaste, use a smaller, rice-grain sized amount until he or she gets the hang of spitting it out. Excessive fluoride can lead to a condition called fluorosis, which may result in white lines or discoloration on developing adult teeth.

In addition to getting fluoride from toothpaste, your child may get fluoride from your tap water if you live in a community that has fluorinated water or your well water has levels of naturally occurring fluoride. Unfortunately, bottled water doesn't supply adequate amounts of fluoride.

If your child's dentist feels your child may be at an increased risk of cavities

MOUTH GUARDS: HELP PROTECT TEETH FROM INJURY

Just as pads and helmets are essential protective gear for young athletes, so, too, are mouth guards. These devices can help protect children from injuries that can break teeth or damage the jaw. Contact sports, such as football and hockey, typically require that players wear them for practices and games. For other sports, such as soccer or gymnastics, they're usually not mandatory but can be beneficial. If your child is into recreational activities that have a higher risk of falls and facial injury, such as skateboarding or in-line skating, you may want to consider a mouth guard for these activities, too.

The American Dental Association (ADA) recommends mouth guards that have been custom-made by a dentist to ensure proper fit and full protection. However, because custom-made mouth guards can be expensive, you may opt to purchase mouth guards for specific sports available in stores. Typically, these are sold by size or are the kind you boil in water to soften and then mold to your child's mouth. Look for the ADA Seal of Acceptance on the packaging, which means the product was tested and shown to provide protection from injuries to the mouth if used properly. You'll want a mouth guard that has some flexibility but isn't so soft that it tears easily. Look for one that's comfortable, doesn't affect how your child talks or breathes, and is easy to clean.

Tooth injuries can be expensive to fix, so any investment you make in protecting your child's teeth is a good one.

and you don't have fluorinated water, he or she may recommend applying fluoride directly to the teeth during a dental checkup. This fluoride treatment may be a rinse, or it may be applied via a gel or foam. Another option is daily fluoride supplements, which are prescribed by your child's dentist and come in various forms, including tablets and liquid drops.

Because many young children find it difficult to spit without swallowing, rinses containing fluoride aren't usually recommended for those under the age of 6.

Flossing Though some experts have questioned the benefits of doing so, the Department of Health and Human Services and professional organizations such as the ADA recommend flossing once a day. Start when your child has two teeth that touch. Flossing removes food that may have gotten stuck between teeth. It also helps remove plaque, a sticky substance that forms on teeth and can contribute to cavities and gum disease.

Because flossing effectively can be a little tricky at first, you'll most likely need to help your child. The ADA recommends guiding the floss between the teeth, then using a gentle up-and-down rubbing motion to the gumline. Products called flossers are designed to make it easier for children to floss and are available in fun shapes and colors. They may help encourage your child to keep up with this healthy habit.

If your child is having difficulty flossing, discuss it with your child's dentist or hygienist. He or she can give you and your child flossing pointers or recommend an alternative method. For example, water flossers, which are devices that pulse water out to clean between teeth, may be a more convenient option if your child is having trouble flossing with braces.

Dental sealants It can be tricky for little hands to maneuver a toothbrush to the very back teeth. The uneven surface of these teeth also makes it easy for food and bacteria to collect. To protect back teeth from decay, the dentist may recommend applying a dental sealant to seal off the grooves in the tooth's chewing surface. According to the Centers for Disease Control and Prevention, sealants may help reduce the risk of cavities in treated teeth by 80 percent for two years after they're applied.

The process for applying sealants is simple: After cleaning and preparing the teeth, your child's dentist paints on the sealant, which takes only a few minutes. The sealant is clear or white and won't be visible when your child is smiling or talking. This method of protection typically lasts several years, though that can vary depending on whether your child regularly eats hard foods or other foods that may cause stress or damage to the sealant. Your child's dentist will check the sealant at each visit to see if it needs to be replaced.

Eating habits Candy, sweets and other foods rich in sugar or starches are prime fuel for tooth decay. You don't have to institute an outright ban on sweet treats in your house to protect your child's teeth, but try to limit candy and other sweets to special occasions.

Another common source of tooth decay in children is juice. Because of the high sugar content, the American Academy of Pediatrics (AAP) recommends no more than 4 to 8 ounces of juice daily, depending on your child's age.

When and how often your child eats plays an important role as well. Experts recommend limiting snacks between meals to reduce the frequency of acid attacks on the teeth and give teeth a chance to repair themselves. If your child has already brushed his or her teeth for the night, veto any last-minute bedtime snacks he or she may request. Saliva production, which helps protect against cavities, decreases at night and may not be enough to counteract acid production resulting from the snack.

TACKLING DENTAL CONCERNS

Try as you might, you can't prevent every dental concern your child may have. Your child may habitually suck his or her thumb. A tooth may get knocked out in a softball game. You may find yourself with an anxious child who is terrified of the dentist. You're not alone. Here are some tips for handling issues many parents face in managing a child's dental care.

Thumb sucking For young children, thumb sucking is often a way to self-soothe or bring on sleep. By age 4 or 5, most children have stopped sucking their thumbs and found other coping methods. However, an older child may continue or even revert back to this behavior if he or she is feeling stressed or anxious. If thumb sucking continues as adult teeth begin emerging, it can affect the roof of the mouth or lead to misaligned teeth or jaw problems — especially if the sucking is vigorous.

In children age 5 and older, the AAP recommends trying to stop the habit. Though it can be a difficult to break, there are ways to help your child, depending on the nature of the habit:

- *Ignore the thumb sucking.* If you think your child may be doing it to get attention, your best bet may be to pay no attention to it.
- *Offer reminders.* If your child seems to be sucking his or her thumb ab-

sent-mindedly, gently remind him or her to stop. Don't scold or criticize.
- *Identify triggers.* If your child seems to suck his or her thumb during stressful situations, find alternate means of soothing, such as offering a hug or a stuffed animal to squeeze.
- *Use positive reinforcement.* Small rewards can go a long way — for example, offer your child a trip to the playground when he or she successfully avoids thumb sucking for a certain amount of time. A sticker chart that records the days your child doesn't suck his or her thumb can also provide a great visual incentive.
- *Enlist expert help.* Your child may be more receptive to advice from someone other than you, such as your child's dentist or even a grandparent. The dentist also may recommend a special mouth guard or other dental appliance that interferes with sucking.
- *Avoid pressuring your child.* It may only delay the process. If you're not successful, wait a little while, and then try again.

Early loss of a tooth One of the functions of baby teeth is to save space for adult teeth until they are ready to emerge. The process of losing baby teeth usually starts by age 6 or 7, beginning with the teeth that came in first. However, sometimes a baby tooth is lost to trauma (see page 177) or needs to be removed because of decay. This can result in shifting and realignment of the remaining teeth.

If your child has lost a tooth prematurely, the dentist may recommend placing a temporary spacer. These devices, typically made of metal or plastic, are placed in the spot of the missing baby tooth, keeping the space open for the adult tooth. Once the adult tooth emerges, the spacer is usually removed.

BABY TOOTH LOSS

Upper Teeth	Shed
Central incisor	6-7 yrs
Lateral incisor	7-8 yrs
Canine (cuspid)	10-12 yrs
First molar	9-11 yrs
Second molar	10-12 yrs

Lower Teeth	Shed
Second molar	10-12 yrs
First molar	9-11 yrs
Canine (cuspid)	10-12 yrs
Lateral incisor	7-8 yrs
Central incisor	6-7 yrs

PERMANENT TOOTH ERUPTION

Upper Teeth	Eruption
Central incisor	7-8 yrs
Lateral incisor	8-9 yrs
Canine (cuspid)	11-12 yrs
First premolar (first bicuspid)	10-11 yrs
Second premolar (second bicuspid)	10-12 yrs
First molar	11-12 yrs
Second molar	12-13 yrs

Lower Teeth	Eruption
Second molar	12-13 yrs
First molar	11-12 yrs
Second premolar (second bicuspid)	10-12 yrs
First premolar (first bicuspid)	10-11 yrs
Canine (cuspid)	11-12 yrs
Lateral incisor	8-9 yrs
Central incisor	7-8 yrs

'Bad bite' (malocclusion) When teeth don't line up properly, a child's overall bite is affected. Ideally, a child's top teeth should come down slightly over the lower teeth, and an upper molar's grooves should fit the grooves of the molar underneath it. When a misalignment occurs, your child may experience tooth overcrowding, abnormal bite patterns, difficulties biting or chewing, mouth breathing and, in some cases, problems with talking, such as a lisp. There are varying degrees of misalignment, from mild to more severe. Most often, this condition is hereditary, but it may also be caused by birth defects, extended thumb sucking, lost or extra teeth, and injury to the teeth or jaw.

Your child's dentist will look for problems with your child's bite and tooth alignment during regular dental exams and, if necessary, refer you to an orthodontist who can further evaluate and treat the problem. If your child's misalignment is minor, no treatment may be needed.

Dental anxiety Fear of going to the dentist is pretty common — it happens in both children and adults. Most dental offices these days are adept at making visits pleasant, however, and some kids even enjoy going to the dentist. Many offices offer perks, such as the choice of a toy from a treasure chest after an appointment. Some places offer distractions in treatment rooms, such as TV and movies.

Still, children may be fearful of going to the dentist because they worry that treatment will result in pain, don't know what to expect at an appointment or have bad memories of a prior dental visit. Children with developmental delays or special needs may experience heightened anxiety when it comes to dental visits. In such instances, you may want to consider specifically seeking the care of a

pediatric dentist. Pediatric dentists are trained to assess and carefully manage young patients who may be frightened and uncooperative.

For your part, you can help ease your child's anxiety by explaining what happens at the visit and why it's important to keep teeth healthy. Videos are available online that can prepare children for what to expect at the dentist's office. Regular cleanings and exams will also help familiarize your child with the dentist and lessen the chance that future visits will involve treating cavities.

If your child is going in for treatment of a dental problem, keep your explanation simple and upfront. While you want to be honest with your child about what the dentist or hygienist will do, consider avoiding words that may sound scary or be misunderstood. For example, instead of "drill the tooth," a more generic description such as "remove the cavity" may work better. For younger children, it may be helpful to play "dentist appointment" at home and recreate what will happen. Bringing a favorite book or stuffed animal to the appointment may also provide comfort.

IF YOUR CHILD NEEDS BRACES

Problems with tooth alignment are easier to fix when you're young and teeth can be more easily moved. Most people get braces between the ages of 8 and 14, when the majority of their baby teeth have fallen out and permanent teeth have come in. If your child doesn't have enough adult teeth yet the orthodontist may recommend waiting before applying braces.

A first visit to the orthodontist typically involves a thorough exam of the teeth, jaws and mouth, as well as X-rays that show the upper and lower teeth in biting position and any teeth still developing under the gumline. To further evaluate your child's bite, the orthodontist will create a plaster model made from soft material that your child bites into.

In severe cases of overcrowding, your child's orthodontist may recommend removing one or more permanent teeth to make room for the remaining teeth as they come in. Surgery combined with braces also may be recommended for children whose bites are significantly out of alignment.

After a treatment plan has been agreed upon for your child, you can expect things to proceed in three phases: placement of the braces, periodic adjustments and wearing of a retainer after the braces come off. Braces usually are fixed on the teeth but sometimes removable aligners are used.

Fixed dental braces These braces use the pressure of an adjustable wire running through brackets and bands temporarily fixed to the teeth to correctly align teeth and jaws. Brackets may be made out of stainless steel, ceramic or other materials. If your child requires additional pressure, the orthodontist may recommend special headgear, usually worn at night, or elastic bands stretched between the upper and lower jaws.

As part of your child's evaluation, your child's orthodontist will discuss risks involved with fixed dental braces. For example, braces can make it difficult for children to properly clean teeth, leading to trapped food particles and the growth of bacteria. This, in turn, can lead to a loss of minerals in the teeth's enamel and permanent white marks on the teeth. Cavities, gum disease and a drifting of teeth back to uncorrected positions may occur.

To reduce the risk of damaging teeth and braces:

- Advise your child on cutting down on sugary or starchy foods — particularly sticky and hard foods, which can pull off or break braces.
- Make sure your child brushes regularly, preferably after every meal, and rinses teeth thoroughly.
- Ask the orthodontist to show your child how to floss with the assistance of a floss threader, which can help get between braces and under wires.
- Schedule regular dental checkups for your child.
- Stress the importance of following the orthodontist's instructions. Not listening to the orthodontist could extend treatment time, lead to complications or result in less than optimum results.

Periodically during treatment, the orthodontist will adjust the braces by tightening or bending the wire, resulting in mild pressure on the teeth and gradual shifting of teeth into a new position. Your child's teeth may be sore for a day or two after an adjustment. An over-the-counter pain reliever should be all that's needed to relieve discomfort. If pain is more severe, speak with your child's orthodontist.

Removable clear aligners Removable aligners are worn as a series of appliances to gradually move teeth to the desired positions. Each set is worn for two to three weeks, then replaced by the next set. To work properly, it's recommended that removable aligners be left in the mouth most of the time.

Unlike fixed braces, these devices are removed when eating, brushing or flossing. Care must be taken when drinking anything other than water to avoid trapping sugary or acidic fluids next to the teeth, which can lead to decay.

A potential disadvantage of removable aligners is that they can be lost or misplaced. You may wish to take this into consideration when deciding on the best option for your child.

Retainers Retainers are a critical part of follow-up care. These custom-made appliances are typically made from plastic or a combination of plastic and metal wires. They help keep teeth from shifting back to their original position. Depending on your child's needs, your orthodontist may recommend a removable retainer to be worn for a certain amount of time every day; a fixed retainer, which is cemented behind teeth; or a combination of the two.

On average, you can expect braces to be on for one to three years. Retainers may be worn indefinitely to help maintain the position and alignment of the teeth.

SEDATION FOR DENTAL PROCEDURES

In some cases, sedation or anesthesia may be needed to keep a child calm or still long enough to perform necessary dental work — particularly for longer, more-involved procedures. You'll want to discuss with your child's dentist the pros and cons of using sedatives or anesthesia and the risks involved. Sedation and anesthesia, especially if not monitored vigilantly, can cause serious complications such as inhaling food particles or liquid (aspiration), trouble breathing, heart problems, allergic reactions, vocal cord spasms, loss of oxygen to the brain and even death.

If your child has special needs, a chronic illness, or airway or facial abnormalities, he or she may be at increased

QUESTIONS TO ASK BEFORE DENTAL SEDATION

If your child requires sedation before a dental procedure, discuss it with your child's dentist or sedation or anesthesia provider beforehand. Here are some questions to ask, based on recommendations from the American Dental Association:

▶ In addition to local anesthesia (numbing), what level of sedation or anesthesia will be given to my child? Will it be mild, moderate or deep sedation, or general anesthesia?

▶ Where will the sedation and procedure take place?

▶ What training and experience does the sedation or anesthesia provider have in providing the level of sedation or anesthesia that is planned for the procedure? Does he or she have experience with sedation in children?

▶ Does the assisting staff have current training in emergency resuscitation procedures?

▶ What do I need to do to prepare my child for the procedure? How long should my child be without food or drink prior to the procedure (except for necessary medications taken with a sip of water)?

▶ How will my child be monitored before, during and after the procedure?

▶ Are the appropriate emergency medications and equipment immediately available if needed, and does the office have a written emergency response plan for managing medical emergencies?

▶ Will the sedation or anesthesia provider give me instructions and emergency contact information in case there are any concerns or complications after returning home?

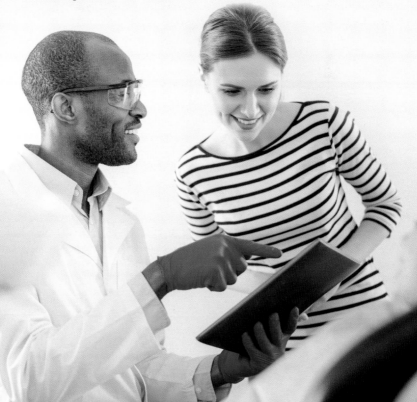

risk of complications related to sedation. In such cases, sedation and anesthesia services should be provided at a facility that offers monitoring under the care of a pediatric anesthesiologist. Be sure to discuss your child's health history, as well as any concerns you may have, with your child's dentist.

Sedation options for dental procedures include:

Mild sedation Typically this involves the use of "laughing gas" (nitrous oxide), a mild sedative that's inhaled along with oxygen via a nose mask during the procedure. Your child remains awake but is more relaxed.

Mild sedation may be used for procedures such as treating a deep cavity or pulling a tooth. Using nitrous oxide along with a local numbing agent, but without any other sedative medications, is common practice in dental offices. In this case, continual observation by the dentist and staff of your child's responsiveness, color, and breathing rate and pattern is recommended. The dentist will occasionally speak to your child to make sure that your child is only mildly sedated and that his or her airway remains clear.

Moderate sedation This is where a child is sleepy but awake and able to follow directions. Moderate sedation at low doses is sometimes done in a dentist's office. But because extra monitoring is required, the procedure may be performed in a hospital setting staffed with professionals trained to provide sedation to children and equipped with the necessary monitoring equipment and rescue protocols should an emergency arise.

Moderate sedation requires monitoring of vital signs such as heart rate, oxygen levels, breathing rate and blood pressure before, during and after the procedure. It's recommended that a qualified person separate from the dentist, as well as extra support staff, be involved in the sedation to monitor these factors. The sedation provider should be trained not only in the administration of appropriate sedative medications to children but also in the basic management of the pediatric airway.

Deep sedation and general anesthesia During deep sedation, medication is given intravenously (IV) and your child will sleep through the procedure, though he or she may still move around a little. During general anesthesia, your child is unconscious. These options are more likely for surgical procedures such as removing multiple teeth or setting a broken jaw.

Deep sedation and general anesthesia require close monitoring of vital signs including heart rate, oxygen levels, breathing rate and blood pressure. If your child requires deep sedation or general anesthesia for his or her dental procedure, the procedure should be performed in a hospital or clinic with experience caring for children. These facilities will allow your child to be appropriately monitored by a pediatric anesthesiologist or nurse anesthetist and trained staff during the procedure.

Such facilities will also have the necessary equipment to monitor vital signs, make sure your child's airway is kept free from obstruction, offer supplemental oxygen and respond rapidly to a medical emergency. Staff should be trained in lifesaving skills.

Don't be afraid to ask questions about the anesthesia specialist's experience, the staff's training or the facility's ability to handle an emergency.

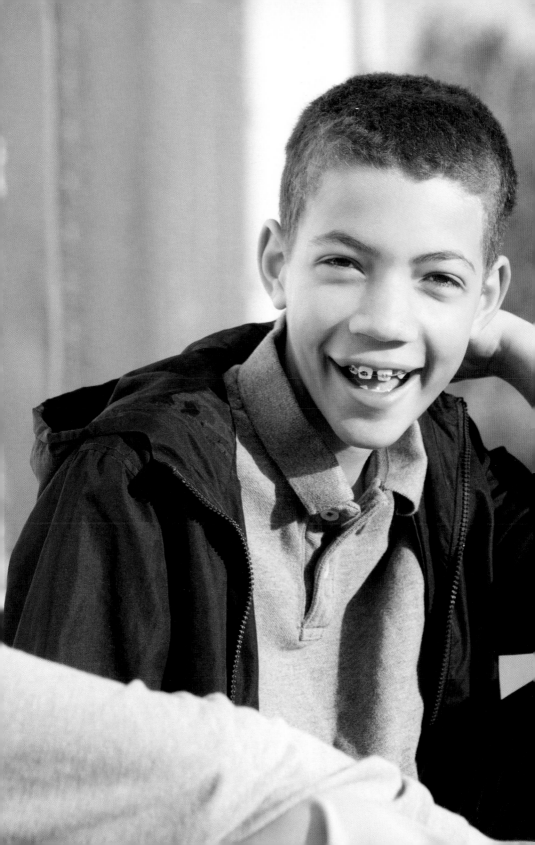

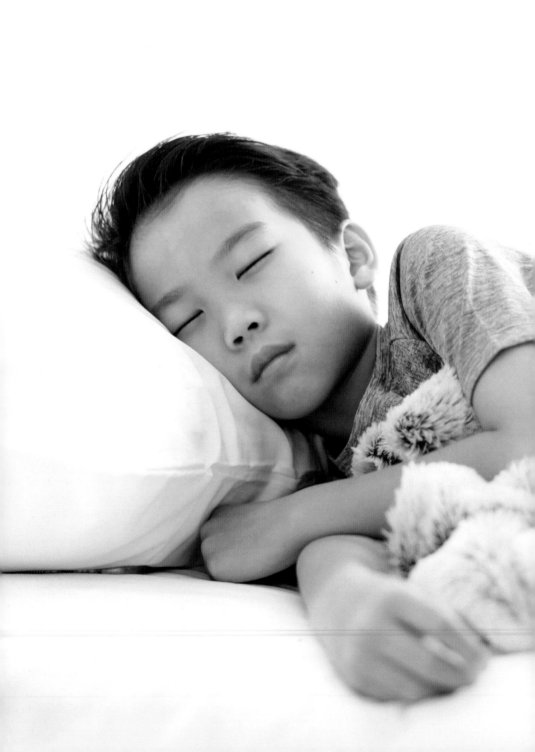

CHAPTER 8

Good night, sleep tight

Does this sound familiar? You start get-ting your 6-year-old ready for bed so he can be asleep by 8:00 p.m. But by 9:30, you're no closer to achieving that goal than when you started. In between, there have been numerous trips to the bath-room, pleading for a few extra minutes of playtime and requests for "just one more" bedtime story. One thing is for sure: Your child may not seem exhausted, but you sure are.

While parents more frequently asso-ciate the newborn and baby years with sleepless nights, the early childhood and pre-adolescent years can rob you of a good night's rest, too. However, you can take some comfort in knowing that, like those sleepless nights you faced when you were a new parent, these too shall eventually pass.

In the meantime, there are many things that you can do to try to develop a bedtime routine so that your child gets a good night's rest. One of the best ways to help maintain your child's health is to en-courage good sleep habits from the start.

GOOD SLEEP HABITS

While your child is sleeping, a complex cycle of events is taking place. During slumber, the body is alternating between one of two states: no-rapid eye move-ment (NREM), which is the quieter stage of sleep, and rapid eye movement (REM), which is when dreams typically occur. By the time your child is preschool age, he or she is alternating between these states about every 90 minutes.

Getting enough sleep — and properly cycling through these stages — is critical because it's the time in which the body gets to do some "housekeeping." During sleep, your child's body is recharging en-ergy levels, repairing tissue and releasing hormones that are critical to develop-ment. Regularly getting enough sleep re-sults in improved attention, behavior, mood, learning, memory, quality of life, and mental and physical health.

Many sleep problems can be prevent-ed by establishing good sleeping habits (sleep hygiene) early on. To promote a good night's rest, develop a routine that allows your child to set aside the activities and anxieties of the day and rest undisturbed until the next morning. Here are recommendations from sleep experts:

Stick to a sleep schedule Help your child get up and go to bed at the same time every day. Try to limit the difference in your child's sleep schedule on weeknights and weekends to no more than one hour. Being consistent reinforces your child's sleep-wake cycle.

To make bedtime predictable and smooth, use the same routine every night. Generally, try to avoid vigorous exercise in the two to three hours before bedtime. Stop playtime, games, and television, computer, video game or cellphone usage an hour before bedtime. During that hour, have your child wind down by preparing for bed, brushing teeth, and focusing on reading or other quiet activities.

Your child's bedtime routine might include a variety of soothing rituals, such as bathing, getting into pajamas and reading bedtime stories. It shouldn't last much more than 20 to 45 minutes.

Pay attention to when and what your child eats and drinks Serve dinner a few hours before bedtime and offer a small snack in between if necessary. Feeling full or hungry can interfere with falling asleep.

Be aware of the caffeine content in what your child drinks. Caffeine can take hours to wear off. In general, caffeine-containing beverages, including sodas and energy drinks, should be avoided in children. Energy drinks pose potential health risks to children because of the stimulants they contain and are inappropriate beverages for children and adolescents at any time.

Create a comfortable sleep environment Ideal sleeping environments are cool, quiet and dark. Make sure that the sheets and blankets are comfortable and that your child isn't too hot or too cold.

Darkness not only helps you fall asleep, it also aids in production of melatonin, a hormone that helps regulate sleep cycles. If your child isn't completely comfortable in a dark room, a small nightlight can ease fears and won't disrupt sleep. Room-darkening shades or curtains can keep out unwanted light from the outside.

Try to minimize noise in the bedroom. If noise is an issue that can't be controlled, try putting on some relaxing music for your child to fall asleep to or bring in some white noise, such as a fan.

Remove distractions Too many toys, books and gadgets in the bedroom can be mentally activating and interfere with falling asleep. Specifically avoid having electronic devices such as TVs, cellphones and computers in the bedroom. Light from screens contains "blue light" that can interfere with melatonin production.

You can remove the temptation of using electronic devices at bedtime by placing them all in a central spot, such as on the kitchen counter.

IS YOUR CHILD GETTING ENOUGH SLEEP?

How much sleep is "enough"? Ideally, you want your child to get enough sleep that he or she is bright and alert during the day. Each child varies in his or her individual sleep needs. While you know your child best, experts offer these recommended ranges within a 24-hour period, including naps:

- **Ages 3 to 5.** Your child should get about 10 to 13 hours of sleep
- **Ages 6 to 11.** Your child should get about 9 to 12 hours of sleep

Getting the recommended amount of sleep isn't always easy. Sleep disruptions are common during the preschool and school-age years, as demands on your child's time and attention increase. He or she may find it difficult to get to bed on time when there's homework to do and sports practices and club events to attend. From a parent's perspective, making sure your child gets enough sleep can be taxing at times, particularly if you or your partner work late or you're putting multiple children to bed.

Nonetheless, getting enough sleep is vital to your child's health and well-being. Children, like adults, suffer the consequences of inadequate sleep. A sleep-deprived child is more likely to have attention, behavior and learning difficulties.

A well-rested child is better able to focus, follow instructions and process information on a daily basis. Sleep also helps improve mood and behavior. Getting enough sleep can mean the difference between a good day and a bad day, so making sleep a priority benefits everyone.

BEHAVIORAL SLEEP ISSUES

Sleep issues are common in preschool and school-age children. The most common problems include difficulties falling

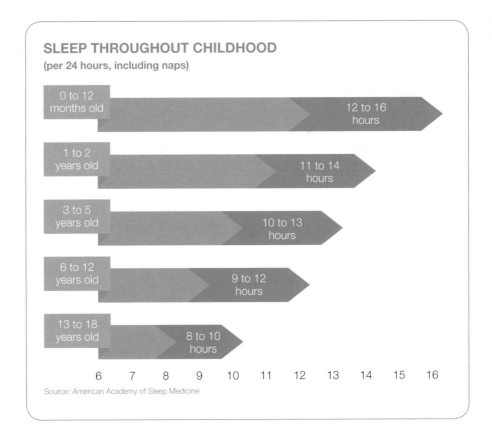

SLEEP THROUGHOUT CHILDHOOD
(per 24 hours, including naps)

0 to 12 months old	12 to 16 hours
1 to 2 years old	11 to 14 hours
3 to 5 years old	10 to 13 hours
6 to 12 years old	9 to 12 hours
13 to 18 years old	8 to 10 hours

6 7 8 9 10 11 12 13 14 15 16

Source: American Academy of Sleep Medicine

asleep or staying asleep (insomnia). The good news is that these kinds of problems are often behavior-related. As a result, they tend to be correctable.

Following are some common stalling tactics kids use to avoid going to bed and what you can do about it:

Comfort me It's a familiar situation faced by many parents: Your child wants comforting so he or she can fall sleep, and you want to eventually go to bed yourself, so you do what you can to check off the boxes. Maybe this involves a song, a gentle backrub or a glass of water.

Unfortunately, children can become so used to these soothing measures that falling asleep or going back to sleep without your assistance during the night is a struggle.

What you can do Learning to fall asleep independently is an important, positive developmental achievement for a child. You can help your child reach this milestone by removing yourself from the picture and helping your child transition to self-soothing measures.

A technique based on ignoring a child's requests for bedtime assistance, called systematic ignoring, is one of the most effective ways to make the break, and there are two approaches. One is to let your child "cry it out." With this method you put your child to bed and don't return until it's time to get up in the morning. However, this cold-turkey technique isn't for the faint-hearted, and many parents find it difficult to carry through.

A second method called the fading technique involves weaning your child from your presence: Put your child to bed drowsy, but still awake, and promise to check in on him or her. Your visits should be brief — one to two minutes — and re-assuring, with no cuddling and minimal physical contact.

In the beginning, check-ins may be frequent. With each night, increase the minutes between visits by a set amount of time with the goal of eventually eliminating all check-ins.

How you time your visits is up to you and also depends on how your child seems to be handling the situation. If more-frequent visits seem to upset your child, consider scaling them back right off the bat. If your child is getting out of bed or calling out, consider returning only when he or she is calm and quiet.

As an alternative to your presence, try offering a new stuffed animal or blanket selected by your child. It may also be comforting to your child if you leave his or her bedroom door partly open as he or she goes to sleep.

For some children, positive reinforcement in the form of rewards — such as a sticker chart — can give your child the incentive to become a more independent sleeper.

The weaning method works for children who need help self-soothing when they wake up during the night. The exception is when your child has nightmares (see page 124). To these you'll want to respond quickly. Reassure your child that it was just a bad dream, and when your child is ready, gently encourage him or her to try to go back to sleep.

The bedtime resistance Fighting the inevitable bedtime is a common occurrence among preschool-age and older children. Your child may outright refuse to go to bed or find ways to delay the process, ultimately resulting in an insufficient amount of sleep.

Children who are more strong-willed, those who don't have a regular bedtime or bedtime routine, those who still nap,

A WORD ABOUT CO-SLEEPING

Co-sleeping is a hot-button topic in the world of pediatric sleep medicine, with plenty of supporters and detractors.

There are many different reasons why parents may share a room or bed with their child. In some parts of the world, such sharing with a toddler or older child is common and part of the culture. Elsewhere, a child may have to share a bed with a parent or other sibling out of necessity if there isn't enough space in the home. Other times, sharing a bed may be done because the parent wants to stay close to his or her child or simply thinks it's the right thing to do. Such examples are referred to as "intentional bed-sharing."

More commonly, children end up sharing their beds with their parents as the result of a sleep problem. For example, your child is too afraid to sleep alone after a string of bad nightmares. Or your child flat out refuses to sleep in his or her own bed. Tired of battling your child on this, you let him or her sleep with you. This is called "reactive bed-sharing," and most parents of children who fall into this category aren't happy about the sleeping arrangement.

Some research has associated bed-sharing with sleep problems, including more difficulties sleeping alone, frequent nighttime awakenings, shorter sleep durations, problems with transitioning between sleep phases and sleep-breathing disorders. Children who co-slept also were less likely to have a regular bedtime.

The American Academy of Pediatrics discourages co-sleeping and recommends helping your child to develop healthy sleep habits with consistent bedtime routines and a healthy sleep environment instead. If your family has circumstances that may hinder your child's sleep, make sure to discuss these with your child's medical provider.

and those who have natural sleep cycles that predispose them to night owl tendencies are more likely to try "bedtime stalling."

What you can do Be consistent in following and enforcing a regular sleep schedule. Many children don't need naps after age 4 or 5. If your child naps, make sure it's for no longer than 45 minutes and not too close to bedtime. Most children need at least four hours to get sleepy again.

If these naps are still causing a disruption, this is likely a sign it's time to get rid of them. Being physically active throughout the day can also help your child fall asleep easier at bedtime.

Sometimes, kids stall bedtime by asking for a snack at the last minute. A glass of water and a few crackers or a bit of fruit is probably fine but avoid feeding your child heavy food or anything that contains caffeine (soda, tea, chocolate), which can disrupt sleep.

Realistically, your child's bedtime behavior will probably get worse before it gets better after you introduce a new set of rules. This increase in negative behavior is called an extinction burst and it's very common when you try to alter behaviors. But stick with the changes you've made and know that you're helping your child establish healthy sleep habits that will serve him or her well into adulthood!

Early to bed, early to rise Sleep needs are highly individual. For one child, 10 hours of sleep may be adequate while for another, 12 hours is ideal. If you're putting your child to bed too early, you may find he or she gives you a hard time about getting ready to go to sleep, wakes up too early or wakes up during the night.

What you can do Tailor bedtimes to your child's needs by delaying bedtime or moving up the wake time. For example, if he or she thrives on 10 hours of sleep and needs to be up at 7 a.m. to get ready for school, set lights-out for 9 p.m. To get your child on a schedule, ease into it by adjusting slowly: Delay bedtime or advance wake time by 15 minutes every few nights till you get to the desired time range.

Suddenly sleepless If your child is normally a good sleeper but lately has been waking up during the night or having trouble falling asleep, this is likely the result of a short-term problem. For example, your child may be stressed about something, such as an upcoming test or a dance recital. Illnesses such as colds or the flu can keep your child up with coughs, aches and pains, and stuffy noses.

While these sleep problems usually correct themselves in due time, they can become chronic if you find yourself resorting to comfort measures to get your child to bed.

What you can do If your child's anxious about something, encourage him or her to offload concerns before going to bed. Sleep tends to come faster when the mind is clear. Let your child know he or she can talk to you about his or her worries. Older children may find it helpful to make a list of concerns and put it aside until the next day when they can look at it with fresh eyes.

For colds and coughs, remedies such as over-the-counter nasal saline drops, humidifiers, plenty of fluids and a half-teaspoon to a teaspoon of honey — taken as needed for nighttime coughs in children over the age of 1 — can help. See page 320 for recommended cold remedies.

OTHER NIGHTTIME PROBLEMS

Most causes of sleep problems in children are behavioral in nature. However, there are other nighttime disruptions that are beyond your child's control. Some of these incidents can be scary or upsetting to witness or deal with as a parent, such as sleep terrors or sleepwalking. However, these episodes are generally harmless and usually don't cause a negative impact on sleep.

SLEEP EVALUATION AND TESTING

If your child still doesn't seem rested, despite adopting good sleep habits, ask your child's medical provider about an evaluation by a sleep specialist. Problems during the day, such as difficulty concentrating, hyperactivity, irritability, and mood swings, can be signs of sleep disruption that warrant further investigation.

To understand your child's sleep difficulties, the sleep specialist may ask how frequently problems occur, how long they've been going on, and if they've come on suddenly or more gradually. The specialist may also ask questions about sleep strategies you've attempted and what, if any, medications have been used.

A complete sleep history is often key to getting to the root of the problem. Sleep histories include when your child goes to bed and when he or she falls asleep and wakes up, as well as any problems encountered — for example, difficulties falling asleep or staying asleep, abnormal movements while asleep, snoring, or prolonged pauses or gasps during sleep.The specialist may recommend that you keep a written sleep log for your child. Other valuable information includes a daily summary of hours your child slept and his or her mood upon awakening.

Bedtime resistance or problems falling or staying asleep are often caused by behavioral issues, and a sleep specialist can help you devise a solution. However, the specialist may also recommend more in-depth sleep testing if he or she suspects a medical cause. Testing may include:

Polysomnography During testing, a person spends the night in a sleep lab while hooked up to special sleep-recording equipment. Sensors are placed on the scalp, temples, chest and legs. The sensors are connected by wires to a computer. Brain waves, limb movements, respiratory and heart functions, and nighttime noises, such as snoring or vocalizations, are some of the things polysomnography records. These recordings can help determine whether a sleep disorder is present. If your child's medical provider suspects a condition such as obstructive sleep apnea or narcolepsy, he or she may order this test.

Multiple sleep latency test Used to assess excessive daytime sleepiness, this test is performed after a nighttime polysomnography test. To test how sleepy a child is, the child spends the day at the sleep lab and is offered five chances every two hours to take a 20-minute nap. How quickly the person falls asleep may indicate how severe his or her excessive daytime sleepiness is. This test is also used to help diagnose narcolepsy.

Actigraphy To monitor sleep patterns and wakefulness, your child wears a device on his or her wrist for about one to two weeks to evaluate nighttime movements. The advantages of this method of data gathering are multiple days of recording, and it's performed in the comfort of the child's home. This test may also be used to evaluate the success of interventions.

Parasomnia is the medical term for sleep events that occur sporadically, usually during the transition between sleep phases. Examples of parasomnias include disorientation or confusion on wakening (confusional arousals), sleep terrors, sleepwalking, and sleep talking. Nightmares also are a type of parasomnia.

If your child has one or two parasomnia events a month or has episodes that are triggered by short-term events such as an illness, your child likely won't require any treatment. Sleep deprivation can trigger parasomnias, so make sure your child is getting enough sleep. Consistent bedtime routines, good sleep hygiene, reducing stress and avoiding heavy meals before bedtime can go a long way to help eliminate sleep issues. Many children outgrow parasomnias over time.

Persistent parasomnias may be triggered by problems such as anxiety, restless legs syndrome, acid reflux or sleep apnea, which increase your tendency to wake during the night. If your child experiences a parasomnia for more than a month or two, check in with your child's medical provider. The provider may recommend testing to rule out an underlying problem.

The most common parasomnias include the following:

Confusional arousals About two or three hours after falling asleep, your child awakens, sits up in bed and appears confused, crying or moaning, while rejecting your attempts to soothe him or her. This may last for five minutes or up to a half-hour. Your child shows no other symptoms, such as sweating or facial flushing, and cannot remember the incident the next day. Children usually outgrow this type of nighttime awakening by the time they're in school.

What you can do While confusional arousals can be upsetting to deal with, there's not much you can do but ride it out. Avoid trying to touch your child or provide comfort, as this may only upset him or her more.

WHEN IS BEDWETTING A PROBLEM?

By the age of 5, most children have enough bladder control to avoid bedtime accidents, though it's not uncommon for problems to continue. About 15 percent of 5-year-olds still wet the bed at least twice a week.

Some children have yet to get through the night dry (primary enuresis) while others develop a bedwetting habit after long periods of not having an accident (secondary enuresis). Primary enuresis tends to run in families, and when family members stopped wetting the bed can be an indication of when your child may outgrow bedwetting, too.

In some children, the ability to sense a full bladder and wake up just needs more development. This isn't unusual and he or she will outgrow it eventually. Secondary enuresis tends to come on because of conditions such as urinary tract infections, sleep apnea, diabetes and stress. See page 315 for more on bedwetting.

Sleep terrors Your child awakens with a scream and appears to be upset. He or she is sweating and may have a flushed face. His or her heart may be racing and he or she may appear to be fleeing from something. Despite your best attempts, your child can't be consoled, and the episode can last up to 20 minutes.

As with confusional arousals, sleep terrors typically occur during the earlier portion of sleep and may repeat several times in the same night. However, your child won't remember the incident in the morning. Sleep terrors are most common between ages 4 and 12.

What you can do Much like confusional arousals, trying to awaken or comfort your child during a night terror will likely only upset him or her more, so it's best to just wait in your child's room while the episode plays out.

Avoid turning on the lights and make sure that his or her sleeping area is free from hazards, should your child decide to get up during the night terror. If you find your child does tolerate your touch, gentle cradling or whispering comforting words may help soothe him or her, as well as yourself.

Sometimes, being overtired can trigger these episodes. If you think this may be the case, try putting your child to sleep about a half-hour earlier than you normally do.

Sleepwalking Your child gets up in the middle of the night to stand by your bed or makes a trek downstairs with the intention of leaving the house. His or her eyes are open, and he or she may appear to be awake, but nothing you say to your child seems to register. This sleep disorder tends to occur earlier in the night, or about two or three hours after going to bed, and can last up to a half-hour.

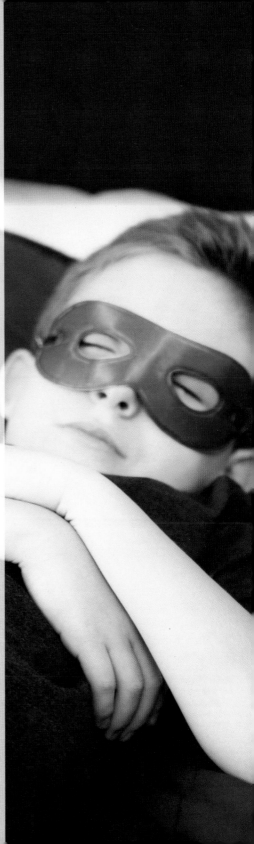

What you can do Sleepwalking at this age is usually not associated with any behavioral or other disorders, although sleepwalking may become more frequent if your child is experiencing stress in his or her life.

Unless your child is in immediate danger because of the wanderings, it's best if you don't attempt to wake up your child. Instead, try to guide him or her back to bed.

If your child's sleepwalking jeopardizes his or her safety, you'll need to take protective measures. This may include installing additional locks to prevent him or her from leaving the house or putting in safety gates at the top of stairs to block access.

Sleep talking Your child seems to be carrying on a conversation while he or she sleeps. Sometimes the dialogue sounds like gibberish, while other times it seems to be a normal conversation.

What you can do Sleep talking is very common among children and adults, and you don't have to take any measures to prevent it. Just remember that your child has no idea what he or she is saying and won't remember any conversation, so don't be too concerned about what is being said or bother to question him or her about it the next day.

In some cases, sleep talking can be a sign of an underlying problem, such as stress, sleep deprivation or depression. It can also be disruptive to the sleep of those around him or her. If it persists beyond a month or two, talk with your child's medical provider.

Nightmares Your child awakens in the early morning hours upset about an unpleasant dream he or she had. To your child, the dream seemed very real, and the feelings it created have left your son or daughter feeling fearful or anxious. Despite your reassurance that "it was just a dream," your child remains very disturbed and is having a difficult time getting back to sleep.

What you can do Understandably, your child may be afraid to go to sleep if he or she thinks the nightmare will keep recurring. In such a situation, offer hugs and comforting words.

You may opt to sit with your child for a bit as drowsiness sets in but avoid making a habit of it. Put your child to bed and promise to return to check in on him or her at a specified time. Holding a favorite stuffed animal, having a nightlight on, leaving the door ajar or softly playing some soothing music can also help quell your child's fears.

Sometimes children want to talk about their bad dreams when they awaken. Allow your child to discuss them and reassure him or her that there's nothing to be scared of and the nightmare wasn't real. If it's less frightening for your child, encourage him or her to talk about the nightmare during the less-scary daylight hours. Children may also take comfort in drawing or rewriting happier endings for their nightmares.

While nightmares are common and normal, some children, such as those with anxiety disorders, may get them more frequently than others. It may help to have a soothing bedtime routine, such as reading a calming story. Avoid watching TV or using electronic devices before bedtime, which can be stimulating.

Bullying and other upsetting life experiences can sometimes trigger more frequent nightmares. In these cases, nightmares can become a problem, and you'll want to discuss them with your child's medical provider.

SLEEP DISORDERS AND OTHER MEDICAL CONDITIONS

In some instances, sleep problems may be a symptom of an underlying or undiagnosed medical condition.

Obstructive sleep apnea (OSA) As in adults, children with sleep apnea stop breathing repeatedly throughout the night, causing the child to briefly startle awake — though usually the incidents aren't remembered. You may notice snoring or abnormal breathing while your child sleeps. These occurrences can greatly disrupt the quality of your child's sleep.

Though obesity can contribute to OSA in both children and adults, it doesn't mean that children who aren't overweight or obese don't develop OSA. The most common cause of OSA in children is enlarged tonsils and adenoids, which is the tissue located high up in the throat, behind the nose and behind the tongue. This can obstruct breathing.

The effects of sleep apnea in children are more likely to present as trouble concentrating or as a behavior problem, rather than daytime sleepiness.

Depending on the severity and cause of the condition, prescription and over-the-counter nasal sprays, continuous positive airway pressure therapy or surgery to remove enlarged adenoids may be treatment options.

Delayed sleep-wake phase disorder Delayed sleep-wake phase disorder is a malfunction of the body's circadian rhythm, or internal sleep clock. If your child has this disorder, you may notice that he or she falls asleep much later than what's considered a reasonable hour and wakes up later in the morning, as well. Usually, the sleep itself is normal — it just occurs on a delay. If your child has to get up at an earlier time than he or she might otherwise, such as for school, it can lead to daytime sleepiness and fatigue.

In this case, your child's medical provider may recommend small doses of melatonin several hours before bedtime to help your child feel sleepy earlier.

Movement disorders Involuntary arm or leg movements while a child sleeps can make it hard to stay asleep or get quality rest. These movement disorders may be diagnosed alongside neurological issues such as ADHD, mood and anxiety disorders, and other sleep disorders, such as sleep terrors and sleepwalking.

What causes movement disorders is unclear. Associated factors include a family history of movement disorders, iron deficiency and problems related to a chemical messenger in the brain called-dopamine.

Movement disorders — and the loss of sleep they contribute to — can have a major impact on how your child functions at school. Types of movement disorders include:

Periodic limb movement disorder (PLMD) This disorder is characterized by repeated limb movements while your child sleeps. As a result of the disruption, your child may have daytime sleepiness, loss of concentration and trouble paying attention.

Restless legs syndrome (RLS) Children who have restless legs syndrome have their sleep disturbed by frequent jerking of their legs, which can look like they're kicking in their sleep. Children with RLS typically feel leg discomfort and an urge to move their legs. Your child may describe the sensation as similar to bugs crawling on the skin. These feelings worsen while not moving and are relieved once your child starts moving again. Though this disorder shares many similarities with PLMD, the two are separate conditions.

Because iron deficiency is common in children with RLS and PLMD, your child's medical provider may recommend assessing your child's iron levels. If needed, the provider may prescribe iron supplements — taken in conjunction with orange juice or vitamin C for better absorption — for several months to help stop the nighttime limb movements.

Also, observe how much milk your child drinks every day. More than 2 or 3 cups a day can make it difficult for your child's body to absorb iron, which can lead to an iron deficiency.

Other types Nocturnal leg cramps, foot tremors, nighttime teeth clenching and grinding, and rhythmic movements — such as body rocking, head rolling and head banging — are also movements that can occur during the nighttime.

Most often, these are harmless and don't require treatment. However, if you find they're disrupting your child's sleep, talk with your child's medical provider.

SLEEP MEDICATIONS

Most children's sleep issues can be resolved through behavioral interventions. In rare cases where these interventions aren't effective on their own, a medical provider may suggest adding a sleep medication to the regimen.

There are no medications approved by the Food and Drug Administration (FDA) to specifically address sleep problems in children. Yet it's not uncommon for medical providers to prescribe a medication "off-label," which means using a medication to treat a condition for which the medication hasn't received FDA approval.

Prescription medications are almost always a last resort when treating sleep problems in children, as they often carry significant risks.

Any medications considered should be used only after other behavioral interventions have been tried for several weeks and failed, and always after a thorough discussion of risks and benefits with your child's medical provider.

Care also needs to be taken to match the sleep medication to the specific sleep complaints. For example, if your child has trouble falling asleep, a medication that makes him or her fall asleep faster but doesn't remain in the system for a long time might be an acceptable option. Longer-acting medications may help a child who has trouble with waking up during the night.

If your child's medical provider feels medication might be helpful, he or she may recommend an over-the-counter option first. These include:

Melatonin Nonprescription melatonin is a synthetic version of a hormone that plays a pivotal role in the natural sleep-wake cycle. Natural levels of melatonin in the blood are highest at night. Some research suggests that melatonin supplements may be modestly helpful in treating sleep disorders involving difficulty falling asleep and insomnia from jet lag.

Research suggests it's well-tolerated in children with and without special needs, isn't habit-forming and doesn't appear to lose its effectiveness over time. However, keep in mind that the quality of melatonin supplements can vary substantially from product to product. It has

not been shown to be effective in helping children stay asleep. Melatonin is typically given about a half-hour to an hour before bedtime.

Antihistamines Available over-the-counter, antihistamines such as diphenhydramine hydrochloride (Benadryl) are commonly used to treat short-term causes of sleeplessness, including jet lag and illnesses, and speed up the time to fall asleep and reduce nighttime awakenings.

Antihistamines aren't recommended for long-term sleep issues because they tend to require increasing dosages as a tolerance for the medication develops. In some children, antihistamines can actually have a stimulating effect.

If your child has an underlying condition that is causing or worsening sleep problems, treatment may require medication that's specific to his or her condition and doesn't interfere with any other medications he or she takes.

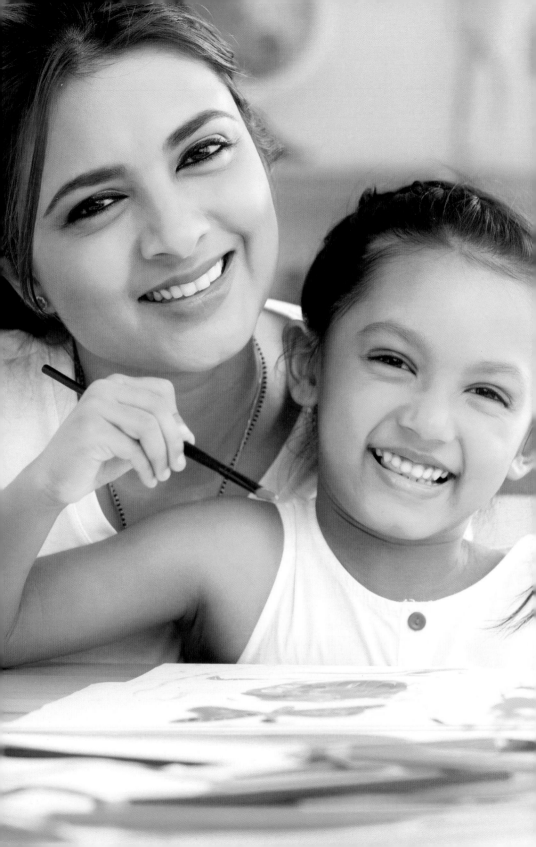

CHAPTER 9

Child care when you're not there

In today's society, many parents work outside of the home and require some form of supplemental care for their children. Working parents often rely on a variety of care providers to meet their needs.

With preschoolers, it's often convenient — and reassuring — to place them in a child care center that's close to work in case an issue or emergency arises.

As kids get older, some parents enlist the help of a neighbor or loved one to get their children to school in the morning. A good number enroll their children in a before- or after-school program or both. Others engage the help of nannies.

There's no right, wrong or straightforward answer to the child care conundrum. You'll probably find that the type of care your child needs evolves over time, shifting from close monitoring to care that allows him or her to take steps toward being more independent.

Depending on the age of your child and your needs, you have a number of ways you can tackle gaps in child care.

The key is to formulate a plan that fits your family's schedule and budget, while providing a safe and enjoyable high-quality environment for your child.

CHILD CARE OPTIONS

Parents have a number of options when it comes to child care, including babysitters, nannies, child care centers and after-school enrichment programs.

Things to consider when looking for high-quality child care include the safety and well-being of your child, the reliability of the caregiver, and how well the care option fits into your budget and schedule. You might also want to consider what activities your child enjoys and whether he or she seems to do better in a group setting or receiving individual attention.

Friends and family can be good sources of recommendations. Their personal experience with a particular caregiver or child care center can offer you great insight. So can visiting a facility and seeing firsthand how the staff interacts with their charges and if the children seem content.

The information that follows isn't exhaustive but can help you weigh the pros and cons of each type of care.

Child care centers Sometimes referred to as day care centers or child development centers, these are facilities that are located in a building — not a home — and regulated by the state. They may be nonprofit, for-profit, receive funding from the state or be a part of a federal program, such as Head Start.

Child care centers are typically organized into separate classrooms or groups based on a child's age. Groups are overseen by staff members who have training in early childhood development, CPR and first aid.

Some centers may have a formal preschool or prekindergarten (pre-K) program and may also provide after-school care for older children.

You'll likely be invited to take a tour of the child care facilities you're considering. During your visit, look for or inquire about the following:

- Proof of licensing and a recent health certificate.
- Accreditation, which requires a center to meet standards that are higher than most state licensing requirements. Accreditation is voluntary and is usually through organizations such as the National Association for the Education of Young Children (NAEYC) or the National Association for Family Child Care.
- Staff training and turnover. High turnover can be hard on children, who may find frequent staffing changes disruptive, and may indicate a chaotic or unstable work environment.

- Adult-to-child ratio. The NAEYC recommends ratios of 1-to-8 or 1-to-10 for 4- and 5-year-olds and classroom sizes of no larger than 16 to 20 children.
- Handling of sudden illness or injury and health matters. Find out what happens if your child becomes ill while at the center, how staff notify parents if a communicable disease is going around the center and how frequently they clean and sterilize toys and surface areas.
- Arrangement of quiet time and naps, and what alternatives are available if you don't want your child to nap or your child doesn't want to sleep.
- Safety and security measures, such as security systems to keep strangers out of the building, secured playgrounds and criminal background checks for staff.

Periodic inspections are conducted by the state to ensure child care centers are in compliance with regulations. Depending on where you live, you can get the results of these inspections either online or by requesting the information from the appropriate state agency. The government-funded program Child Care Aware has compiled state-by-state resources, including links to inspection reports, on their website.

The child care director should be able to provide you with an outline of how your child will spend his or her day, what curriculum is followed, and how the center's planned activities will help foster your child's learning. What your child learns at the center should follow state guidelines for early learning.

Overall, choose a child care center that's generally on the same page as you when it comes to discipline, learning, nutrition, playtime and other key ingredients to raising a healthy child.

5 CHILD CARE BUDGET TIPS

Child care costs can add up quickly. But there are ways to save:

1. *Create a budget.* Write down all of your monthly expenses, including big-ticket items such as mortgages, car loans and student loans. Also note what you pay for necessities, such as groceries and gas, and nonessentials, such as dining out and trips to the movies. Once you have your budget laid out, you'll have a better picture of how child care expenses will fit in and where you might find ways to cut costs.

2. *Shop around.* Compare pricing of various child care options. Contact your local Child Care Resource and Referral (CCR&R) agency to get an idea of average costs of child care in your area.

3. *Consider payment structures.* Some child care providers may offer you the option to pay for services in a lump sum at the beginning of the month or to break up the total cost into smaller, weekly charges, which you may find more manageable. When figuring out your monthly child care costs, don't forget to factor in "hidden costs," such as registration fees, meal costs and late fees.

4. *Save elsewhere.* If your budget comes up short, think about other areas where you can cut costs. This might include planning meals around what's on sale at the grocery store, carpooling or packing your lunch instead of eating out when you're at work.

5. *See if you qualify for assistance.* Find out if you qualify for help paying for child care, such as state subsidies or assistance from your employer, including employer discounts or dependent care spending accounts. Visit Child Care Aware of America online for more information. If you're a military family, you may also qualify for certain programs.

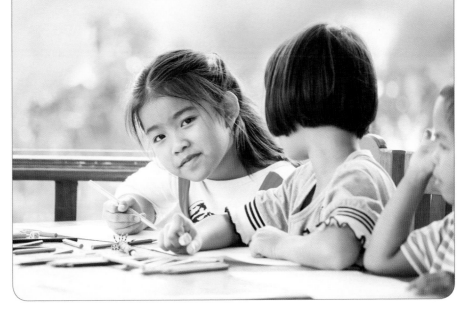

CHILD CARE OPTIONS

Pros	Cons
Child care centers	
• Generally governed by state and other local standards for operation; may be accredited • More likely to have structured programs geared toward specific ages • Formally trained staff, with certifications in CPR and first aid • Reliable care • Socialization opportunities • May have extended hours and flexible commitments	• Can be expensive • May require keeping a sick child at home • Increased risk of exposure to contagious illnesses • May feature less individual attention • May charge a fee for late pickup • Potentially long waiting lists for popular centers
Relatives or friends	
• Greater individual attention • Care may occur in the comfort of familiar surroundings • Reduced risk of exposure to outside illnesses • Sick child care • More flexible hours • May be less expensive than some other options	• Lack of a formal curriculum • Caregiver may not have training in CPR or other emergency care • Requires backup care if the caregiver is unable to care for your child
Family child care	
• Home-like setting • Opportunities for socialization • Often less expensive than other options • May be required to meet state and local regulations, depending on state guidelines • May provide more flexibility in terms of schedule	• Quality of setting and care can vary widely • Providers may not have to undergo background checks or enroll in ongoing training • Transportation may not be provided for older school-age children • May not offer a formal learning program

Pros	Cons
Nannies or au pairs	
• Care occurs in your own home	• Not well-regulated
• May allow for parent travel or a longer work schedule	• Usually more expensive than other care options
• Individualized attention	• Potential agency fees
• Reduced risk of exposure to outside illnesses	• Caregiver may not have training in child development or have training in emergency care, such as CPR
• Sick child care	• May entail responsibilities such as paying a minimum wage, providing health insurance and tax reporting
• Caregiver duties may include light housework or meal preparation	
• In-home care costs may be less or comparable to other options if you have multiple children	• Not as many socialization opportunities for preschool-age child
	• Requires backup care if caregiver becomes sick or takes vacation

Pros	Cons
Before- and after-school programs	
• Usually more affordable than some other care options	• Depending on the state, regulation may not be required
• Opportunity for socialization	• Transportation may be an issue if your child is attending a program outside of his or her school
• Familiar environment for your child	
• Possibility of enrichment programs	

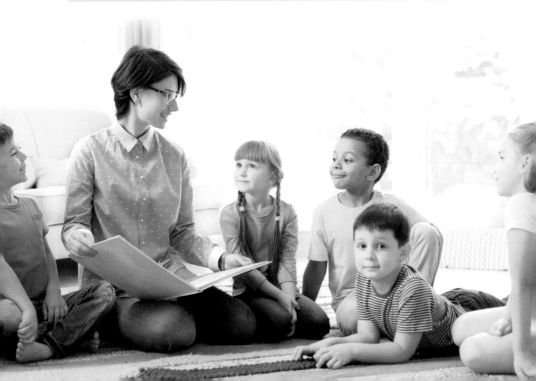

Relatives or friends Many people recruit friends or family to provide part- or full-time care for their children, either in the child's home or the caregiver's home.

It can be comforting to know someone who really knows your child is looking after him or her. But it can also present some challenges.

Although your child may not get as many colds and infections as at a child care center, he or she may not have as many opportunities to socialize with other children.

Backup care options may need to be set up for those times when your child's caregiver gets sick or goes out of town.

GUIDELINES FOR BABYSITTERS

Virtually every parent dreams of the perfect babysitter for those occasional nights out. You've done your homework — checked references, made sure CPR training was up to date — and you've found someone who's responsible and gets along great with your child.

However, even the most responsible and experienced babysitters require guidance. If this is the first time you're using a particular babysitter, have him or her arrive early so that you have plenty of time to go over the rules and guidelines:

▶ *Contact info.* Share emergency contact numbers with the sitter. Your list should include how to reach you directly, as well as the numbers for neighbors, your child's health care provider, the fire and police departments, and the Poison Control Center (800-222-1222 in the U.S.). Also include your home number and address, and your child's full name and date of birth, in case the babysitter is asked to provide this info in an emergency.

▶ *House tour.* Familiarize your babysitter with the kitchen and bathroom, the exits in your home, safety gates, and other areas or features important to your child's care.

▶ *House rules.* Discuss when to serve meals and what beverages or snacks are allowed. Outline screen time limits set for your child. Explain your child's bedtime routine — such as baths, tooth brushing and bedtime stories — and what time your children should be in bed. Address acceptable ways to handle poor behavior.

▶ *Babysitter rules.* Talk about what rules the babysitter must follow — for example, not using his or her cellphone while watching your child or not having friends over.

▶ *Safety first.* Go over any allergies your child has and how to respond if he or she has a reaction. Instruct the sitter on what to do in certain safety situations, such as answering the door. Show the babysitter where the emergency supplies are, such as first-aid kits and flashlights.

When you return home, ask your child what he or she thought about the babysitter and what they did while you were away. If all went well, you've found yourself an invaluable child care provider!

Also, to avoid confusion and potential misunderstandings, you may need to be clear about your expectations of the caregiver in terms of preparing meals and snacks, managing behavior, allowing enough playtime, and minimizing screen time.

Family child care Many people provide child care in their homes for small groups of children, sometimes in addition to caring for their own. These groups usually cover a range of ages, from infants to school-age children. An advantage of this type of care is that it may offer a smaller, more home-like setting than a child care center.

Often, state guidelines will dictate the size of licensed family child care groups. Generally, this includes a limit on the total number of children a single person can care for, as well as limits on the number of infants and toddlers. For example, a family child care group may have a limit of seven to 12 children total, and a further limit of no more three children under age 2.

When considering home-based child care, look for a place that's certified and licensed. Bear in mind that, depending on what state you live in and how many children are being cared for in the home, licensing may not be required.

Other factors to consider include:

- The ratio of care providers to children
- Background checks on care providers
- Care provider's references
- Care provider's training in childhood development and safety response, including CPR and first aid
- Care provider's approach to learning, discipline, nutrition and other issues
- Who lives in and visits the home, and how that person might interact with your child
- What measures are in place to keep your child safe
- What happens when the care provider takes a vacation

The care provider should be able to provide you with a snapshot of a typical day at the home and how activities may help support your child's learning and development.

Nannies or au pairs With this type of arrangement, a nanny or au pair either lives in your home or comes there daily to provide child care. Au pairs are people who typically come to the United States on a student visa and provide child care in exchange for room and board and a small salary.

Checking references for a nanny or au pair candidate is crucial. You'll want

---

NEED HELP?

If you're having difficulties finding appropriate care for your child, Child Care Resource and Referral (CCR&R) agencies can put you in touch with child care providers located near your home or work. Visit the website for Child Care Aware to search for your local agency.

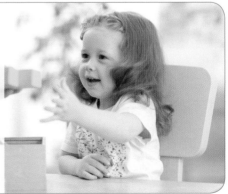

SUMMER CARE: OFF TO CAMP WE GO!

Summertime can present a particular challenge for working parents of school-age children. Suddenly, you're left trying to find a day care solution that fills the hours your children would have been at school. From your child's perspective, summer means goodbye to teachers and homework for a couple of months and a lot more fun kid stuff. Summer camps are a popular option for many families to fulfill the needs of both parents and children.

Some parents choose to send their children to a day camp program offered through a local park and recreation department, community organization or day care center. Some zoos, museums and nature centers offer day camps, as well.

Day camps may be focused on specific areas, such as science, sports or drama, or offer a sampling of activities, from crafts to swimming. Many camps offer half-day and full-day options. If you have a younger child or a child who isn't yet ready to spend nights away, this may be your best bet, supplemented by child care if needed.

Parents may also choose to send their children to a sleepaway camp where a child spends a week or more away from home. Some may have a specific theme, such as soccer, cheerleading, nature or computers. Others are structured for specific purposes, such as camps for kids with special needs.

When choosing a summer camp, think about the setting your child will feel most comfortable in and what activities he or she would most like. Then, you can narrow down your options by asking the camp director some key questions:

▶ **Can I see the camp first?** Ask about tours and to see a daily schedule before putting down a deposit. Do the setting and schedule fit your child's personality?

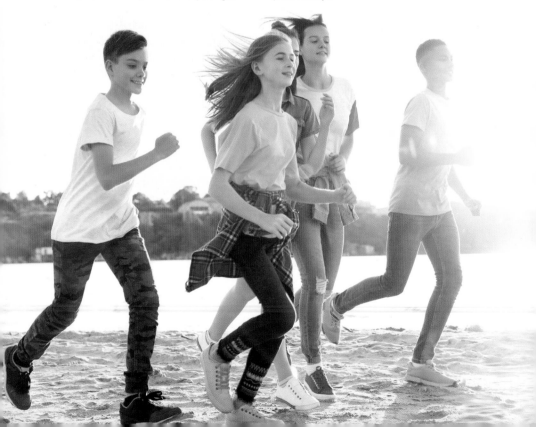

▶ **Is this camp licensed and accredited?** Licensing is through the state where the camp is located and looks at health and safety issues, and program standards. Requirements for licensing vary from state to state, and not all states require licensing. Accreditations obtained through organizations such as the American Camp Association are voluntary and are earned by meeting guidelines and standards set by the accrediting organization.

▶ **What do others have to say?** Personal recommendations are helpful, but if you can't get a recommendation, go online and search for reviews of the camp. Ask the camp director if references are available.

▶ **Are there hidden fees?** Is everything included in the price, or do some activities, such as field trips, cost extra? Are lunches provided or will you need to pack a lunch each day?

▶ **What are the staffing standards?** Check out the camp's website or contact staff to learn about the staff's training, counselors' ages, staff background checks and camper-to-staff ratios. The American Camp Association requires its accredited camps to maintain specific staff-to-camper ratios:
  ➤ *Sleepaway camps:* 1-to-5 for ages 4 to 5, 1-to-6 for ages 6 to 8 and 1-to-8 for ages 9 to 14
  ➤ *Day camps:* 1-to-6 for ages 4 and 5, 1-to-8 for ages 6 to 8 and 1-to-10 for ages 9 to 14

▶ **What happens in an emergency?** How does the camp handle emergencies? Is there a camp nurse available, or medical facilities nearby? Staffers should have CPR and other safety training, such as courses taken through the American Red Cross.

▶ **How will the camp keep my child safe?** The camp should be able to provide you with a set of written rules for the camp and details on how rules are enforced — for example, how they deal with bullying. If your child has a special health concern, such as asthma or a food allergy, find out how this will be handled. Make sure the camp has any medications your child needs.

▶ **How will my child and I keep in contact?** Find out the camp's policy on children contacting parents, or if you're allowed to visit your child while at camp. A little distance between parent and child during summer camp can be beneficial in helping a child establish independence and develop resilience. For example, some camps have rules banning cellphones to allow children to immerse themselves in the camp experience. But know how to contact the camp in case of an emergency.

Day camps tend to be the most economical of the camp options, although even these can be a budgetary burden. However, many camps offer resources that may help make summer care more affordable — for example, discounts for paying early, payment plans, scholarships and other forms of assistance. Don't hesitate to ask.

to talk to several of the care provider's former employers to find out his or her strengths and weaknesses, as well as any issues the employer may have had.

You may be able to get a sense of the person's caregiving style by asking certain questions, such as how he or she would correct behavior or soothe an upset child. In addition, it's important to hammer out the particulars of the job, including expectations regarding:

▶ Normal work hours
▶ Additional household duties
▶ Time off
▶ Salary range
▶ Health insurance
▶ Tax withholdings
▶ Length of service

To ensure that you find someone who's a good fit, consider using a nanny or babysitting agency. Although you'll likely have to pay a fee, you'll have the comfort of knowing that the candidates have already been vetted. You can also browse vetted caregivers by joining online caregiver referral sites.

Before- and after-school programs
School and work schedules don't always match up neatly, as many parents know. If your school-age child needs care before or after school, check to see whether your child's school offers a before- or after-school care program on-site.

Other possibilities include community programs run by local recreational or religious centers or organizations such as the Boys and Girls Clubs and YMCA. Sometimes a school will partner with such an organization to offer before- or after-school care.

These programs are often offered in a time frame that meets most working parents' schedules. During this time your child may have a snack, take part in learning activities, do homework or socialize.

Schools may also offer before- and after-school enrichment programs that focus on learning or improving skills in areas such as sports, art, music, math and science. Enrichment programs may only cover an hour or so after school, so you may need to combine these classes with another program to meet your child care needs.

HOME ALONE

As your child gets older, you may wonder when it's appropriate to let him or her stay home alone. Maybe you want to make a quick run to the pharmacy. Or maybe it's for those few hours after your child gets home from school and before you get home from work.

Most experts recommend waiting until age 11 or 12 before leaving a child home alone. If your child is younger and spending a regular amount of time unsupervised, you may want to consider finding child care for the time you're away from home until your child is older.

Factors to consider But even for occasional times, age is just one factor in your decision. You'll also want to consider other factors, such as:

Legal issues Only a handful of states have laws that specify a minimum legal age for a child to be home alone. While most states rely on parents using their best judgment, many offer guidance on this topic on their official websites.

If you're unsure about your state or local guidelines, do a quick internet search for your state, county or municipality and "home alone resources," and you should easily find your state's specific laws or recommendations.

Safety issues One of the biggest concerns with leaving a child home alone is safety. Your child needs to know how to follow an emergency plan, where to find the first aid kit, and how to contact you or another designated adult and call 911 if there's an emergency. Your child should be able to recite his or her full name, home address and telephone number. Additional factors to consider include hazards in the home and the safety of your neighborhood.

Your child's maturity level Before leaving a child home alone, consider whether he or she is developmentally ready to handle this responsibility. Does your child obey rules and follow directions? Would she feel OK being home alone? Does he make good choices? Does she respond well to unfamiliar situations? How do you think he would react to an emergency? These are just some of the questions to consider.

If you think your child is ready If you think your child is responsible enough to stay home alone, there are several things you can do to prepare for this milestone:

- *Do a trial run.* Use that pharmacy run, trip to the grocery store or other short errand as a trial. This can give you a good sense of how your child will handle being left home alone for a longer period.
- *Set house rules.* Be clear about what your child is allowed to do and what's not OK. Make a list of chores, homework or activities to be done. Provide healthy snacks that are easily accessible. Talk about rules for going outside, having friends over and using social media.
- *Prep for emergency.* Talk about what constitutes an emergency and how to handle one. Post a list of emergency numbers where your child can see them, or program them into a cellphone used by your child. Create and practice an emergency plan. Being able to coordinate with a trusted neighbor is helpful. For example, if your child smells smoke or gas or hears a smoke alarm go off, have them go to the neighbor's house to call the fire department.
- *Address how to handle strangers.* This might include not answering the door for anyone not previously agreed upon, knowing how to answer the phone without letting the caller know the child is home alone, and not talking to strangers or revealing whereabouts online. Some parents find it helpful to establish a code word with their child. The code word can be required to communicate through another person when needed.
- *Clear hazards.* Don't leave safety to chance. Make sure potentially dangerous items are properly stored or locked away. Examples include weapons, power tools, poisonous household items, matches and lighters, medications, and alcoholic beverages.
- *Check in frequently.* Call your child and have him or her call you to check in — such as when he or she gets home from school. It's good practice for getting a hold of you. The Red Cross also offers apps for smartphones and tablets that feature emergency preparedness features for parents and children, as well as basic first-aid information, which children can refer to if needed.

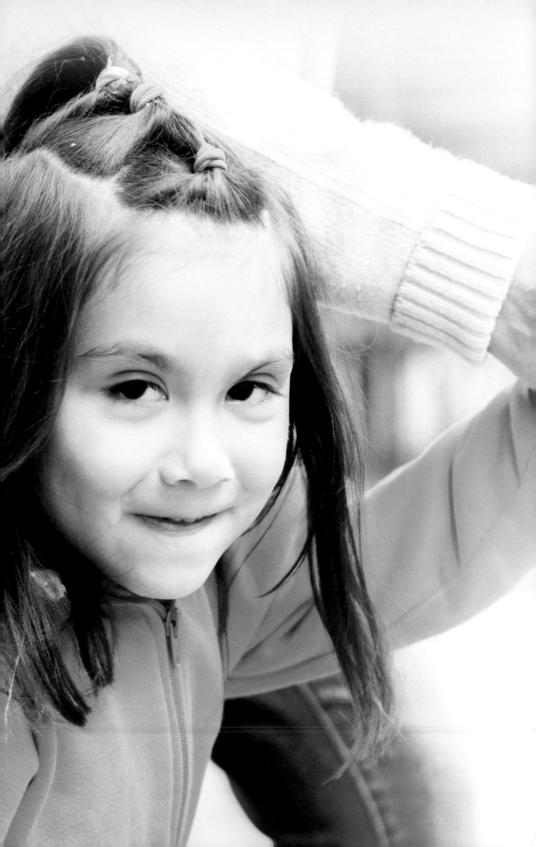

CHAPTER 10

Staying safe

To a child, the world is filled with new and exciting adventures around every corner. And while you do your best to let your child experience the wonders of his or her world, you also recognize that there are hazards out there, as well.

Accidents often happen when a child's skill set doesn't match up with his or her desired activity. Think of a curious preschooler who tries to climb a ladder or a couple of fourth-graders who decide to swim across a pond when they're not yet strong enough to do so. Keeping your child's developmental stage and environment in mind when setting limits can help prevent or reduce the risk of harm.

Personality also comes into play. If you have multiple children, you may be surprised to see just how different they are when it comes to safety — how you can't assume that because your oldest child played it safe, your youngest will, too.

Although you won't be able to prevent every mishap, there's a lot you can do as a parent to help your child avoid everyday risks and injuries. This chapter offers you a foundation for building that prevention plan.

HOUSEHOLD HAZARDS

Though most parents do their best to childproof their homes, the reality is that most houses are still geared toward adults. Because of this, where a child lives is the most likely place he or she will be injured. To help prevent childhood injuries, look at your home through the eyes of your child to identify areas that need attention. As your child gets older, you can re-evaluate the precautions you take.

If you have multiple children in your home, plan around those who are most vulnerable, based on age but also, importantly, developmental abilities.

A thorough assessment of home safety can be especially important for grandparents or others who might be caring for children after an extended period of having no kids in the house.

Cleaning and other household products Kids are explorers by nature, so it's not surprising that they can find their way into closets and under bathroom and kitchen sinks, where hazardous items are typically stored. Cleaners, laundry detergent, furniture polish, antifreeze and other household items may have pleasing scents and packages that are visually appealing to children, enticing them to play with the contents or taste them, exposing their skin, eyes and digestive systems to caustic chemicals.

Any household product you store in your home has the potential to be harmful to your child. Prevention centers recommend the following safety strategies:

- Keep household products in an out-of-reach place in your home. If you have to store them in a place your child can access, such as under the sink, install child safety locks.
- Store household products in their original, child-resistant containers. This can help prevent access and avoid confusion about what your child was exposed to in the event of an accidental ingestion or exposure. Never store products in empty food containers because it can confuse your child, who may think the contents are safe to eat or drink.
- Purchase only those products or other hazardous materials you need to use soon to avoid having to store them.
- Be vigilant when in the homes of other people, particularly those who may not have taken child safety precautions in their houses.

Medications Medications help relieve pain or fight infection, but they also pose a risk of overdose or poisoning. Unfortunately, accidental medication overdoses happen all too often in children. To prevent this from occurring, pay special attention to the way you store, administer and dispose of medications. This can be especially important for grandparents or other older adults who may have more medications in their homes.

Storage Store medications where your child can't see them, even those you may use regularly for your child. Having a designated area for medications can help you keep them organized, easy for you to find and out of the reach of children.

Cabinet and dresser locks are a good idea for keeping young children away from medications. Child-resistant caps provide a second line of defense.

It can be tempting to leave medication on a kitchen counter or bedside table for the sake of convenience. But because young children may find the bright colors or packaging irresistible, it's important to avoid the habit of leaving medications out.

If you have a medication that must be refrigerated, put it on a high refrigerator shelf so that young children can't reach it or in a place where it's not visible.

Administration Unintentional drug overdoses may occur when parents are giving medication to their children and accidentally give them too much. To avoid this:

- Always check the label each time you give a medication to ensure you're giving the right medication in the right dose. Dosing should be based on your child's weight. See dosage charts for acetaminophen (Tylenol, others) and ibuprofen (Advil, Motrin, others) on pages 478 and 479. If it's the middle of the night, turn on the light so you that can see the medication better.
- Avoid alternating acetaminophen and ibuprofen so that you don't accidentally give the same medication

twice. Stick to one medication and write down the time and dose that was given to keep track.

▶ If using a liquid medication, only use the dispenser that came with the medication. To avoid dosing confusion, don't use cooking utensils, such as teaspoons or tablespoons, for measuring medication.

▶ Don't allow older children to take medications unsupervised. Also make sure you see exactly what they're taking and how much. Teach your child to double-check the label for appropriate dosing instructions.

You can further discourage children from taking medication that's not theirs by taking yours in private, when your child can't watch and be tempted to imitate you.

Disposal A crucial way you can help prevent medication overdosing is to properly dispose of leftover or expired medications. To do so safely:

▶ Find a drug take-back program or authorized collector — typically local police departments, pharmacies and hospitals. The Drug Enforcement Administration (DEA) hosts events annually where prescription-drug collection sites are set up in local communities. To find out more about events or find a DEA-authorized collector in your area, visit the DEA's Diversion Control Division website.

▶ If a medicine take-back program isn't nearby, you can throw medications in the trash. To do this, the Food and Drug Administration recommends these precautions: Mix the medication with something inedible such as coffee grounds, dirt or kitty litter. Seal it in a plastic bag or container and place it in the garbage. Scratch out any personal information on the prescription label before disposing of the original container.

▶ Some prescription medicines may be especially harmful if taken inappropriately. These may come with instructions for flushing unused portions immediately down the toilet, if no take-back program is readily available.

▶ Keep the phone number for Poison Help (800-222-1222 in the U.S.) handy in case your child accidentally ingests or is exposed to medication. The staff at the poison help center can provide reliable and timely information on the need for medical care and the potential administration of antidotes.

Choking Food accounts for more than half of all choking incidents. Button-type batteries, coins, beads and other small objects also are choking hazards. To prevent choking:

▶ Insist that your child stay seated while eating.

▶ For children younger than age 4, cut up foods such as grapes, hot dogs and baby carrots for easier chewing and swallowing.

▶ Also avoid giving foods such as hard candy or peanuts that are smooth and slide easily toward the throat.

▶ Follow the age recommendations on toy packages.

▶ Keep younger children away from small objects they might inadvertently swallow, such as buttons, marbles, small toys, pen caps and rubber bands.

▶ Supervise play with latex balloons, another choking hazard.

Burns There are many home goods and appliances that can pose a burn risk for your child — not just ovens and stoves, which are some of the first things that come to mind. Hot water, food and electrical outlets also can injure your child.

To prevent burns at home, consider the following:

- Set your home's hot water heater at or below 120 degrees Fahrenheit.
- Always check your child's bathwater before putting him or her in it. Bathwater should be around 100 degrees Fahrenheit.
- Teach your child about kitchen safety and keep him or her a safe distance from the oven while you cook. Hot liquids, foods and grease can spill on your child and cause serious burns. Use the back burners on the stove

CREATE YOUR OWN MEDICAL SUPPLIES KIT

A well-stocked medical supplies kit can help you respond quickly and effectively to common injuries and emergencies. You can buy kits at many drugstores or assemble your own. Keep your medical supplies in a place that's easily accessible but out of the reach of young children. Make sure that children who are old enough to understand the purpose of the kit know where the kit is stored.

Remember to replace items after their use to make sure the kit is always complete. Check your supplies yearly for outdated items that may need replacing. Check expiration dates on medications twice yearly. Also make sure to include a first-aid manual. Here's what you need to be prepared for accidents and common illnesses:

- *Cuts.* Bandages of various sizes, gauze, paper or cloth tape, an antiseptic solution to clean wounds, and an antibacterial ointment to prevent infection.
- *Burns.* Cold packs, gauze, burn spray and an antiseptic cream.
- *Aches, pain and fever.* A thermometer, a nonsteroidal anti-inflammatory drug and acetaminophen (avoid aspirin use in children).
- *Eye injuries.* Sterile eyewash (such as a saline solution), an eyewash cup, eye patches and eye goggles.
- *Sprains, strains and fractures.* Cold packs, elastic wraps for wrapping injuries, splints and a triangular bandage for making an arm sling.
- *Insect bites and stings.* Cold packs to reduce pain and swelling. Hydrocortisone cream (0.5 or 1 percent), calamine lotion or baking soda (combine with water to form a paste) to apply to site until symptoms subside. Antihistamines to reduce itching and swelling. If a family member is allergic to insect stings, include a kit containing an epinephrine autoinjector. Your doctor can prescribe one. Check the expiration date regularly.
- *Ingestion of poisons.* Keep the Poison Help phone number, 800-222-1222 in the U.S., near your landline telephone and programmed into your cellphone.
- *General first-aid care.* Sharp scissors, tweezers, cotton balls and cotton-tipped swabs, plastic bags, safety pins, tissues, soap, cleansing pads or hand sanitizer, latex or synthetic gloves for use if blood or body fluids are present, and a medicine cup or spoon.

with pan handles turned inward, if possible. Never leave food cooking on the stove unattended.

▶ Avoid leaving hot food or beverages in places where a young child can easily reach them, such as the edge of a counter or on the kitchen table.

▶ Test any food or beverage that you've heated up in the microwave first before giving to your child. Microwaves are notorious for heating foods unevenly, leaving hidden hot spots.

▶ Keep your child at a safe distance from fireplaces, space heaters, radiators, grills, fire pits and campfires.

▶ Place hot devices such as clothes irons and curling irons out of reach and unplugged when not in use.

▶ Skip the warm-mist humidifiers and opt for a cool-mist version, which can help avoid steam burns and hot water spills.

▶ To prevent electrical burns, use safety protectors for any electrical outlets not in use. Replace damaged, brittle or frayed electrical cords, and don't run cords under rugs or carpets.

▶ Cover your child's car seat with a towel or blanket to prevent buckles or straps from getting too hot during the summer.

Fires Accidental fires can break out for any number of reasons, including candles left unattended and children playing with matches. Because fires can move quickly and leave little time for escape, prevention and planning are crucial to save lives. To protect your family and home:

▶ Store matches and lighters in a secure place, out of sight. Teach your child that matches and lighters aren't toys.

▶ Keep candles out of the reach of children and put them out before leaving a room. Consider using flameless candles, which are battery operated.

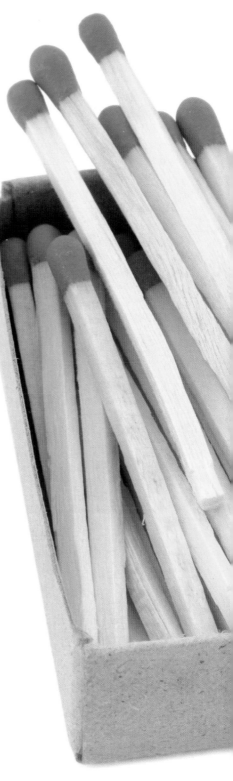

CALLING 911

In some emergency situations, your child may be the one who has to contact 911 for help. If your child is able to recognize when someone needs help and can follow verbal instructions, teach him or her how to call 911:

▶ Explain what 911 is, when is the appropriate time to call — for example, only when police, firefighters or an ambulance are needed — and how to dial the number, which can be practiced on a fake phone. In some instances, your child may not know whether a situation is an emergency. In these cases, your child can call 911 and have the operator assess the situation.

▶ Make sure your child knows how to use a phone, whether it be a landline or cellphone.

▶ Around age 5, your child can do some role-playing with you if you think it's appropriate. Create a pretend emergency and test your child's reaction. Your child should be able to tell a 911 operator his or her name, your name, telephone number, and address. It's natural for anyone to get flustered in an emergency, so keep a list of these important details by your phone for easy reference.

▶ Stress the importance of trusting the 911 operator, answering all of his or her questions, and staying on the phone until told to hang up.

▶ Caution your child about accidentally calling 911. However, if 911 is called by accident, let your child know it's important that he or she doesn't hang up. Instead, stay on the line and explain what happened. This lets the 911 dispatcher know there is no emergency and saves him or her from having to call you back or send emergency help.

- Smoking is hazardous to your health for a number of reasons, but it's also a common cause of fires in the home — another good reason to quit. If you do smoke, don't smoke in the house.
- Keep space heaters at least 3 feet away from flammable items, such as bedding and drapes, and never leave a space heater on while you sleep.
- Maintain your fireplace and chimney with annual inspections and cleanings.
- Install smoke detectors to alert you to danger and give you and your family more time to get out of your home.
- Place at least one smoke detector on each floor of the home, near bedrooms, and test them monthly. Use long-life batteries and change them at least once a year. Replace smoke detectors every 10 years or by the expiration date marked on the device.
- Keep a fire extinguisher in your kitchen, out of the reach of children, and learn how to use it.
- Teach your children to "stop, drop and roll" in the event their clothing catches fire: Stop, drop to the ground and cover the face with hands, and roll on the floor to put out flames.
- Have an evacuation plan in place for your family. Make sure everyone knows how to exit any room in the house. Teach your children to leave a burning building by crawling under the smoke. Determine a meeting place outside, preferably in the front of a house where firefighters can easily find you. If you live in an apartment building, look for posted evacuation routes, such as in stairwells or lobbies.

Carbon monoxide Carbon monoxide is an invisible, odorless gas produced by burning fuel in cars and trucks, small engines, stoves, lanterns, grills, fireplaces, gas ranges, generators, and furnaces. When carbon monoxide gas can't escape, it can build up, poisoning those who breathe it.

One of the most important preventive measures you can take is to install carbon monoxide detectors in your home. Many come combined with a smoke detector, giving you two lifesaving devices in one. These should be placed on each floor, near bedrooms. Check and replace the batteries regularly. Other steps you can take to prevent carbon monoxide poisoning include:

- Have your heating system, water heater, and coal-, wood- or kerosene-burning appliances serviced by a trained service person annually.
- Make sure all your gas appliances are properly vented.
- Never use a generator inside your home or outdoors within 20 feet of windows, doors or vents.
- Never use a gas oven for heating your home.
- Get your chimney inspected and cleaned every year; before lighting and extinguishing a fire in your fireplace, make sure the fireplace damper is open.
- Open the garage door before starting your car.
- Make sure a keyless ignition car is turned off in the garage before going into the house.

If your carbon monoxide detector goes off, don't ignore it or attempt to investigate potential sources. Instead, immediately move your family outside, call 911 or emergency services, and stay out of your home until first responders tell you it's safe to go back in.

Lead exposure Because of their rapid growth rate and a tendency to put their hands in their mouths, children under age 6 are at the greatest risk of lead poisoning — most commonly from coming into contact with soil or dust contaminated with lead-based paint. Although lead-based paint was banned in the United States in 1978, children who live in older homes or apartments may still be exposed to old paint and face an increased risk of lead poisoning.

Even low levels of lead can negatively affect a child's IQ, ability to concentrate and school performance. Once lead poisoning has occurred, its effects can't be reversed, so efforts focus on testing and prevention.

Routine lead testing in children is commonly performed at ages 12 months and 24 months. But it may be done at other times, depending on your child's risk factors, such as lead in the home.

Minimizing your child's exposure to lead sources is crucial. If your home was built before 1978, assume it contains lead paint unless testing shows otherwise. Take the following precautions:

⟩ Keep children away from any areas of peeling lead-based paint, particularly if you're doing renovations, which can disturb old paint. Children should be kept from these areas until proper cleanup is completed by a licensed professional.

⟩ Regularly wash children's hands and toys, which can carry lead-contaminated household dust or soil.

⟩ Wet-mop floors and wipe down windows and other horizontal surfaces every few weeks to cut down on dust, which can contain lead.

⟩ Have your family and visitors remove shoes when they come into the house to prevent transfer of lead-contaminated soil into your home.

⟩ Cover any bare soil with grass, mulch or other ground cover to minimize contact with contaminated soil.

Sometimes, there are less obvious sources of lead exposure. Imported candies, herbal and folk medicines, serving dishes, and cooking pots may contain lead. Pay attention to toy and costume jewelry recalls for lead contamination. Consider eliminating or avoiding older toys, such as those found at garage sales.

Additional tips: Use only cold tap water for drinking and cooking, as hot water is more likely to contain lead. Shower and change clothes if you've been exposed to lead-based products, such as stained glass or bullets at a firing range.

Furniture and appliances According to the Consumer Product Safety Commission (CPSC), thousands of furniture- and appliance-related injuries occur in children each year. A child may attempt to climb a dresser or TV stand, causing the furniture and appliance to topple over on top of the child. In some cases, these injuries can be fatal.

Childproofing is key to preventing tip-over tragedies. The CPSC recommends:

⟩ Placing televisions on furniture that was designed for this use, such as TV stands and media centers.

⟩ Anchoring televisions to the wall or to furniture.

⟩ Anchoring furniture to walls with anti-tip brackets, which don't cost much and are available at hardware stores. If you've purchased new furniture, such as a dresser, anti-tip hardware should be included. Install it immediately.

⟩ Eliminating the temptation to climb by removing toys, remote controls and other objects from the tops of televisions and furniture.

Lawn mowers Lawn mowers pose a serious risk of injury for many reasons.

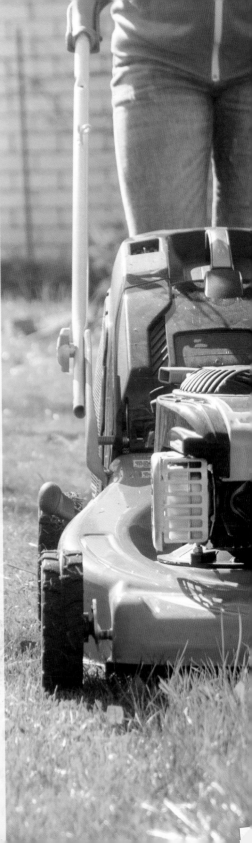

They have hot surfaces and powerful, spinning blades. They can send rocks and other objects flying. And they're the most common cause of amputation in children. Riding mowers are associated with a higher injury rate than push mowers.

To prevent lawn mower injuries in children, take these precautions:

▶ Don't allow your child to be in the yard when you're mowing or let your child ride on a mower with you.

▶ Don't allow your child to operate a lawn mower. Children should be at least 12 before using a push mower and at least 16 before using a riding mower.

▶ Teach your child about the dangers of lawn mowers and to stay away from running mowers, which should never be left unattended. Reinforce how critical it is that hands should never be put near the motor or blades, even if something is caught in there.

▶ Remove debris from your yard that could become projectiles if run over with a mower.

▶ Avoid mowing in reverse. If you have to back up, look for children behind you first.

▶ Never rig your lawn mower to override important safety features — for example, those that turn the mower off when you take your hands off the handle.

Guns Gun sports are popular in the U.S., and many families choose to own guns. Having a gun in the home poses safety risks, however. Among young children accidentally killed by guns, wounds are typically self-inflicted or inflicted by another child while at home.

Not having a firearm in the home is one of the most effective ways to prevent firearm injuries in children. If you own one or more guns, make sure you're properly trained in the safe use of firearms. Importantly, take steps to keep firearms safely away from children and other unauthorized users:

- Store firearms unloaded and in a locked cabinet, safe, vault or storage case. Cartridges should be stored in a separate locked location. Consider hiding the keys or combinations somewhere your child can't find them.
- If you remove your gun from storage, never leave it unattended. When returning from a hunting trip or firing range, unload, clean and store firearms right away. Don't leave them lying around.
- A variety of gun safety devices — such as loaded-chamber indicators, magazine disconnects and others — are available and can be helpful. "Smart guns" are able to identify accepted users and block those who don't have permission to use the gun.
- Locks and safety devices can fail. Most importantly, know how to handle a gun safely: Always point the firearm in a safe direction, and never place your finger on the trigger unless you intend to shoot. Educate your child about gun safety, and allow him or her to attend a gun safety class at a reputable school or shooting range when appropriate.
- Be wary about whether other people follow proper gun safety protocol. Don't be afraid to ask whether there are guns in the home before your child visits a friend.
- Reconsider having a gun in your home if someone who lives there has a mental illness, including severe depression, or has the potential to be violent. There is an increased risk that this person will use the gun for self-harm or to hurt others.

SEXUAL ABUSE

Although sexual abuse is a serious crime, it's unfortunately common. By teaching your child about appropriate and inappropriate touching, you can help protect your child from sexual predators. Help your child understand that he or she has the right to forcefully say no to anyone who threatens him or her, and to tell you about it right away.

Know what it is Sexual abuse involves any sexual contact or sexual behavior with a child, including showing him or her pornography or taking pornographic pictures of the child. It affects both girls and boys. In most cases, a child who is sexually abused knows his or her abuser — for example, a family member, caregiver or coach — and the abuser will use manipulation and intimidation to get the child to engage in sexual acts, as well as keep it secret. In many cases, the abuse goes on for a long time.

Indications that a child may be sexually abused include fear of a particular person or place, withdrawal from friends and family, marked changes in behavior, sleep problems, loss of appetite, inappropriate sexual behavior, and self-destructive tendencies such as getting in trouble repeatedly. In most cases of sexual abuse, physical signs aren't apparent but sometimes may include anal and vaginal bleeding, genital infections, repeated bladder infections, or wetting accidents after having been toilet trained for a while.

Reduce your child's risk To reduce your child's risk of molestation:
- Teach your child the correct names for genitalia. Give honest answers to questions about sex. Addressing the topic in a straightforward manner and

using accurate terms shows your child that sex isn't a taboo subject.

▶ Make sure your child knows that it's always OK to tell you of any "weird" or inappropriate sexual contact, even if he or she feels guilty or ashamed, and that you will never punish your child for telling you. Perpetrators often

MISSING CHILDREN

It's every parent's worst nightmare: Your child is missing. Though you may feel frightened and overwhelmed, act immediately to increase the odds you're successfully reunited with your child. If you believe your child is missing, it's important to start by alerting the authorities. Though it's a natural instinct to want to start looking for your child right away, you may be losing crucial time. Remember: Look for your child only after you've called local law enforcement. Don't worry if it turns out to be a false alarm. It's better to be safe than sorry.

What you can do If your child is missing, take these steps:
▶ Immediately call local law enforcement to report your child missing. Provide key information, including a physical description of your child, what he or she was wearing, and whether he or she has any defining characteristics, such as a birthmark. Also provide information on when your child was last seen and who may have seen him or her. Ask that your child be added to the FBI's National Crime Information Center Missing Persons File.
▶ After filing a report with local law enforcement, consider contacting the National Center for Missing & Exploited Children (NCMEC) at 800-THE-LOST (800-843-5678) if law enforcement hasn't already done so. This nonprofit organization offers families and local law enforcement support in finding missing children.
▶ If you're at home, search through areas where your child may have fallen asleep, may be hiding, or may have been injured or trapped, including under beds or in closets, laundry hampers or large appliances such as dryers. Check vehicles and nearby outdoor spaces, such as abandoned wells and creeks.
▶ If you're in a store, school or hospital, alert staff, managerial or security personnel that your child is lost, then call police. Many places have a missing-child protocol in place and will act immediately to secure the building.
▶ Make sure any computers or other devices your child may have used to go online are secured until law enforcement can examine them. Avoid conducting your own search. Secure your home, as well, until law enforcement has had the chance to search it.
▶ Ask law enforcement whether an Amber Alert will be issued for your child. This is an emergency alert system that notifies residents in specific areas that a child is missing via texts, road signs and other methods.
▶ For more information, visit the NCMEC website at *www.missingkids.org.*

groom their targets by telling them that they'll get in trouble if they tell anyone or that no one will believe them if they do tell.

- Teach your child about privacy and respect. Let your child know that no one has the right to touch the private parts of his or her body without permission, and that he or she needs to respect other people's right to privacy, too.
- Talk about potential scenarios where a molester might try to draw a child in, such as offering gifts or special outings. Encourage your child to exercise caution and to always check in with you first before accepting gifts or money from others. Warn your child to never enter someone's home or vehicle unless accompanied by a trusted adult. Exercise vigilance when it comes to adults who pay extra attention to your child, such as buying your child gifts or offering to watch your child without others around.
- When you provide love and attention to your child, you establish an open and trusting relationship between you and your child. This eliminates the need for your child to seek attention elsewhere. Be involved in your child's activities. Be aware of whom your child spends time with and where, and what they're doing.

If your child is molested If your child tells you he or she was sexually abused, take this seriously. Make sure that your child understands that the abuse isn't his or her fault and that you will do everything you can to protect your child.

Call your child's medical provider or contact the nearest child advocacy center, which is staffed by professionals trained in assessing child abuse. The staff at the center can provide coordinated care and help avoid scenarios where your child has

to share his or her story multiple times. They may interview your child, perform a physical, look for signs of injury, collect evidence (if possible) and file the necessary reports, as well as offer other resources, such as referrals for psychological counseling for you and your child.

To search for an advocacy center near you, visit the National Children's Advocacy Center's website. You can also call the Childhelp National Child Abuse Hotline in the U.S. at 800-4-A-Child (800-422-4453).

SUBSTANCE USE

When kids are young, it may seem as if it's too early to talk about drug and alcohol use. But talking to your child about drugs and alcohol before he or she is widely exposed to them is the ideal time to start an ongoing discussion. Consider these strategies.

Be open Though children can sometimes be stubborn when it comes to listening to their parents, the reality is that parents can have a huge impact on how children ultimately respond when drugs are offered to them. Often, your influence starts with being open to discussing difficult topics and really listening to your child's response. Let your child know you're there and fully supportive.

Clarify family rules It can be tempting to put off discussing drugs, thinking your child already knows that drugs are bad and not to use them. But don't let rules about drug use go unspoken. Be very clear about what you expect from your child and offer praise when he or she makes good decisions. Consider some role-playing exercises that will test what your child will do when — not if — he or she is offered drugs. Don't shy away from telling your child about the harsh realities of what drug use can do to his or her health, particularly since drugs are sometimes mixed with other chemicals that make them even more dangerous.

Set a good example Equally important, set a good example by not using tobacco or drugs, or engaging in excessive drinking yourself. Drinking several glasses of wine after a hard day, for example, may give your child the wrong idea about how to properly deal with stress. Avoid allowing your child to watch TV and other media programs that downplay the dangers of using drugs, alcohol and tobacco.

Keep track of friends and activities Talk with your child if you notice concerning behavior from a peer. Let your child know that he or she doesn't have to do something to be accepted. Encourage your child to get involved with school clubs, sports and other activities that offer structure and foster positive behavior.

Empower your child Teach your child to say no in different ways. Maybe this involves declining drug offers and offering to do another activity, such as playing basketball or a video game instead. Let your child know it's OK to just walk away, too, and it's always OK to call you for a ride home whenever he or she feels uncomfortable.

Know the signs Though there are no guarantees that your child will avoid drugs, starting your prevention efforts early can certainly help reduce that risk. Unfortunately, some children will start experimenting with drugs early on. If you think this may be the case for your child, look for signs, such as:

- Red eyes
- Dilated or constricted pupils
- Frequent nosebleeds
- Problems sleeping
- Sudden weight loss or weight gain
- Messy appearance
- Smell of alcohol or tobacco on your child's breath or clothing
- Troubling behavior, such as stealing money, acting up at school, withdrawing from family and friends, angry outbursts, problems focusing, and poor school attendance and grades

If your suspicions are confirmed, prepare to discuss it with your child and get help. Your child's medical provider or school guidance counselor can help you get the resources you need.

VEHICLE AND TRAFFIC SAFETY

Vehicle-related accidents — as passengers or pedestrians — are the leading cause of childhood deaths. Taking appropriate safety precautions, such as always using car seats and seat belts appropriately, will help you reduce this risk.

Car safety Car seats and booster seats can protect your child from serious injury if he or she is ever in an automobile accident. However, to get the maximum safety benefit, your child needs to be in a proper seat that's correctly installed.

The National Highway Traffic Safety Administration (NHTSA) and the Centers for Disease Control and Prevention (CDC) recommend that children ride in the back seat of an automobile through at least the age of 12, using the proper car seat, booster seat or a seat belt. Depending on where you live, your state may have specific laws governing when a child can legally sit in a front seat.

To maximize safety, follow these research-based guidelines for using a forward-facing car seat, booster seat and seat belt.

Forward-facing car seat Keep your child in a forward-facing seat that has a harness and tether until he or she reaches the maximum height or weight limit for that particular seat — typically between ages 4 and 7. Check the car seat's instruction manual for this information. Forward-facing seats come in various designs:
- Convertible seats change from rear facing to forward facing.
- Combination seats change from forward facing to booster.

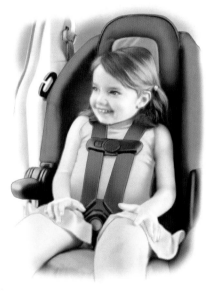

- All-in-one seats can be used rear facing, forward facing or as a booster seat.

Winter coats or bulky clothing can prevent harnesses or seat belts from fitting properly. In cold weather, keep jackets off until you arrive at your destination. Use blankets over the car seat if needed to keep your child warm.

Belt-positioning booster seat Once your child outgrows a forward-facing car seat, you can move him or her to a booster seat, with the car's seat belt placed across his or her chest. Make sure the seat belt lies snug and flat across the chest. Booster seats come in various styles, including ones with high backs, which are

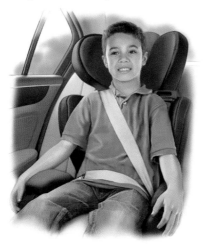

good for cars that don't have headrests or high seat backs, and backless ones, good for vehicles with headrests.

Seat belt A child can begin using a seat belt by itself when the belt fits correctly — typically when he or she reaches 4 feet 9 inches tall and is between the ages of 8 and 12.

A seat belt's lap belt must lie snugly across the upper thighs, not the stomach. The shoulder belt should lie snugly across the shoulders and chest and not across the neck or face.

If you're unsure of which seat to use, search the NHTSA's website for its Car Seat Finder, an easy-to-use tool that uses your child's age, height and weight to find the right seat.

Once you've selected your child's seat, make sure to follow the manufacturer's directions for proper installation. The NHTSA's website has videos that demonstrate how to do this. You can also get your car seat inspected at certain locations, such as your local fire or police station.

After selecting and installing your child's seat, make sure to register it with the manufacturer or the NHTSA. This will ensure you get recall notices and other updates.

WHEN TO REPLACE A CAR SEAT

Because crashes can damage car seats and reduce their ability to protect children in future accidents, the National Highway Traffic Safety Administration recommends replacing a car seat after any moderate or severe crash.

Minor crashes may not require that your child's car seat be replaced. To be considered minor, all of the following must apply:

▶ You were able to drive away from the accident
▶ The door located nearest to the car seat wasn't damaged
▶ There were no injuries in the crash
▶ No airbags were deployed during the accident
▶ There's no visible damage to the car seat
   If you're ever unsure, err on the side of caution and replace the car seat.

Pedestrian safety "Look both ways" is sound advice when teaching children how to safely cross a street. Children should make eye contact with drivers before crossing and continue to look both ways until safely across.

When is the right time to allow your child to cross the street alone? Consider your child's developmental stage and his or her personality. For example, is he or she a big risk-taker? If the answer is yes, you may want to keep helping your child get safely across the street. In addition, consider these pedestrian safety tips:

▶ Have your child avoid using phones, headphones or other distracting devices until he or she is safely across the street.

▶ Encourage use of sidewalks or paths, if possible. If there are no sidewalks, walk facing traffic, on the shoulder of the road, and as far away from traffic as possible.

▶ Tell your child to cross at street corners, where traffic is guarded by traffic lights and crosswalks. He or she shouldn't try to cross between parked cars, which limit visibility and can catch a motorist off-guard.

▶ Wear brightly colored or highly visible clothing when walking at night.

▶ Teach your child to be cautious around cars that are backing up or turning in a parking lot, but also your home driveway. Take extra precautions around larger vehicles, trailers and boats.

RIDING THE SCHOOL BUS

If your child rides a school bus and has to cross in front of the bus to get home, reinforce some common safety rules:

▶ Walk on the side of the road until he or she can see the driver and the driver signals that it is safe to cross.

▶ Look left, right and then left again to ensure no vehicles are coming, and then cross the road, continuously looking for any oncoming vehicles.

▶ Stay away from the back of the bus.

RECREATIONAL DANGERS

Play is a great way for children to be physically active and decompress after a long day at school. As with any activity, there may be some risk of injury involved.

Bikes, skateboards, scooters and skates Learning to ride a bike, roller skate or perform tricks on a skateboard is an enjoyable part of childhood. Many of the injuries linked to these activities can be prevented by wearing the proper protective gear and following safety rules.

Always wear a helmet A helmet should fit securely to the person using it, so take your child along when purchasing one. Some helmets have fun colors and designs. Let your child choose and he or she may be more inclined to wear it. If your child does multiple wheeled sports, make sure to buy a multisport helmet. Helmets should be worn down over the forehead, not pushed back. If you also participate in these activities, set an example by wearing the proper helmet, as well.

Don't forget protective pads Pads that cover the elbows and knees, as well as gloves and wrist guards, can protect bones in the event of a fall while skateboarding, riding a scooter, roller skating or in-line skating.

Follow basic traffic safety rules Have your child stop and look both ways to check for cars and other hazards when pulling out into an area where there is traffic. When riding or skating, he or she should keep as far to the right of the road as safely possible — being on the lookout for any uneven pavement or other surface problems — and ride with traffic. Obey all traffic signals and stop signs, just as a car would. Wear brightly colored

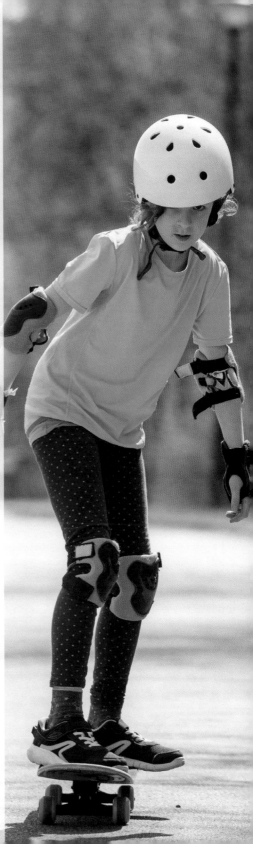

clothing for better visibility. Use hand signals to indicate turning or stopping.

Teach balance and falling techniques
Teach young skateboarders how to fall properly to minimize injuries. To lessen the chance of breaking a bone, have your child:

▶ Stay loose, rather than stiffen up
▶ Crouch down to reduce the distance of the fall
▶ Roll to keep the arms from absorbing all the force
▶ Aim to land on more cushioned parts of the body, such as the buttocks

Skateboarders should never grab onto bikes, cars or other vehicles when riding. Skateboarding tricks should be reserved for designated areas.

All-terrain vehicles (ATVs) The American Academy of Pediatrics (AAP) discourages the operation of all-terrain vehicles (ATVs) by children under age 16 due the potential for serious injury and death. Children this age are often not developmentally ready to drive a vehicle, making them particularly susceptible to crashes. As a general rule, the AAP recommends limiting driving an off-road vehicle only to those who have a license to drive a car, and also advises against allowing your child to ride as a passenger on an ATV.

If you allow your child to use an ATV, follow these guidelines from the AAP to help prevent serious injury:

▶ Always supervise your child when he or she is using an ATV.
▶ Don't let your child drive or ride on an adult-size ATV. Look for warning labels on individual ATVs, which state minimum age requirements.
▶ Inspect the ATV to ensure tires are properly inflated and brakes are working. Check for any damage that could pose a safety issue when riding before your child uses it.

▶ Insist on all riders wearing helmets, eye protection and reflective clothing. Look for a helmet that's meant for motorcycle use and has safety features that protect the eyes, such as visors or face shields.
▶ Don't allow your child to use an ATV on streets or at night.
▶ Make the ATV more visible by adding items such as reflectors and lights.
▶ Consider an ATV safety course. Check for classes offered through the ATV Safety Institute, the National 4-H Council, local rider groups, state agencies or ATV manufacturers.

Trampolines and bounce houses
Trampolines and bounce houses have become staples of backyards, community and family events, and children's birthday parties. Their softer surfaces can lead you to believe that they're safe for your child. However, each year children sustain injuries on trampolines and in bounce houses ranging from sprains and broken bones to traumatic head and neck injuries. These injuries can stem from children landing on a hard part of the trampoline — such as the frame — or attempting difficult moves, such as flips. The vast majority of these injuries are in children between ages 5 and 14.

You can help reduce the risk of serious injuries by taking some preventive steps:

▶ Check your trampoline to make sure the frame, surface and protective padding are in good condition.
▶ Supervise trampoline and bounce house use at all times.
▶ Limit trampoline activity: No children under the age of 6 and only one person at a time.
▶ Don't let safety netting give you a false sense of security. Netting may

only prevent your child from taking a tumble off the trampoline. The majority of injuries happen while on the trampoline.

- Consider banning flips, somersaults and other high-risk jumping, unless your child has received proper instruction in how to do them and has protective equipment, such as a safety harness.
- Remove ladders to the trampoline when they're not in use to discourage children from bouncing without your supervision.
- Follow the same rules for bounce houses as you would for trampolines, as bounce houses can produce injuries similar to those that occur on trampolines. If your child is playing with a small group of children in a bounce house, make sure all the participants are roughly the same age and size.
- Make sure bounce houses are securely attached to the ground. Avoid using them when high winds or storms are present.

Water safety Swimming is great exercise and a fun way to beat the summer heat. But it can be dangerous if children are left unsupervised or without proper safety precautions. The same goes for other water activities, such as boating.

Watching your child while he or she swims or plays in water is one of the most important things you can do to help prevent drowning. It's a good idea to take an American Red Cross water safety course, as well as first-aid and CPR courses. If your child doesn't know how to swim, enroll him or her in a swim class.

Children and inexperienced swimmers should wear a life jacket whenever they are near any body of water, including while on boats, at waterparks and in

---

GET TRAINED IN CPR

Reading about cardiopulmonary resuscitation (CPR) and learning to recognize when it's needed is important, but it's no substitute for hands-on knowledge, especially when it comes to children. Experts strongly recommend that parents and other child care providers get trained in CPR. Taking a pediatric CPR course is an excellent way to invest in your child's safety. In the event of an emergency it can save your child's life.

Local chapters of the American Red Cross, American Heart Association and other organizations offer courses in pediatric first aid and CPR to the public. Portions of the course may be taken online, and many chapters offer classes at various times of the day to provide greater flexibility.

---

pools, even if there are lifeguards present. Bear in mind, life jackets are not a substitute for adult supervision.

Always stay within arm's reach of young children and avoid distractions, such as cellphones, when watching them. Never consume alcohol while supervising children near water.

To ensure a life jacket will provide your child with the most protection:

- Look for a life jacket that's for your child's intended activity and that has a U.S. Coast Guard stamp on it. Floatation devices that fit around the arms and inflatable toys aren't a substitute for life jackets and aren't meant to be lifesaving devices.

Make sure your child fits within the jacket's specified weight range.

Check the jacket for any damage that can compromise safety; make sure the buckles work properly.

Teach your child how to be a safe swimmer by swimming only in areas that are patrolled by lifeguards. Advise your child to never swim alone. If in a pool, children should also avoid certain areas that have suction, such as drains.

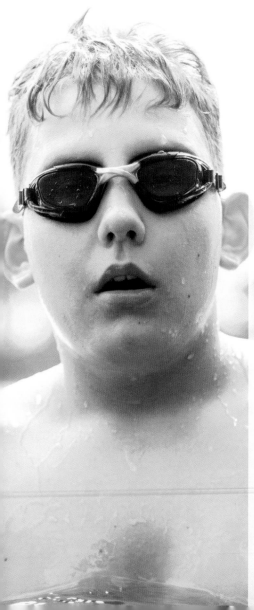

Though you may have strict rules about no swimming in a home pool without an adult, children can still be tempted to go swimming unsupervised. In general, good safety measures to have in place include:

Fencing that is at least 4 feet high and has a self-closing and self-latching gate that a child can't reach. Fencing should be hard to climb (not chain-link fences).

Safety covers and pool alarms that alert you to when someone opens the gate or enters the water.

Rescue equipment, such as a life preserver or shepherd's hook.

A large storage container for pool toys. This helps to keep toys out of sight so young children aren't tempted to enter the pool area to get to them.

Removable access ladders that can be stored away when above-ground and inflatable pools aren't in use.

Inexpensive kiddy pools and inflatable pools are a popular option for summertime. It's important to remember that just because these are temporary and often much shallower than your typical in-ground or above-ground pool, they still present a very real drowning risk for children. Use the same water safety precautions as you would with any other size pool.

The municipality where you live may have specific laws on safety measures for home pools. Your local building code may require a fence around larger, inflatable pools, as well. Check with your local authorities for more safety guidelines.

WEATHER HAZARDS

Children often don't quite understand that weather can pose a risk to their health. You've probably seen evidence of this when your child wants to run out in the snow without a jacket or balks at putting sunscreen on. A few simple precautions will help you keep your child safe.

Cold Warm clothing forms the basis for comfort and safety when it's cold outside. Dress your child warmer than you would yourself. Boots, gloves or mittens, and a hat are must-haves. If you're traveling with your child by car, have him or her wear several thin layers and bring a coat along. Wearing bulky clothing can make it difficult to properly tighten a restraint or seat belt around your child.

Additional ways you can keep your child safe during winter in cold climates:

Make time to warm up Set time limits on how long your child is outdoors to avoid conditions such as a severe drop in body temperature (hypothermia), and skin and tissue damage from exposure to the cold (frostbite). Schedule regular "check-ins" for your child to come in and warm up before heading back outside.

Be safe while active Supervise your child's activities such as skating, sledding, skiing and snowboarding. Sledding should be done feet first to help prevent head injuries, and in non-crowded, obstacle-free areas.

Skiers and snowboarders should always wear helmets and sport-specific protective gear, such as safety bindings, goggles and gloves with wrist guards. Children should not attempt a course that they aren't comfortable with or is above their skill level. Consider enrolling your child in a skiing or snowboarding class first.

Exercise caution with snowmobiles The AAP advises against children and teens under age 16 operating a snowmobile, and children under age 6 riding on one.

If your child rides a snowmobile, have him or her wear appropriate protective gear, such as goggles and a helmet designed for motorcycles or other motorized vehicles.

Teach your child basic safety rules, such as driving at reasonable speeds and staying in areas without trees or other hazards.

Heat When playing outside on days with temperatures in the 90s and high humidity, be sure to take breaks to cool off. Keep an eye on your child for signs of heat exhaustion and heatstroke. To beat the heat:

▶ Encourage your child to drink water regularly.
▶ Opt for lightweight, light-colored clothing that can wick away sweat.
▶ Let your child have downtime. Heat can sap strength.
▶ Have your child take a cool bath, run through a sprinkler or go for a swim.
▶ Seek out air conditioning. If your home doesn't have it, find a space that does. Some towns and cities designate spaces as "cooling centers," such as libraries or recreation centers.
▶ Never leave a child in a closed car in the summer. Temperatures in the vehicle can quickly rise and be fatal.

Seek emergency care if your child starts exhibiting unusual symptoms that could be heat related, such as faintness, lethargy, headache, fever, nausea, vomiting, irregular breathing, muscle discomfort, skin tingling or numbness.

If you're unsure of your child's symptoms but think they may be heat related, call your child's medical provider who can tell you what steps to take next. Or take your child to the nearest emergency department.

Sun A few serious sunburns in childhood are all it takes to increase a person's risk of skin cancer as an adult, making sunburn prevention critical. Sunburns can occur before you see any changes in your child's skin, so don't wait for skin color changes to take protective steps.

For the best protection, combine multiple methods of sunburn prevention:

Be diligent about sunscreen Sunscreen should be applied to all exposed areas at least 30 minutes before sun exposure, even on cloudy days. Choose a broad-spectrum sunscreen with a sun protection factor (SPF) of at least 30. Apply generously and make sure to reapply every two hours — or more often if your child is swimming or perspiring. Lip balm that contains sunscreen will help protect those often-overlooked lips.

Cover up Have your child wear a hat and suitable clothing. Hats should cover the face, scalp, ears and neck. Some clothing has SPF built in. As a rule of thumb, tightly woven fabrics offer the most protection.

Avoid the harshest rays Ultraviolet A and B (UVA and UVB) rays are the ones that damage skin. These rays are strongest between 10 a.m. and 4 p.m. When possible, try to plan outdoor activities for morning or early evening.

Wear sunglasses Protecting children's eyes from UV light can help prevent cataracts from developing later in life. Opt for sunglasses that are a wraparound style and block both UVA and UVB rays.

Natural disasters Preparation is key to handling emergencies due to natural disasters. Have a plan in place that addresses how you and your family will handle an emergency, so you aren't left figuring it out in a chaotic or stressful environment. Having an organized plan in place can also help ease some of your child's fears about potential disasters. The American Red Cross offers tips for formulating an emergency plan:

Review emergency scenarios Talk with your family about the different emergencies that could happen in your home or community — for example, a hurricane or tornado — and what can be done in response. Knowing what to do in such a situation can give children some sense of security.

Assign tasks Talk about how your family will work together in an emergency situation and the responsibilities for each family member. Reassure your child that there isn't currently an emergency, but you're just preparing.

Decide evacuation routes Choose several alternate routes and where you will end up — for example, at a specific hotel. If you have pets, it's a good idea to research accommodations that will accept them.

Choose meeting places This is important in case you and your family are separated. This may be the front lawn in the event of a fire or a public space outside of your neighborhood if you're ordered to evacuate.

Practice Rehearse as many elements of your plan as you can. The American Red Cross recommends doing this twice a year.

Set up an emergency contact person Identify a relative or close friend who doesn't live in the area. Have this number saved in every family member's cellphone and in writing. To reconnect with loved ones after a disaster, you can register your family as "safe and well" at the American Red Cross website. You can also search for loved ones on the list.

Put together an emergency kit Make sure to include water, nonperishable food, a battery-powered radio, a flashlight and extra batteries, as well as other emergency and first-aid supplies. Store enough for at least three days or more. Consider scanning important documents to store in a secure place online.

TRAVEL SAFETY

Traveling as a family is a great way to show your child the wonders of nature, participate in the energy of big cities and experience different cultures. But it can also present unfamiliar environments, changes in routine and hazards you may not find at home. A little bit of preparation and planning can eliminate a lot of the headaches and at least some of the risks parents encounter while traveling with children.

Air travel Flying with your children may not always be stress-free, but certain precautions can make it go more smoothly and safely.

Pack an essentials bag Bring plenty of snacks, entertainment, and hand sanitizer or wet wipes; an extra set of clothing; chewing gum or something to suck on if your child is prone to ear pain during descent; and any medication regularly taken.

Avoid the rush Allow plenty of time to get to the airport. The Transportation Security Administration recommends being

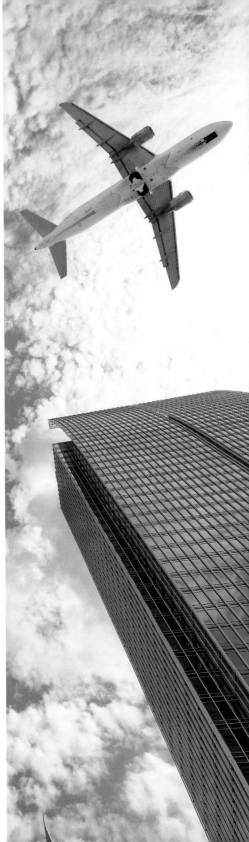

at the airport two hours before a domestic flight and three hours before an international one.

Keep your family's outfits simple This helps get through security checks with minimum fuss. Wear layered clothing and shoes that can easily be removed and put back on. If your child is under age 12, he or she shouldn't have to remove his or her shoes during the security screening.

Offer reassurance If your child is particularly attached to his or her belongings, reassure him or her that anything you carry on the plane needs to be screened but will be returned quickly.

Keep it neutral Make sure your child knows that inappropriate jokes, such as saying "I'm going to blow up the plane," will be taken seriously by airport security.

Consider car seat accommodations If your child is still in a car seat, you can bring your own and check it as you would luggage or, if you're renting a car, have a car seat reserved at your destination. Make sure that any checked or rented car seat is free of damage before using it.

If your car seat is government approved for use in aircraft, you may be able to bring the car seat onto the plane and attach it to the seat. Ask your airline what its policy is on this. Visit the Federal Aviation Administration's website for more information on flying with children.

Minimize jet lag Similar to adults, children can have a tough time adjusting to different time zones. To help curb jet lag, adjust your child's sleep schedule a few days before your trip. Once you arrive at your destination, encourage your child to play outdoors during the day to help his or her body adjust its internal clock.

International travel Traveling abroad with children can be an exciting adventure. But the last thing you want to do is spend all of your time in a hotel — or worse, in a hospital. There are things you can do to help your family have a safe and healthy trip. For more detailed information, talk to your child's medical provider or visit a travel clinic.

Before you travel Make sure you and your child receive any vaccinations that may be needed before your trip. Have any needed dental work done before you go.

Plan ahead for medication needs. For critical medications, bring an extra supply. Put some in your checked baggage and keep some with you. If your child has a history of severe allergic reaction (anaphylaxis), make sure to bring his or her epinephrine autoinjector. Consider bringing several doses, as refills in another country may not be possible.

Check with your insurance provider about coverage while you travel. Ask whether there are any rules about getting medical care in another country. Help your child get plenty of sleep before you travel to prevent jet lag.

What to bring Items that will come in handy include hand sanitizer gel and wipes, sunscreen, pain relievers, mosquito repellent containing up to 30 percent DEET, and antihistamine medications for itching, hay fever and other allergies. Bring water purification tablets or a portable water treatment system if there's a possibility that the drinking water supply may be tainted.

While you're there Don't pet or feed dogs, cats, monkeys or other animals. The risk of being bitten by an animal that might have rabies is too high. If you or your child is bitten, this is an emergency.

In areas that don't have clean, drinkable water, use water from sealed bottles for drinking and brushing teeth. Drink sealed, commercially canned or bottled carbonated beverages. Avoid using tap water for rinsing toothbrushes or using ice unless you know it's made from treated water. Don't drink or eat unpasteurized dairy products, such as milk and yogurt.

Wash your hands often. Avoid eating street food or uncooked food, raw fruits or vegetables that don't need to be peeled, or food that may have been stored unrefrigerated.

As a general rule, avoid swimming in lakes and rivers in developing countries due to the risk of acquiring a parasitic or bacterial infection. Swimming in the ocean is usually safe, but be aware of dangerous ocean currents. Watch out for stings from jellyfish, sea anemones and coral. Protect your child against sunburn. Never allow your child to swim alone or at night.

Always keep your child close. Be aware of strangers in busy areas due to the potential for kidnapping and trafficking.

After you return See your child's medical provider if your child was sick or in the hospital at any time during your trip. If your child experiences fever, persistent diarrhea, skin rash or any other unusual signs or symptoms within three months of getting home, make an appointment to see your child's provider.

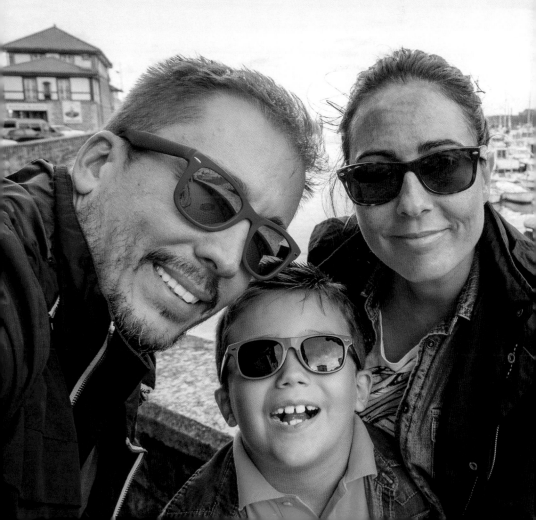

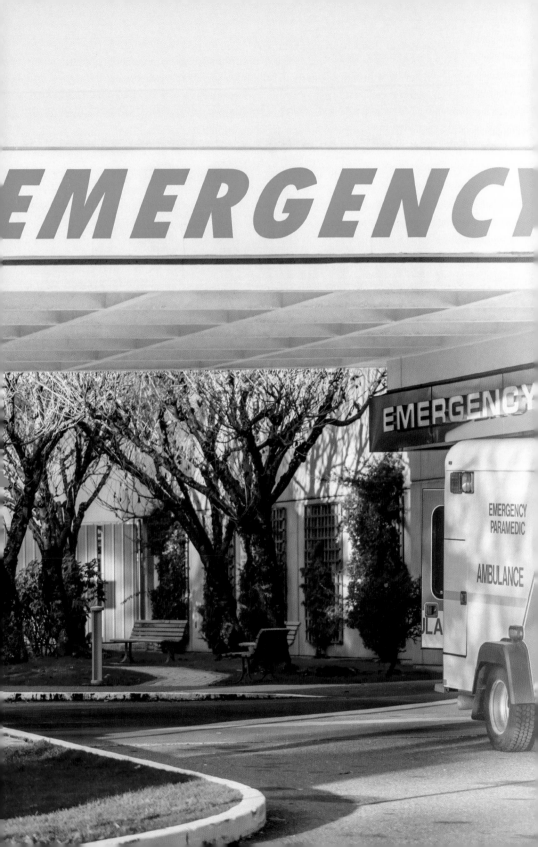

CHAPTER 11

First aid and emergency care

Kids are naturally active, curious and eager to explore their surroundings. But because children at this age are still developing the skills needed to take on the world, sometimes that curiosity can lead to injuries and, at times, emergencies.

As a parent, the best plan of action is to anticipate the dangers your child may encounter and take steps to safeguard against them. It's also important to be prepared if an emergency occurs. Chapter 10 discusses safety measures in depth. In this chapter, you'll learn more about first aid and emergency care.

Reading about safety and emergency care is helpful. Even more effective is taking a class on pediatric first aid, cardiopulmonary resuscitation (CPR) and the use of an automatic external defibrillator (AED). Look for classes at local chapters of accredited associations such as Red Cross, American Heart Association and others. Better yet, gather a group of parents and do it together. It may mean the difference between life and death someday.

IS IT AN EMERGENCY?

Not every injury is an emergency. In fact, many injuries or conditions can be treated in a medical provider's office or at home. But how do you know when to call 911? Here are signs and symptoms of an emergency situation:

- Bleeding that can't be stopped
- Head injuries followed by loss of consciousness, confusion, change in personality, severe headache or vomiting
- First-time seizure
- Trouble breathing or skin or lips that look blue, purple or gray
- Loss of consciousness or inability to respond
- A sudden inability to move
- Severe burn
- Inability to move the neck, especially when accompanied by fever
- Inability to drink or swallow
- Eye pain
- Vomiting or coughing up blood
- Bone that looks deformed or is at an odd angle after a fall or other accident

WHEN A CHILD NEEDS CPR

If a child is unconscious or unresponsive, cardiopulmonary resuscitation (CPR) can make a critical difference in saving the child's life. It can supply additional oxygen to a child's brain and other organs, helping to prevent permanent damage or death.

CPR in children achieves the best results when performed by a trained individual. That's why it's important for parents to take a course in CPR. Check with your local chapter of the American Heart Association or Red Cross for a listing of classes.

The sooner you start CPR, the greater the chance of saving your child's life or preventing permanent injury.

911 or CPR first? If you're alone and didn't see the child collapse, perform five cycles of compressions and breaths on the child — this should take about two minutes — before calling 911 or your local emergency number and getting an automatic external defibrillator (AED), if one is available.

If you're alone and you did see the child collapse, call 911 or your local emergency number and get the AED, if one is available, before beginning CPR. Or dial 911 while on speakerphone and proceed with CPR. The 911 responder can help guide you through the process.

If another person is available, have that person call for help and get the AED while you begin CPR. To perform CPR, remember the acronym C-A-B, which stands for **C**ompressions-**A**irway-**B**reathing.

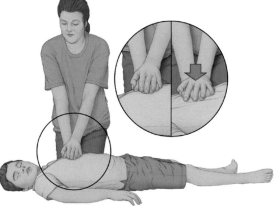

Compressions Chest compressions help restore blood circulation. Do these first unless it's a drowning emergency. In that case, ventilation is most important and you need to do rescue breathing first (see Breathing).

1. Put the child on his or her back on a firm surface.
2. Kneel next to the child's neck and shoulders.
3. Use two hands, or only one hand if the child is very small, to perform chest compressions. Keeping your elbows straight, press down on the chest about 2 inches. Push hard at a rate of 100 to 120 compressions a minute.
4. If you haven't been trained in CPR, continue chest compressions until there are signs of movement or until emergency medical personnel take over. If you have been trained in CPR, go on to opening the airway and rescue breathing.

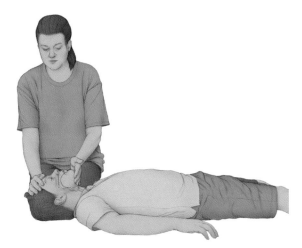

Airway If you're trained in CPR and you've performed 30 chest compressions, open the child's airway using the head-tilt, chin-lift maneuver. Put your palm on the child's forehead and gently tilt the head back (don't do this part if you're concerned there might be a neck injury). With the other hand, gently lift the chin forward to open the airway.

Breathing Breathe for the child. Use the same compression-breath rate that's used for adults: 30 compressions followed by two breaths. This is one cycle.

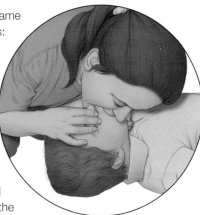

1. With the airway open, pinch the nostrils shut for mouth-to-mouth breathing and cover the child's mouth with yours, making a seal.

2. Prepare to give two rescue breaths. Give the first rescue breath — lasting one second — and watch to see if the chest rises. If it does rise, give the second breath. If the chest doesn't rise, repeat the head-tilt, chin-lift maneuver and then give the second breath. Be careful not to provide too many breaths or to breathe with too much force.

3. After the two breaths, immediately begin the next cycle of compressions and breaths. If there are two people performing CPR, conduct 15 compressions followed by two breaths.

4. As soon as an AED is available, apply it and follow the prompts. Use pediatric pads if available, for children up to age 8. If pediatric pads aren't available, use adult pads. Administer one shock if prompted to do so by the AED, then resume CPR — starting with chest compressions — for two more minutes before administering a second shock if prompted by the AED. If you're not trained to use an AED, a 911 or other emergency medical operator may be able to guide you in its use.
Continue until the child moves or help arrives.

In emergency situations — or any situation where you believe your child's life is in danger or your child is at risk of permanent harm — call 911 or your local emergency services. If it's not possible to get emergency help to come to you, take your child to the nearest emergency facility.

If you're not sure whether your child's injury is serious enough to warrant a trip to the emergency department, call your child's medical provider first. He or she will be able to provide guidance. If emergency care is needed, the provider may call ahead to the hospital to let staff know you're coming, which can help speed up the process when you get there. As a general rule, according to the American Academy of Pediatrics (AAP), if your child can walk, talk, interact and play, the situation is likely not an emergency.

In the event of a possible poisoning in the U.S., call the Poison Help line at 800-222-1222. Have this number by your telephone. If an ingestion is causing emergency signs or symptoms, call 911.

ANIMAL OR HUMAN BITES

The vast majority of bites are caused by household pets, such as dogs and cats. However, bites from humans and wild animals also can occur. Rabies is a life-threatening disease that can be transmitted by a bite from a wild animal, as well as unvaccinated dogs and cats. If your child sustains a bite, do your best to find out the source of the bite.

How serious is it? Infections are the most common complications stemming from bites. Animal bites can cause scars, especially if the bite is on the face. Cat bites carry the greatest risk of becoming infected because cats have long, sharp teeth that can more easily penetrate skin and transmit bacteria to deeper tissue.

Bite wounds that occur on the hand have the greatest chance of causing complications because bones and joints aren't far beneath the skin's surface in this area and risk becoming infected. Bites by animals carrying rabies can be fatal without proper treatment.

What you can do Treat any animal or human bite that breaks the skin as a serious injury. Bites by a wild animal such as a skunk, raccoon, fox or bat should receive immediate medical evaluation for rabies risk, as should bites from cats and dogs whose vaccination status is uncertain.

Also seek medical help right away if you think a bone may be broken, the child has an underlying condition such as diabetes or cancer, or the child takes a medication that weakens the immune system. He or she may need antibiotic treatment.

If the bite was caused by an animal that may carry rabies, your child's medical provider may administer a series of shots to prevent rabies infection. Once an infection takes hold, there is no effective treatment.

Finally, it's important that your child is up to date on his or her tetanus immunization. Your child's medical provider may recommend a tetanus shot if your child has received fewer than three doses of the vaccine or the wound is dirty and your child's last dose was more than five years ago.

Minor bites If the wound is superficial or barely breaks the skin and there's no rabies danger:
▶ Wash the wound thoroughly with soap and large amounts of water.
▶ Apply an over-the-counter antibiotic cream or ointment.

- Cover with a clean bandage.
- Call your child's medical provider if the bite broke the skin. Your child may need evaluation or antibiotics.

Deeper wounds If the wound is a deep puncture, or if the skin is torn or bleeding badly, take the following measures:
- If the wound is still bleeding, apply gauze or a clean cloth to it and apply pressure to help stop the bleeding. Wrapping a wound snugly can also help stop the bleeding.
- Seek help from your child's medical provider or local emergency services.

For both minor and more-serious bites, monitor the wound for signs of infection, including redness or warmth, fever, pus drainage and worsening pain in the days that follow the injury. For wounds near a joint, look for pain, swelling or problems moving the joint, which can be signs of an infection that requires antibiotics.

BLEEDING

Cuts, punctures and abrasions can lead to bleeding. This may be a result of an injury to a vein or small blood vessel (capillary), or to an artery.

How serious is it? The rate of blood loss is a good indication of how serious the bleeding is. Minor bleeding — a slow, steady flow of dark red blood — usually indicates injury to a vein or capillary. Blood that is spurting out of a wound is usually a sign of an injury to an artery, which can quickly become life-threatening. If bleeding is profuse, won't stop, or is accompanied by confusion or loss of consciousness, call for emergency help right away.

What you can do A bleeding wound can be a little scary at first. The important thing is to stop or slow the bleeding. To do so, follow these steps:
- Reassure your child that everything will be OK and remain calm yourself.
- If necessary, remove clothing to get a better look at the extent of the wound.
- Cover the wound with gauze or clean cloth. If the wound is large and deep, try to insert the gauze or cloth into the wound. Don't attempt to first clean the wound or remove any embedded objects.
- Place both hands directly on top of the wound and apply continuous pressure, pushing down as hard as you can. Hold this continuous pressure until the bleeding stops, or, in the case of more-serious injuries, until emergency help arrives.
- If the bleeding stops, cover the wound with a tight dressing and tape the area securely. If the bleeding eventually soaks through that bandage, place a more absorbent material over the first bandage.
- If possible, elevate the area of injury.
- If bleeding doesn't stop, call for emergency assistance or bring your child to the nearest emergency department.
- Talk to your child's medical provider to make sure your child's tetanus immunization is up to date.

BREATHING PROBLEMS

Having breathing problems (respiratory distress) means your child isn't adequately breathing and he or she isn't getting enough oxygen. Respiratory distress is the leading cause of cardiac arrest and the most common life-threatening problem for a child. There are a number of

OFF TO THE EMERGENCY DEPARTMENT

If your child needs to be seen in the emergency department, here are some steps you can take to make the visit go a little smoother. In some situations, your child may need to be seen immediately and you may not have time to prepare.

- *Project calm.* Do your best to calm your child's fears. Tell your child what he or she may expect, that this is the place that will help make him or her better, and take along a comfort item, such as a favorite blanket or toy. Remaining calm yourself can help your child do the same.
- *Gather up necessities.* This might include medications your child takes, medical records, insurance information, specific treatment plans and any supplies you use at home for treating a medical condition, such as a gastrostomy or tracheostomy tube.
- *Avoid food.* Hold off giving your child any food in case a procedure needs to be performed.
- *Enlist help.* If your child has siblings, try to find someone to watch them while you're at the ER.
- *Provide pain relief as needed.* If your child is uncomfortable or in pain, it's OK to give him or her a pain reliever. Just make sure to note the medication, time and dosage.
- *Be patient.* Trips to the emergency department can be lengthy, especially if your child needs to have imaging or other tests done.
- *Follow up.* Plan to schedule a follow-up visit with your child's health provider after the emergency trip.

factors and conditions that can cause your child to have difficulty breathing: chronic conditions such as asthma, an object lodged in the airway, chest injuries that result in a collapsed lung (pneumothorax) and viral illnesses such as the flu.

How serious is it? It doesn't take long for a lack of oxygen to become life-threatening for a child. This is why respiratory distress should be treated as a medical emergency.

What you can do If your child is having difficulty breathing, call 911 or emergency services right away. Warning signs of respiratory distress include:

- Rapid breathing
- Breathing with increased effort; you might notice retractions, which appear as the pulling in of the muscles below the rib cage, between the ribs or above the collarbone when your child breathes in
- Unusual body position, such as leaning forward with the hands on the knees to help breathing
- Restlessness, anxiety and agitation
- Pale or bluish coloring to the skin
- Drowsiness and lethargy as breathing becomes more difficult

Though it's understandable for your child to be upset, try to keep him or her calm. Crying can increase the need for oxygen and place an even greater demand on breathing. Position your child in a way that allows him or her to breathe more comfortably until help arrives — for example, on your lap or in a more upright position, instead of flat on his or her back.

If respiratory distress is triggered by asthma, use of medication such as a rescue inhaler (bronchodilator) can quickly improve symptoms. If the treatment you normally use to control your child's asthma isn't working, seek help immediately. Don't hesitate to call 911 or take your child to the emergency department. See page 310 for more on asthma care.

If your child isn't breathing at all, call 911 and begin CPR (see page 168).

BROKEN BONE

A broken bone (fracture) is a common injury in children, particularly those under the age of 6. In most cases, a broken bone occurs because of a fall or motor vehicle accident. A bone may completely break, bend or buckle. There may be swelling and pain, and your child may not be able to walk on or use an affected arm or leg. However, a broken bone can be present even without these signs and symptoms.

How serious is it? Some breaks are obvious, but others may require imaging tests to determine if a fracture has occurred. If your child is in pain or can't use a limb or extremity, make an appointment with your child's medical provider promptly to determine the extent of the injury.

For a simple fracture, keeping the bone immobile by using a cast is all that's needed for proper healing. If the fracture has caused misalignment of the bone pieces, your child's medical provider may need to gently move the pieces back into place so that the bone heals properly.

In some instances, a break can damage the bone's growth plate. This is the area at the ends of the bone that helps dictate future growth. If this doesn't heal correctly, the bone may become deformed or experience abnormal growth. If there is potential growth plate damage,

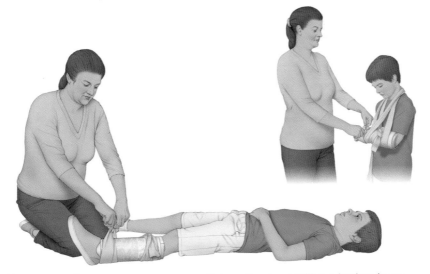

Use a magazine or newspaper as a splint or sling to stabilize a broken bone.

your child's medical provider will likely recommend monitoring the injury for a specific amount of time to ensure there is proper healing. Depending on where the injury is located, your child's provider may also recommend surgery to reduce the risk of problems down the road.

A more complicated fracture, such as an open fracture or a fracture where the bone is broken into several pieces, typically requires surgery to realign the broken bone and to implant wires, plates or screws to keep the bone in place during healing.

A compound fracture is a type of serious break in which the bone sticks out through the skin. A fracture that has broken through the skin increases the risk of infection and must be treated promptly.

What you can do If you think your child has a broken bone, call his or her medical provider right away. He or she can advise you on immediate relief measures, such as giving your child a pain reliever or using a cold pack, and may recommend calling 911 to transport your child to an emergency department for evaluation and treatment.

In the meantime, use a sling or splint to help stabilize the bone — a rolled up magazine or newspaper will work (see page 173). If your child can't move, don't try to move him or her. For a compound fracture, don't attempt to reposition the bone. Apply firm pressure to the wound and cover it with gauze. Call 911 or your local emergency number.

BURNS

When skin is exposed to extreme heat — whether from a hot stove, hot water or hot sun — the layers of skin can be burned and damaged, sometimes beyond repair. Taking proper precautions can help minimize the chances that a burn will occur (see page 143). If your child does experience a burn, here's what to know.

How serious is it? Injuries can range from mild to serious and are classified according to their severity. The amount of

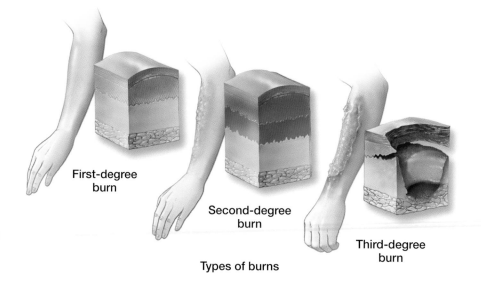

First-degree burn

Second-degree burn

Third-degree burn

Types of burns

damage or degree of the burn depends on how many layers of the skin are affected.

First-degree burns These are superficial burns. They're the mildest and affect only the outer layer of the skin. They can cause redness and slight swelling of the skin.

Second-degree burns With these burns, the top layer of skin has been burned through, and the second layer is also damaged. Superficial partial and deep thickness burns cause blistering, intense reddening, and moderate to severe swelling and pain.

Third-degree burns These burns are the most severe. Full thickness burns appear white or charred (brown or black) and involve all the layers of the skin. There may be little pain with these burns because of substantial nerve damage.

What you can do If your child's burn is minor, you can usually take care of it at home with first-aid measures. To care for a minor burn:

▶ Remove constricting items. Since burned areas can swell, you'll want to take off any jewelry, belts and similar items. Try to do this quickly and with care.

▶ Hold the burned area under cool (not cold) running water for several minutes until the pain subsides. You can also immerse the burn in cool water or cool it with cold compresses. This helps stop the burning and reduces the swelling. Do not put ice on the burn.

▶ After cooling the burn for comfort and cleaning, cover the burn with an antibiotic ointment. This will prevent bandages or dressings from sticking to the burn. Avoid breaking any blisters, as these provide protection from

infection. If a blister does break, wash gently with water and apply an antibiotic ointment.

▶ Make sure the burn is clean and covered with a sterile gauze bandage. This provides comfort by keeping air off of the injury, and it reduces the risk of infection. Don't use fluffy cotton or other material that may get lint into the wound. Wrap the gauze loosely to avoid putting pressure on burned skin.

▶ Give pain relievers as needed. If your child's burn is causing discomfort, consider giving him or her acetaminophen or ibuprofen. Avoid the use of aspirin in children because of the risk of complications.

▶ Though home remedies such as applying butter, honey or similar products to burns have been advised over the years, these aren't recommended because they may increase the risk of infection.

Minor burns will usually heal without the need for further treatment. However, you'll need to keep an eye on the burn for signs and symptoms that an infection could be developing. These include increased pain, redness, fever, swelling or oozing. If an infection develops, seek medical help.

When a burn is severe Call 911 or your local emergency number. Don't submerge the burn in cold water, as this can cause a decrease in body temperature (hypothermia), resulting in a drop in blood pressure and impaired circulation (shock). Until help arrives, take these steps:

▶ Check for signs of breathing, coughing or movement. If breathing is absent and there are no other signs of consciousness, begin CPR (see page 168).

▶ Remove any jewelry, belts or other items. Burned areas can swell rapidly, and these items can quickly become restrictive.

- Cover the burn using a cool, moist, sterile bandage; clean moist cloth; or moist towels.
- Elevate the burned body part or parts, raising them above heart level, if possible.
- Watch for signs and symptoms of shock, including fainting, pale skin or shallow breathing.

Minimize scarring Whether a scar forms after a burn depends on the severity of the burn. In general, deep burns and those that blister are more likely to scar. You can minimize your child's risk of scarring by keeping the burns covered until new skin has formed and the burn no longer leaks fluid. After the burn heals, make sure to apply sunscreen over the area or cover the scar with clothing when your child is outdoors for a year afterward.

CHOKING

Most childhood choking incidents occur in the infant and toddler years, when children don't have enough teeth yet to chew properly and try to swallow something too big for their windpipe. In older children, choking tends to occur because of swallowing small items such as a pencil eraser or a piece of a toy. Doing other activities, such as laughing or running, while eating also can lead to choking.

How serious is it? Choking can be life-threatening if the object that's lodged in the windpipe remains there. The longer your child is deprived of oxygen, the greater the chance of permanent brain damage or death. If you can't clear the

airway, call for emergency help or ask someone nearby to call.

What you can do If your child is able to cough, cry or make noises with force, let him or her do so until his or her windpipe is clear. Keep a watchful eye on your child and be ready to help at a moment's notice.

If your child can't make sounds, stops breathing or turns blue, act immediately. Look into your child's mouth. If you see an object, use your finger to carefully remove it but be careful to not push the object into the throat. If you don't see an object, don't put your fingers in your child's throat.

The American Red Cross recommends a "five-and-five" approach to choking (this approach should not be used for infants):

- *Give five back blows.* Stand or kneel behind your child. Place one arm across your child's chest for support. Bend your child over at the waist so that the upper body is parallel with the ground. Deliver five separate back blows between the child's shoulder blades with the heel of your hand.

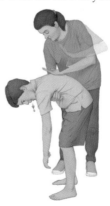

- *Give five abdominal thrusts.* Perform five abdominal thrusts (also known as the Heimlich maneuver). Make a fist with one hand and position it slightly above your child's navel. Grasp your fist with your other hand and press hard into your child's abdomen with a quick, upward thrust — as if trying to lift the child up.

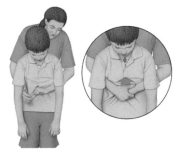

▶ *Alternate between five blows and five thrusts.* Do this until the blockage is dislodged.

If your child becomes unconscious, begin CPR or call 911. If you're alone, attempt CPR for two minutes, and then call 911. If someone is with you, have that person call for help while you continue to administer CPR. Continue doing CPR until your child starts coughing, crying or speaking. If your child resumes breathing within a minute or two, he or she will most likely not suffer any long-term effects.

After your child is breathing again, look for continued coughing or choking. This may mean that something is still preventing him or her from breathing properly. Call 911 or local emergency services.

DENTAL INJURIES

Dental injuries are common in children. If not cared for appropriately, injury to a permanent tooth can result in the loss of the tooth. This can impact your child's appearance, self-esteem and ability to chew. Falls and sports-related injuries are some of the most common causes of dental injuries in children.

How serious is it? Most dental injuries are minor, such as a chipped tooth with cracks that affect only the surface of the tooth. Other times, fractures may damage structures and soft tissue that anchor the tooth to the bone. Dental injuries may cause little to no pain or be highly sensitive to touch or temperature. Depending on the injury, there may be an increased risk of infection. Dental trauma can also occur alongside other injuries, such as brain injury, injuries to the spine and jaw fractures. In general, serious tooth injuries include:

▶ A broken, loose or missing tooth
▶ Spontaneous tooth pain
▶ Tenderness when touched or during eating
▶ Sensitivity to hot or cold temperatures
▶ Change in bite or the way teeth fit together
▶ Bleeding that can't be stopped after 10 minutes of applying pressure
▶ Pain when opening or closing the jaw
▶ Problems breathing or swallowing

What you can do Determine whether the injury is to a baby (primary) tooth or a permanent tooth. The loss of a baby tooth is generally less serious than the loss of a permanent tooth. For children 5 and younger, most if not all teeth are baby teeth. Children ages 6 to 12 tend to have a mixture of baby and permanent teeth. The tooth's appearance can also offer clues: Baby teeth are smaller than permanent teeth, and permanent teeth tend to have a smoother edge.

If a baby tooth is knocked out, putting it back in isn't recommended because of the risk of injury to the permanent tooth under the gums. For most children, having a baby tooth knocked out won't negatively impact the way your child speaks or the development of the tooth

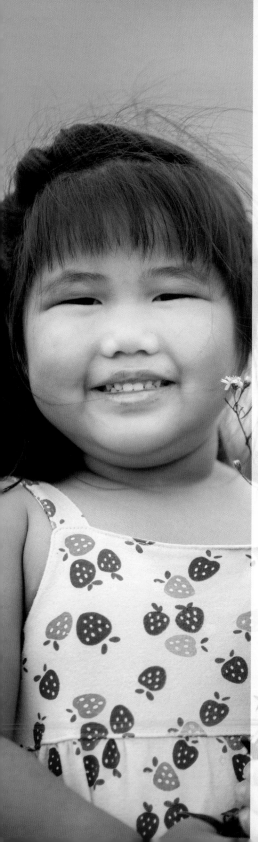

underneath. A loose tooth can be left in place, or it may be removed if there's a risk that it could be swallowed or it's interfering with the way your child bites.

If your child has a broken baby tooth, his or her dentist can determine if nerves or blood vessels in the tooth are damaged. Your child's dentist may be able to smooth down the broken piece of tooth or repair it with resin material. It may also be left alone or removed.

If a permanent tooth is knocked out, consider it an emergency. Permanent teeth need to be put back into place quickly to increase their chance of survival. Placing a tooth within 15 minutes is ideal, but you may have up to one hour. Because of time constraints, it's recommended that you attempt to temporarily place the tooth yourself until you can get your child to a dentist.

When implanting a permanent tooth, make sure you handle it by the top of the tooth (crown). Quickly rinse the tooth with saline or tap water to remove any food or debris. Don't use any other cleaning methods. Put the tooth back in its empty spot (socket) and place a clean cloth or towel in your child's mouth. Have your child hold the tooth down with his or her tongue to keep the tooth from shifting. Call your child's dentist to make an emergency appointment. Your child's dentist will likely be able to guide the tooth back into its original position. Braces or splints may be necessary to ensure the tooth stays in place.

If you can't get an emergency dental appointment right away, storing the tooth in cold milk can extend the treatment window. If milk is unavailable, place the tooth in a small container of your child's saliva. Don't store a tooth in water, as water can damage cells in the tooth's root and increase the risk that the tooth won't survive.

If your child breaks a permanent tooth, and he or she is experiencing sensitivity to hot or cold temperatures, this is also a dental emergency. Unlike teeth that have been knocked out, a broken piece of your child's tooth can be stored in tap water until your child's dentist can evaluate whether reattachment is an option. Otherwise, resin may be used to fill in the missing portion of the tooth.

If your child is experiencing pain or discomfort, offer ice, a frozen treat or over-the-counter pain medications such as ibuprofen or acetaminophen to provide relief. Your child may also have to adjust his or her diet after a dental injury, consuming a soft diet for several days and avoiding salty, crunchy or chewy foods. Have your child brush his or her teeth with a soft-bristled toothbrush during this time.

If a tooth or tooth fragment can't be found, it's possible your child may have inhaled it. See your child's dentist for an evaluation. If undetected, an aspirated tooth could cause partial or complete blockage of your child's airway. It also increases your child's risk of lung damage, pneumonia and asthma.

DROWNING

A child can drown in less than 2 inches of water, which makes close supervision of your child crucial whenever your child is swimming or playing near water. This includes bath tubs, kiddy pools, swimming pools, ponds, rivers, lakes, oceans and other sources of water.

Even if your child is a capable swimmer, be on the lookout for signs of potential drowning, such as uneven swimming strokes, bobbing or treading water, or floating face down.

How serious is it When a child's face is submersed in water, he or she will quickly run out of air to breathe. Emergency rescue is imperative. All near-drowning incidents require a trip to the emergency department, where staff will monitor vital signs and conduct a full trauma evaluation and any necessary imaging tests. If your child has been submersed and emerges choking, coughing, gagging or vomiting, take him or her to the emergency department to rule out any lung complications. In a few cases, lung injuries can show up hours later, which is why your child will likely be monitored for four to six hours after the incident.

What you can do If you think your child is drowning, immediately call emergency services or 911. If you're not a strong swimmer, don't swim out to attempt a rescue, as you're also putting your own life in danger, which will not be helpful. Instead, try other methods, such as extending a long pole or branch, or throwing out a life vest or life ring to your child.

As soon as your child is out of the water and on a stable surface, check for breathing and a pulse. If your child isn't breathing, start CPR but begin with rescue breathing (see page 169). Ventilation is most important at this point. If your child's chest doesn't rise after two rescue breaths, begin chest compressions and perform CPR until help arrives.

First aid for choking shouldn't be used on someone who has been rescued from the water, except in those rare cases where the airway is blocked and all other rescue breathing attempts have failed. First aid for choking can increase the risk of the unconscious person vomiting and choking on the vomit.

If a child is wearing cold, wet clothes, remove them and cover him or her with something warm to prevent hypothermia.

ELECTRICAL SHOCK

The damage that can be caused by an electrical shock varies depending on factors such as the source of electricity that caused the shock, the current's voltage and the length of time your child was exposed to the current.

Most electrical shocks are minor. There may only be a slight "jolt" or a minor burn-like injury at the point of contact. Sometimes, though, an electrical shock can cause a child to stop breathing and the heart to stop beating (cardiac arrest). In some cases of electrical shock, internal organ damage may occur.

How serious is it? Voltage and the length of time a child is in contact with the electrical current can predict how serious an injury is. In general, small electrical shocks, such as from touching an outlet, aren't a serious problem.

What you can do Minor electrical burns, such as from an electrical outlet, may be treated in a way similar to other types of minor burns (see page 174).

If your child is in contact with the electrical current, avoid touching your child, as this may transfer the current to you. First, try to disconnect the source of the electrical current. If that isn't possible, move the electrical source away from your child using an object made of material that won't conduct electricity, such as plastic or rubber. Never touch a live wire with your bare hands.

Call 911 or emergency services for the following signs and symptoms:
▶ A severe burn
▶ Confusion or unusual behavior
▶ Problems breathing
▶ Abnormal heart rhythms
▶ Unresponsiveness
▶ A heart that stops beating

▶ Muscle pains and contractions
▶ Seizures

If your child isn't moving or breathing, begin CPR while you wait for emergency help to arrive (see page 168). Try to keep your child from becoming chilled and, if available, cover any burned areas with a sterile gauze bandage or clean cloth. Avoid using blankets or towels, which may have loose fibers that can stick to burns.

EXPOSURE TO HARMFUL SUBSTANCES

Many common household products and medications can cause harm to children. Poisoning can occur through swallowing, inhaling, touching or injecting a harmful substance. How toxic a substance is varies greatly, and how the exposure is treated depends on your child's symptoms, the type of poison and the amount consumed.

Assume that a poisoning has occurred if there are certain clues, such as

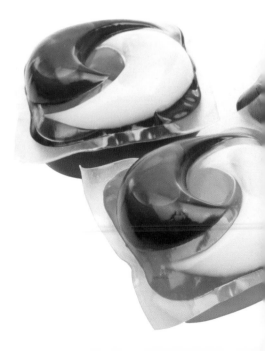

empty pill bottles or packages, scattered pills, burns, stains, or odors on your child or nearby objects. Also look out for items such as medicated patches, detergent pods and button batteries.

How serious is it? Substances vary widely when it comes to the amounts required to do harm and the seriousness of their effects. Remember, though, that it can take a much smaller amount of a product or medication to hurt a child than it would for an adult.

Length of exposure matters too. Active ingredients in extended release medications are designed to be released slowly over time, so your child may not show signs or symptoms of ingestion till much later.

What you can do If your child seems stable and doesn't show symptoms, call Poison Help at 800-222-1222 in the United States. An operator can help you gauge the seriousness of the situation and whether your child needs emergency care. Be prepared to relate as many details as possible. The operator may ask you to read labels, and describe the substance ingested, including how and when your child came into contact with it.

If your child has applied medicated patches, remove them.

If you suspect your child has swallowed a button battery, immediately take him or her to the nearest emergency department for evaluation. Batteries that get caught in a child's esophagus need to be removed before they can cause major tissue damage. You can also call the National Battery Ingestion Hotline at 800-498-8666 in the U.S. for guidance.

When it's an emergency Call 911 or your local emergency services if your child is showing signs and symptoms of poisoning, such as:

▶ Burns or redness around the mouth and lips
▶ Drooling
▶ Breath that smells like chemicals
▶ Vomiting
▶ Problems breathing
▶ Drowsiness
▶ Confusion
▶ Agitation
▶ Seizures
▶ Sweating
▶ Diarrhea
▶ Pupil changes

While waiting for emergency help to arrive, take the following precautions:

▶ *If poison is ingested.* Be careful when trying to remove anything remaining in your child's mouth. If you don't see anything, don't put your finger in his or her mouth. Don't give your child anything to eat or drink as this may provoke vomiting or make the evaluation more challenging.
▶ *If poison is on the skin.* Use gloves to remove contaminated clothing and rinse your child's skin for 15 to 20 minutes in a sink or shower or with a hose.
▶ *If poison is in the eye.* Gently flush the eye with cool or lukewarm water.
▶ *If poison is inhaled.* Move your child into fresh air as soon as possible.
▶ *If your child is vomiting.* Turn his or her head to the side to prevent choking if he or she is lying down. If upright, position his or her head to the side or forward.
▶ *If your child has no pulse or isn't breathing.* Begin CPR immediately (see page 168).

FROSTBITE

Frostbite occurs when skin and underlying tissues freeze after being exposed to very cold temperatures. Kids can get frostbite when they're playing in the cold outdoors for too long without proper clothing. The areas most likely to be affected are the fingers, toes, ears, cheeks and chin.

How serious is it? Frostbite can cause skin damage similar to that of a burn. It can range from mild to severe — or first to third degree — depending on the length of exposure to cold temperatures.

▶ Frostnip is mild frostbite that irritates the skin, causing redness, prickling and a cold feeling followed by numbness. Frostnip doesn't permanently damage the skin and can be treated with first-aid measures.

▶ Superficial frostbite leaves skin feeling warm, a sign of serious skin involvement. A fluid-filled blister may appear within 24 hours after rewarming the skin.

▶ Deep frostbite may cause numbness. Joints or muscles may no longer work. Large blisters may form a day or two after rewarming. Afterward, the area turns black and hard as the tissue dies.

What you can do Mild frostnip can be treated at home. All other frostbite requires immediate medical attention.

▶ *Get out of the cold.* Head indoors as soon as possible.

▶ *Check for hypothermia.* Seek emergency medical help if you suspect hypothermia. Signs and symptoms of hypothermia include intense shivering, drowsiness, muscle weakness, dizziness, and nausea.

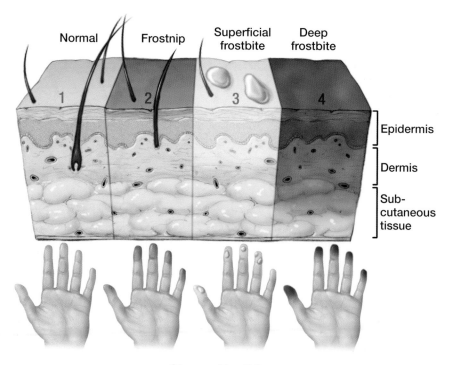

Stages of frostbite

- *Protect skin from further damage.* If there's any chance the affected areas will freeze again, don't thaw them. If they're already thawed, wrap them up so that they don't refreeze. Protect your child's face, nose or ears by covering the area with dry, gloved hands.
- *Don't rub the affected area.* Doing so can damage frozen tissues. Never rub snow on frozen skin. Don't walk on frostbitten feet or toes if possible.
- *Warm up.* If you're outside, warm frostbitten hands by tucking them into your armpits. Once you're indoors, remove wet clothes, dry off and wrap up in a warm blanket. Take care to not break any blisters.
- *Gently rewarm frostbitten areas.* Soak the frostbitten areas in warm water — 99 to 104 F. If a thermometer isn't available, test the water by placing an uninjured hand or elbow in it — the water should feel very warm — not hot. Rewarming should be done gradually and should take about 30 minutes. Stop soaking when the skin becomes its normal color or loses its numbness. Don't rewarm frostbitten skin with direct heat, such as a stove, heat lamp, fireplace or heating pad. This can cause burns.
- *Drink warm liquids.* Offer your child hot cocoa, tea or soup to help warm him or her up from the inside.
- *Consider pain medicine.* If your child is in pain, consider an over-the-counter pain reliever such as acetaminophen or ibuprofen.
- *Know what to expect as skin thaws.* If the skin turns red and your child feels it tingling and burning as it warms, that means normal blood flow is returning. Seek emergency help if numbness or pain persists, or if the skin develops blisters.

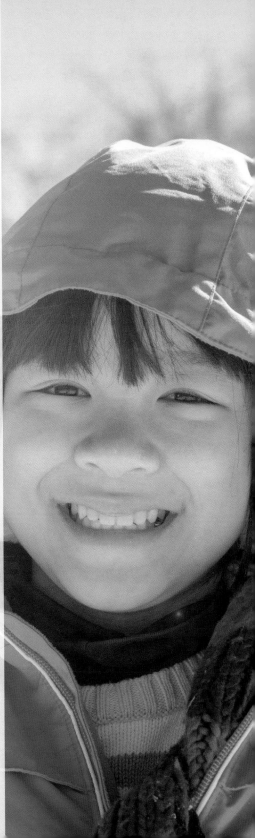

HEAD INJURIES

Head injuries may result from a fall, a sports injury or a car crash. If you're ever in doubt about whether your child needs to be seen by a medical provider after hitting his or her head, don't hesitate to make the phone call. Your child's provider can help you decide whether an office visit or trip to the emergency department is necessary.

How serious is it? In most cases, head injuries are minor. However, depending on the nature of the injury and your child's signs and symptoms, complications such as a concussion or other head trauma may result (see page 322).

For anything more than a light bump on the head, the AAP recommends calling your child's medical provider. If your child is acting normally and can respond to your questions, the head injury is likely mild and your child's provider may not need to do further testing. Your child may be scared, or the resulting bump may hurt, so crying is common.

What you can do In general, head injuries need to be monitored. Watch your child closely for the next 24 hours, looking for any unusual changes, which can signal internal damage to brain tissue and the need for urgent evaluation. Signs to watch for include:
- Problems walking
- Headache that won't go away or gets worse
- Watery or bloody discharge from the ears or nose
- Persistent vomiting
- Slurred speech or confusion
- Persistent dizziness
- Irritability
- Vision problems
- Change in pupil size
- Paleness
- Ringing in the ear
- Arm or leg weakness
- Memory problems

If your child seems to be excessively sleepy or lethargic, has a seizure, or loses consciousness, call 911 or emergency services right away. Begin CPR immediately if breathing stops or if there's no heartbeat (see page 168).

If your child's medical provider recommends monitoring your child at home after a head injury, it's OK to let your child go to sleep. Your child may also need to take a break from electronic devices, homework and other daily activities until he or she has had a chance to properly recover.

In the event your child's condition seems to worsen or new symptoms start, call your child's medical provider or emergency services right away.

SEIZURES

Seizures can be frightening to witness for both parents and medical professionals alike. Seizures occur when there's a sudden, uncontrolled disturbance of the electrical activity in the brain. This may occur as a reaction to a high fever (see "Febrile seizures" on page 336), taking a medication or experiencing a head injury. Recurrent, unpredictable seizures may be a sign of a seizure disorder such as epilepsy.

During a seizure, your child may lose consciousness, stiffen up, have jerky body movements, and bite his or her tongue. Your child's arm may shake, or he or she may appear to be staring off into the distance while making chewing motions or smacking his or her lips.

Seizures usually last no longer than a few minutes, and your child may not be able to recall the incident. He or she may seem tired or out of sorts, have a headache, or complain about feeling weak in the arms or legs. Problems speaking or seeing typically resolve within several minutes of the seizure ending.

How serious is it? While scary to witness, seizures typically don't cause any permanent damage or affect your child's development. Still, if this is your child's first seizure, call 911 or take him or her to an emergency department so that he or she can be evaluated as soon as possible.

Seizures found to be related to a fever, medication or head injury typically don't recur and generally aren't cause for further concern.

If your child has more than one seizure and they occur on separate occasions more than 24 hours apart, your child's medical provider will likely conduct an evaluation for epilepsy, which typically includes a review of your child's medical history, a medical exam and a test to measure the electrical activity in your child's brain (electroencephalogram or EEG). Sometimes other tests are needed.

What you can do If your child is having a seizure, focus on preventing your child from unintentionally hurting himself or herself during the seizure. Don't try to hold your child's tongue or restrain your child to stop the seizure. Instead, move your child onto his or her left side — the side where the stomach is located — to help clear the throat and allow spit or vomit to flow out. Clear the area of furniture and other potentially dangerous items. Don't leave your child alone.

Take note of how long the seizure lasts. If it goes on for more than five minutes, call 911. If possible, have someone else call for help while you stay with your child during the seizure. Also call for emergency help if:

▶ Your child is injured while having the seizure
▶ Your child is having trouble breathing
▶ A second seizure occurs right after the first
▶ You can't wake your child up after the seizure

If your child has been diagnosed with a condition such as epilepsy, treatment with anti-seizure medications can help prevent or minimize future seizures. Some children are prescribed a "rescue" medication to take when a seizure is occuring. Follow the instructions provided by your child's medical provider. The provider can also offer guidance on managing the condition while at school or during other activities.

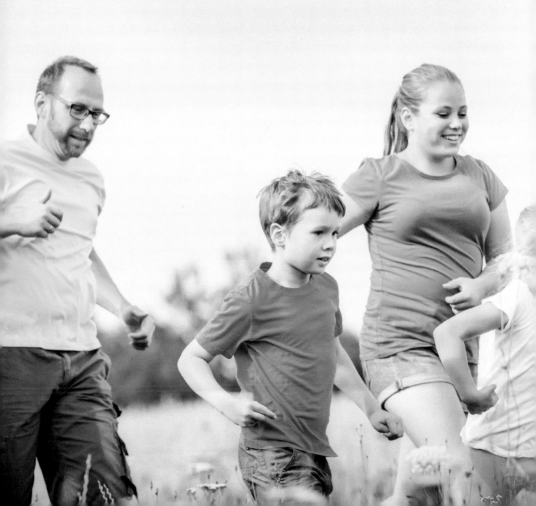

PART 3

Fitness and nutrition

CHAPTER 12

Moving for life

Swinging on the monkey bars at recess, playing tag with neighborhood friends and learning a new tumbling pass in gymnastics class — for your child, these are fun activities and memories in the making. But they're also great ways to reap the benefits of physical activity.

As with adults, children need regular physical activity to stay heathy. And since some adult health problems such as heart disease can take root in childhood, forming good habits now may help prevent these health problems from occurring later.

The Department of Health and Human Services encourages at least one hour of physical activity each day for children, with the majority of this time spent engaging in moderate to vigorous aerobic activity. Guidelines also recommend exercises to strengthen kids' muscles and bones at least three times a week.

At first glance, that may seem like a lot. But don't worry — this isn't as intimidating as it sounds. Physical activity for children isn't like a structured gym routine or exercise program an adult might follow. Instead, your child's regular daily activities help him or her reach the goal. For example, a game of tag would count as vigorous aerobic activity, while gymnastics strengthens bones and muscles.

Also, physical activity doesn't have to be done in an hourlong chunk. For kids, it's often more doable to break up activity in increments — 30 minutes on the playground and 30 minutes riding a bike.

Essentially, your child can meet the recommendations for daily physical activity by just doing fun kid stuff.

CORE COMPONENTS

Physical activity guidelines focus on three main forms of exercise: aerobic exercise, muscle strengthening and bone building.

▶ Aerobic exercise involves moving the body's large muscle groups in a rhythmic fashion. This forces the heart to work harder, pumping more oxygenated blood to muscles, and makes the lungs move more air. With regular aerobic exercise, the heart, lungs and circulatory system become stronger and more efficient. Running, walking, swimming, dancing and riding a bicycle are all examples of aerobic exercise.

▶ Muscle strengthening forces the muscles to work harder than usual, making them stronger over time. Climbing trees, scrambling over rocks, and digging in the sand or dirt are examples of activities that make muscles stronger.

▶ Bone strengthening relies on moving against gravity. This applies force on bones and promotes bone growth. Any activity that results in making impact with the ground can help build strong bones, including running, jumping, and playing hopscotch, soccer or basketball.

Although guidelines do weigh in with recommendations regarding specific factors such as frequency and intensity of activity, research suggests that the total amount of time someone is physically active is the most important factor for improving health.

HOW TO GET MOVING

You've probably heard of the benefits of regular exercise for adults. Children can reap similar benefits. Physical activity:

▶ Keeps the heart working efficiently
▶ Helps reduce the risk of developing heart disease, type 2 diabetes, high blood pressure and obesity
▶ Helps build muscle, which creates a strong frame for the body
▶ Improves bone health, which can reduce the risk of osteoporosis years later

▶ Helps control weight and improve body composition
▶ Offers a mental boost, improving cognition and learning
▶ Reduces stress, anxiety and depression
▶ Improves sleep
▶ May help reduce the risk of certain types of cancers
▶ Relieves boredom

Despite all of the benefits, only about a third of children are physically active every day. But there's a lot you can do as a parent to help encourage this healthy behavior in your child.

A key point to remember is to help your child find something he or she enjoys. As with adults, children will be more likely to stick with an activity if they love doing it. If your child hasn't been as active lately, encourage a gradual increase in activity to reduce the risk of injury.

Also, keep in mind your child's age and what's appropriate for him or her. If your child's younger, he or she may be active in shorter bursts, then rest. That's OK, it still counts! An older child can stay active for longer periods of time or take part in more-structured activities. To get your child moving:

Make it a family affair Get the whole family moving by scheduling walks after dinner or enlisting help with yardwork, vacuuming, planting a garden or other household chores. It's a great way to bond as a family.

Be a role model Children who see adults engaging in physical activity and having fun while doing it are more likely to engage in physical activity themselves. Find an activity you enjoy and share your enthusiasm with your child.

Get rid of distractions The American Academy of Pediatrics recommends that

WHAT'S THE ACTIVITY LEVEL?

Activity level	Type of activity
Moderate intensity aerobics	Skateboarding, in-line skating, bicycling, hiking, brisk walking, raking leaves, baseball, softball, basketball
Vigorous intensity aerobics	Running, jumping rope, bicycling fast or up hills, vigorous dancing, martial arts, games of tag, soccer, ice or field hockey, basketball, tennis, swimming, cheerleading, gymnastics
Muscle strengthening	Climbing a rope, tree or climbing wall; swinging on playground equipment; doing modified push-ups (knees on the floor); using resistance bands, free weights or weight machines; doing situps; performing gymnastics
Bone strengthening	Hopping, skipping, jumping, running, jumping rope, hopscotch, volleyball, basketball, tennis, gymnastics

Source: Centers for Disease Control and Prevention

Note: Some activities appear on both the moderate and vigorous intensity lists; intensity depends on the effort put into the activity.

IS IT TOO EARLY TO LIFT WEIGHTS?

By age 7 or 8, most children have learned how to follow directions. With proper instruction and supervision, those who are interested can usually engage in more-formal strength training with few problems. Strength training might include using light resistance bands, lifting light free weights, working out on machine weights and doing modified push-ups, where the knees are kept on the floor.

This type of training shouldn't be confused with activities such as body-building or powerlifting, which focus on making muscles bigger or lifting maximum weights. Before kids go through puberty and experience hormonal changes it's difficult to gain significantly larger muscles. Strength training at this age focuses on increasing muscle coordination and endurance, not bulking up.

If your child is interested in taking up strength training, ask your child's coach or a personal trainer experienced with youth to offer some pointers and create a safe, effective training program based on your child's individual abilities. Programs should include not only strength training, but proper warmups — such as walking or jogging in place for five to 10 minutes — and cool-downs, such as gentle stretching.

If your child has any health issues, check with his or her medical provider first before embarking on a strength training regimen.

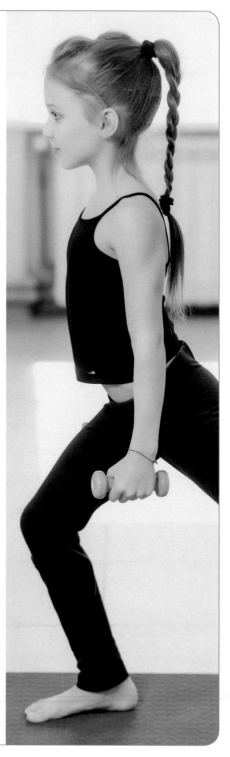

children over age 5 spend no more than two hours daily on cellphones, computers, televisions or video games. When possible, encourage your child to hang out with friends in person, instead of calling, emailing or texting them.

Consider alternate transportation

Encourage your child to bike or walk to school if your child is old enough and you live in an area where it's safe to do so. If safety might be an issue, consider forming a "walk to school" group with other families in the neighborhood.

Also consider fun destinations nearby that your child can walk or ride a bike to, such as a park or library.

Be creative

Some of the best activities are those in which your child doesn't even realize he or she is working toward physical activity goals. Here are some ideas to get you started:

- Birthdays and holidays are a perfect time to purchase items that encourage exercise. Bicycles, kites, jump-ropes and skateboards are all fun ways to get moving. If your child is into video games, consider buying ones that encourage movement — for example, those centered on dancing or mimicking sports, such as tennis or bowling.
- Speaking of birthdays, consider hosting an activity-based celebration for your child. Whether it's a soccer, basketball or gymnastics party at a local gym or a party that simply incorporates open play, fun and exercise are bound to mingle.
- Plan an active getaway. Consider vacationing somewhere that offers ample opportunities for activities — for example, hiking, swimming, skiing or bodysurfing. A visit to a zoo also can help get some walking time in.

- Have fun close to home. Check the calendar listings in your local newspaper or the events in local parenting groups on social media for activities that your family may enjoy.

Don't go overboard Sometimes there's a temptation to sign up children for every activity that they might possibly be interested in. Don't forget that children need downtime, too.

Encourage your child to let you know if he or she experiences pain during an activity. Exercise shouldn't hurt and pain can be a sign to take things down a notch.

Other signs of overdoing it might include a sprain or a strained muscle. If this happens, rest the injured area and take your child to see his or her medical provider. Follow the provider's instructions and pick up activity again gradually after the injury has healed.

SPORTS FOR KIDS

An effective, and perhaps convenient, way to get a child moving is through sports, whether it be through your child's school or a local recreational league.

In addition to all the benefits listed previously for physical activity, participating in sports has been shown to have other positive effects, including:

- Improved motor skills
- Greater likelihood of eating healthy foods
- Improved self-esteem
- Decreased engagement in risky behavior, such as smoking or taking illegal drugs
- Improved social skills and a wider range of friendships
- Better performance in school and increased graduation rates

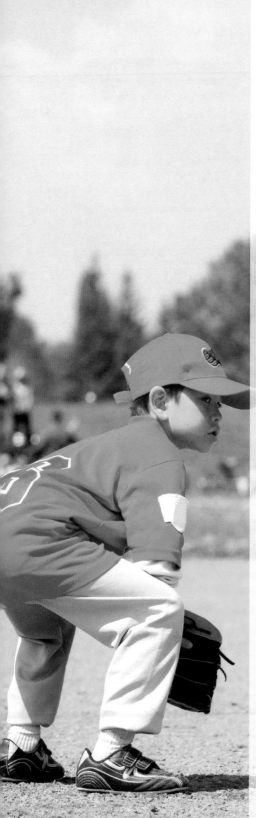

- ▶ Greater likelihood of remaining physically active through adulthood
- ▶ Greater resilience

Starting off right The age at which you decide to sign your child up for a sports program is up to you and whether you think your child is up to it. Children can start being exposed to sports whenever they're developmentally ready.

The focus of sports changes over time. Initially, the focus is on having fun, learning the game and getting the basics of movement. As kids get older, other aspects such as keeping score and playing games tend to be incorporated.

Parents often feel pressure — sometimes self-imposed — to give their kids an early edge in a particular sport.

For most sports, there's little proof that starting a child at a young age will give him or her any sort of additional skills or edge in performance when he or she is older. Ultimately, children may become stressed, frustrated or disillusioned with a sport if they struggle too much with it.

Until about the first grade or so, the focus should be on simple activities such as running, tumbling, catching, throwing or swimming. Even at older ages free play continues to be an important part of healthy physical and mental development. So strive for a good balance between the two.

Finding a good fit If your child isn't particularly interested in team sports, talk about trying an individual sport, such as tennis or bowling. Some children may not enjoy sports because they don't care for competition. That's OK too. Noncompetitive activities such as recreational canoeing, hiking or bicycling are great alternatives that still get them moving, without the pressure to compete.

Sometimes, children lose interest in playing a sport after a while. If your child doesn't want to sign up again or is truly unhappy with a chosen sport, it may be best not to force the issue. However, continue to promote the goal of staying active. This can be done through trying a new sport or other less structured activities.

SPORTS SAFETY

Playing sports isn't without risk of injury. Sprains, fractures and concussions can occur. And while anyone who's physically active runs the risk of injury, kids are more prone to certain types of injuries than are adults. That's because kids' bodies are still developing. During

SPORTS AND DISABILITIES

Physical activity benefits all children, including those with disabilities. If your child has a physical or intellectual disability, talk with your child's doctor, physical therapist or aide about how you can help your child become more active in a healthy and safe way.

For example, a weight-bearing program can help children with cerebral palsy increase muscle strength and endurance. Participating in a specialized aerobics class may help children with Down syndrome increase exercise endurance and improve the ability to accomplish tasks of daily living. In children with autism, exercise can help improve behavior and fatigue, and reduce repetitive movements.

Check offerings at your local recreation center. Many communities have adaptive sports classes and camps for kids with disabilities. Special Olympics is a worldwide organization that offers training and organizes events for athletes with intellectual disabilities. The organization has local branches in every state in the U.S. and also around the world. You can search for a branch near you on the Special Olympics' website.

In children with disabilities, participation in sports and regular physical activity can help:
▶ Improve muscle tone and conditioning caused by impaired mobility
▶ Optimize physical functioning
▶ Enhance social skills and build friendships
▶ Increase self-confidence and independence
▶ Express individual creativity
▶ Improve mental health and overall well-being

With the approval of your child's medical care team, encourage your child to participate in sports he or she enjoys. Some activities may require a little preparation beforehand — such as using an inhaler before a soccer game for children with asthma, or knowing how to recognize early signs of hypothermia in children with spinal cord injuries. But foster a can-do attitude as much as possible. With proper guidance from parents, medical providers and coaches, athletes with disabilities are no more prone to injury than those without a disability.

FOSTERING A HEALTHY PARENT-COACH RELATIONSHIP

When it comes to sports, adults often think of winning as the ultimate goal. But kids tend to look at it a bit differently. According to surveys of children, the ultimate goal of sports is having fun. Positive parent-coach connections can help children do both — develop the skills necessary to flourish in a sport and enjoy doing it.

A healthy relationship between a parent and a coach relies on give-and-take, with expectations for both parties. Below are some typical expectations for coaches and parents. Keeping these in mind can help you forge a meaningful relationship with your child's coach. If you've had a preseason meeting with your child's coach, some of these may sound familiar:

What to expect from a coach
- Clear communication about practice and game schedules, how to practice at home, and what equipment is needed
- Well-organized practices that work on improving skills
- Focus on player safety
- Fair and consistent treatment of players
- Constructive criticism that is focused on improving a skill
- Emphasis on players doing their best, not on winning
- End goal of helping children improve and grow in the sport

What a coach expects from a parent
- Doing drills at home with your child to develop skills
- Arriving to practices and games on time, and picking up on time
- Keeping comments about your child and his or her team positive
- Making sure your child knows the importance of having fun, making friends and improving skills
- Lending your child's coach a hand, such as setting up equipment during practice, keeping players hydrated by bringing them water, or helping keep children safe when on the sidelines or bench
- Letting the coach do the coaching during practices and games — and not shouting out instructions to your child from the sidelines — to avoid confusing your child and other players
- Updating your child's coach on any health or behavioral issues your child may be having, to keep your child safe during practices and games

Sometimes, issues arise during a practice or game that may warrant a conversation between you and the coach. Maybe you feel your child is sitting on the bench too much or is somehow being treated unfairly. Consider contacting the coach the next day to set up a time to discuss the issue. This allows time for emotions to settle and ensures you'll be able to talk about the problem uninterrupted, without your child or other players and their parents overhearing.

In addition, avoid speaking negatively about the coach or the team in front of your child, which can decrease morale and enthusiasm. Take the long-term view — sport seasons are relatively short in the grand scheme of things. Choose to model mature behavior for your child.

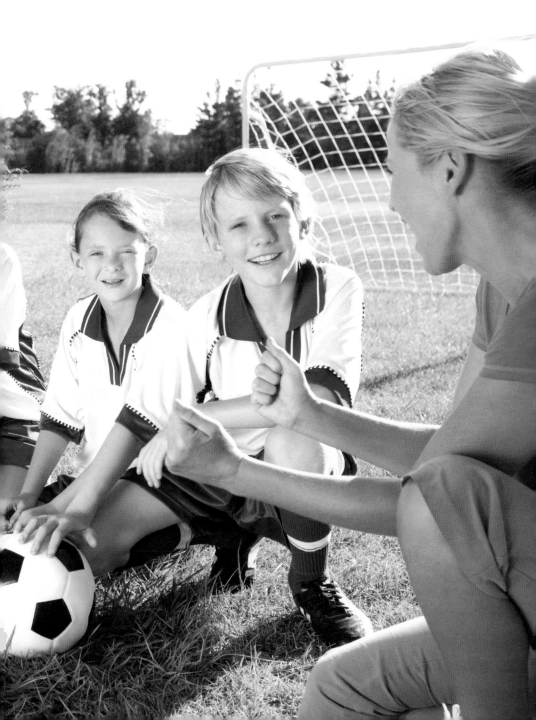

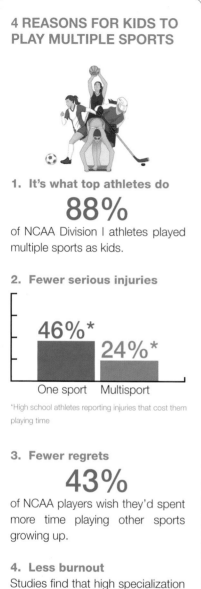

4 REASONS FOR KIDS TO PLAY MULTIPLE SPORTS

1. It's what top athletes do

88%

of NCAA Division I athletes played multiple sports as kids.

2. Fewer serious injuries

46%* **24%***

One sport   Multisport

*High school athletes reporting injuries that cost them playing time

3. Fewer regrets

43%

of NCAA players wish they'd spent more time playing other sports growing up.

4. Less burnout

Studies find that high specialization at a young age carries an increased risk of:

▶ Stress and anxiety
▶ Social isolation
▶ Burnout, and ultimately quitting the sport earlier

Based on Mayo Clinic News Network. Infographic: Playing multiple sports.

---

this period of physical development, kids have:

▶ *Growing bodies.* The natural process of growing or experiencing growth spurts over time can create changes in a child's movement patterns, flexibility, coordination and balance. Together, these can increase the risk of injury somewhat.

▶ S*oft areas of bone.* Growth plates are located at the ends of the body's long bones — for example, the femur in the thigh and the radius and ulna in the forearm. These areas don't fully develop until late adolescence and are more vulnerable to fracture. Often, growth plate fractures occur because of a single event, such as a fall or a blow to the growth plate. But they can also be caused by repetitive stress, such as from overtraining.

Experts agree that the benefits of participating in sports and staying physically active usually outweigh most of the risks. If you and your child follow basic sports injury prevention and keep certain precautions in mind, there's no need to discourage your child from participating in a sport.

Sports specialization If your child shows promise in a particular sport, it's tempting to want to invest time and energy in it. But in elementary school kids, specializing in one sport can be too much of a good thing too soon.

Sports specialization is defined as intensive year-round training in a single sport at the exclusion of other sports. Playing and training year-round may not give your child the proper downtime needed to let his or her body recuperate and may increase the risk of injury.

In sports such as gymnastics and figure skating, a more rigorous training and competition schedule is common when athletes are still young and growing. Research results have been mixed on how this may affect a child long term. Some studies show no effect. Others link intense training during childhood and adolescence to issues, such as an increase in overuse injuries.

In girls — especially those who participate in sports that emphasize weight categories or aesthetics, such as ballet or gymnastics — excessive training can sometimes be harmful. Intense conditioning combined with an inadequate intake of calories necessary to meet energy demands can lead to hormonal changes. Such changes can alter growth and development, as well as increase the risk of certain injuries and conditions.

Not all sports injuries are physical in nature. For children who focus on one sport, not having a break may lead to burnout and stress. This could be one reason why many children stop playing sports by the time they get to high school.

Preventing injury Varying the type, frequency and intensity of activities can keep your child in good health. To help prevent overuse injuries:

▶ Encourage your child to participate in multiple sports
▶ Avoid focusing on a single sport till your child is skeletally mature, typically around late adolescence or near the end of puberty
▶ Take off three or four months a year from a single sport
▶ Take off one or two days a week from a single sport
▶ Spend less than 16 hours a week total on a single sport

A good rule of thumb is to not perform more hours a week in a specific sport than the child's age in years. For example, a 10-year-old baseball player shouldn't play more than 10 hours of baseball a week.

Additionally, your child can prevent other sports-related injuries by:

▶ Wearing properly fitted gear, such as pads, mouthpieces, helmets and other protective items
▶ Doing strength and flexibility training
▶ Taking breaks during games and practice, when needed
▶ Abiding by the rules of the game and not engaging in risky sports behavior, such as tackling headfirst in football
▶ Sitting out if he or she is injured
▶ Staying hydrated before, during and after games and practices

If you're concerned that your child may not develop the necessary skills to compete later on without specializing in a preferred sport, consider this: Research suggests that world-class athletes in many sports share some common characteristics. They played multiple sports when they were younger and typically only started intense training and competition in their particular sport when they were older.

Remember to keep up with regular visits with your child's medical provider. This will help to address any concerns you may have regarding sports participation. As sports training intensifies, usually around middle school and high school, yearly sports physicals become more important to help ensure your child is safe and ready to compete.

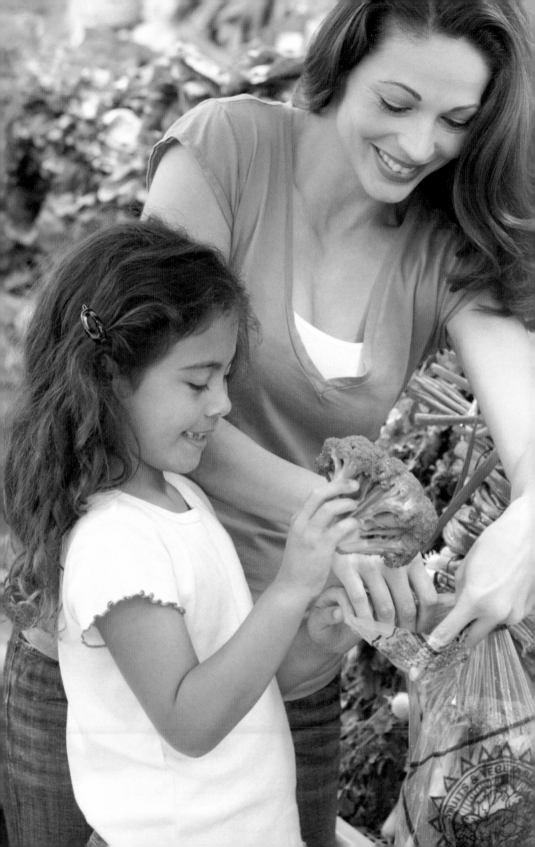

CHAPTER 13

Nutrition for growing kids

Like most parents, you probably wonder about your child's diet and whether you're doing it right. Is it healthy enough? Is your child eating too much or too little? Will a trip through the drive-through make you a bad parent?

It's not always easy to plan — let alone persuade children to eat — healthy, balanced meals that support growth and development. If you've given up trying to find the perfect balance of carbs and proteins, cook only the healthiest meals, or offer only fruits and vegetables for snacks, welcome to the club. You're certainly not alone, and frankly, your child's plate will likely never be picture-perfect. Nor should it be, really.

Feeding your child is about more than just making sure your child eats the right stuff. It's also about establishing long-term healthy eating patterns, teaching your child about balance, and helping your child learn to nourish his or her body. And it's about spending time together, observing the family rituals and traditions that often surround mealtimes.

By providing healthy options as often as you can, getting your child involved in preparing meals, and teaching habits that promote a healthy body and mind, you can make sure your child is getting all of the necessary nutrients and establishing a healthy relationship with food that will last into adulthood.

GUIDELINES FOR HEALTHY EATING

Getting children to eat well — or even eat at all, in some cases — can be one of the biggest challenges for parents. Think of the countless times you may have sat at the dinner table coaxing your preschooler to eat just a few bites, or bribing your older child to eat his or her vegetables.

Feeding the family is often one of the areas where parents feel the most pressure to get it right, and to feel guilty if they don't.

But it may not be as cumbersome as you think. Here are some simple evidence-based guidelines that you can use to encourage healthy eating patterns in your child.

Provide healthy options Encourage your child to eat well by providing a wide variety of healthy options from all of the food groups.

Keep in mind that ultimately, you decide what groceries come in the house. While it's probably not realistic to deprive your family of all junk food, look for ways to include more nutritious foods — such as fruits, vegetables and low-fat dairy — into your daily menus.

Make these healthier foods easily available. Place a bowl of clementines or some bananas on the kitchen counter. Keep the low-fat yogurt at kid-level in the fridge.

Set regular mealtimes Offer your child three nutritious meals and one or two scheduled healthy snacks a day.

Whenever possible, have the entire family sit down to eat together. Sharing a family meal allows parents to model healthy food choices and appropriate portions. Eliminate distractions such as television and phones to encourage the social aspects of the meal, too. Read more on mealtime and snacks later in the chapter.

Make room for choices As a parent, you may want your child to eat a bit of everything being offered. While it's fine to encourage that, avoid forcing the issue.

Let your child choose from the healthy options you've provided. This approach not only encourages your child to enjoy mealtime but also helps your child develop decision-making skills.

Let your child decide how much Don't feel the need to be a part of the "Clean Plate Club." Instead, help your child discern and heed his or her own hunger and fullness cues. Provide small portions and offer seconds if your child is still hungry.

Some kids may say they're full only to turn around and ask for a favorite snack or dessert right after the meal. Discourage this behavior by sticking to your pre-planned meal and snack schedule.

BALANCING HEALTH AND ENJOYMENT

Eating habits developed now form the foundation for future eating patterns. As you feed your child, encourage a balance between health and enjoyment. Placing restrictions on what children can eat, pressuring them to eat certain foods, using food for purposes other than nutrition — such as for comfort or reward — or worrying about things such as a child gaining too much weight can have unintended consequences. Such an approach can create an unhealthy relationship with food and contribute to distorted views about body image. This in turn can lead to problems such as anxiety, depression, weight gain, repeated attempts at dieting and eating disorders later on. See the next chapter, Preventing obesity and eating disorders, for a more in-depth look.

Promote flexible eating Encourage a flexible attitude toward food. Flexible eating means no foods are considered "bad" or off limits. Rather, the focus is on moderation and variety. A flexible diet emphasizes healthy, nutritious meals, but allows room for sweets and treats when appropriate. When portioned appropriately, all foods can be part of a healthy diet.

Be a role model Your child looks to you for cues on how to behave, including how to relate to food. If you enjoy eating healthy foods, your child is more likely to do the same. If you say, "Wow, these strawberries are so sweet" or "I love how crunchy these carrot sticks are," your child might take the same approach.

If you reserve desserts and other treats for special occasions — and avoid using these foods as a reward or as a comfort measure — your child will see that they can be enjoyed in moderation for their own sake.

As your child observes how you eat and the way you nurture your body and self-image through wise choices, positive talk and a willingness to be physically active, he or she will follow along to the same mental "playlist."

CALORIE INTAKE BY AGE

Here's a general idea of how much a moderately active child should be eating daily from each food group based on age and gender:

	Gender	Daily Calorie Intake	Vegetables*	Fruits*	Grains*	Protein*	Dairy*
3-5 years old	Girls	1,200-1,400	1½ cups	1-1½ cups	4-5 ounces	3-4 ounces	2½ cups
	Boys	1,400	1½ cups	1½ cups	5 ounces	4 ounces	2½ cups
6-8 years old	Girls	1,400-1,600	1½-2 cups	1½ cups	5 ounces	4-5 ounces	2½-3 cups
	Boys	1,600	2 cups	1½ cups	5 ounces	5 ounces	3 cups
9-12 years old	Girls	1,600-2,000	2-2½ cups	1½-2 cups	5-6 ounces	5-5½ ounces	3 cups
	Boys	1,800-2,200	2½-3 cups	1½-2 cups	6-7 ounces	5-6 ounces	3 cups

Source: U.S. Department of Agriculture

* Cups and ounces are intended as cup-equivalents and ounce-equivalents. For example:

1 cup-equivalent of fruit = a small apple or large banana

1 cup-equivalent of vegetables = 1 cup of raw or cooked vegetables or 2 cups of raw leafy greens

1 ounce-equivalent of grains = 1 slice of bread, 5 whole-wheat crackers or 1 small muffin

1 cup-equivalent of dairy = 1 1/2 ounces of cheddar cheese or 8 ounces of fat-free yogurt

1 ounce-equivalent of protein = 1 large egg, 1 tablespoon of peanut butter or 1/4 cup of black beans

For more information on cup- and ounce-equivalents for the different food groups, visit www.choosemyplate.gov.

WHAT TO EAT?

No single food or food group provides all the nutrients needed for growth. Focus on providing a variety of foods over the course of the day or the week, drawing from each of the following food groups:

Vegetables Vegetables are important sources of dietary fiber. They also provide a wealth of vitamins, such as A, C, K, E and B6; and minerals, such as potassium, copper, magnesium, folate, iron and others essential for growth and development. Frozen or canned vegetables are easy to prepare when you're in a hurry. Make sure you're incorporating dark green, red and orange veggies — such as spinach, broccoli, sweet peppers and carrots, for example — and beans and peas each week. Choose canned or packaged veggies that are lower in sodium.

Fruits Fruits contribute a host of nutrients to your child's diet, including dietary fiber, potassium and vitamin C. Encourage your child to eat whole fruits – whether fresh, canned, frozen or dried. Whole fruits contain more fiber than fruit juice. For fruits that are canned, make sure they're canned in juice, not syrup. If you're offering fruit juice, look for 100 percent juice. Watch out for added sugar, especially in canned or packaged foods. Check the labels for ingredients such as high fructose corn syrup, corn sweetener, corn syrup and sugar — especially if they're near the top of the list. The higher an ingredient is on the list, the more there is in the food.

Grains Whole grains provide nutrients such as dietary fiber, vitamins A and B6, and a host of minerals. Refined or enriched grains are often fortified with iron and B vitamins. Your child may prefer white breads, pastas and rice, but try to make at least half of your child's daily grain intake whole-grain varieties, such as whole-wheat bread or pasta, oatmeal, popcorn, quinoa, or wild or brown rice.

Proteins Dietary protein is essential for growth. It provides basic building blocks (amino acids) for the structure and function of all of the body's cells. Protein-rich foods also provide a variety of vitamins and minerals. Protein can be found in foods such as seafood, lean meats and poultry, eggs, tofu, beans, peas, unsalted nuts, peanut butter, and other nut butters. Choose meat that is lean and low in fat and sodium — and limit processed meats, such as deli or luncheon meat.

Dairy Dairy products are rich in calcium, an important nutrient for strong bones, as well as minerals and vitamins. Fat-free and low-fat varieties provide the same nutrients but fewer calories. Encourage your child to eat and drink a variety of dairy products, such as low-fat or fat-free milk, yogurt, cheese or fortified soy beverages. If your child isn't drinking milk with meals, incorporate healthy dairy snacks — such as low-fat string cheese or yogurt.

Fats Fats are necessary for brain and nervous system development and are a good source of calories. Vegetable or nut oils and spreads can provide necessary fatty acids and vitamin E. Healthy fats are also found in foods such as avocados, olives and seafood. But added fats — for example, hydrogenated or partially hydrogenated oils, and tropical oils, such as palm oil — in packaged foods such as cookies and chips have little nutritional value. Also, limit saturated fats – fats that come from animal sources such as butter and meats. Opt more often for vegetable oils and lean poultry without skin.

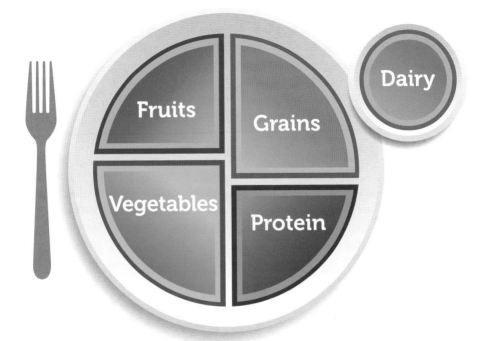

Choose**MyPlate**.gov

Source: USDA Center for Nutrition Policy and Promotion

A healthy eating plan can be illustrated in many ways. The U.S. Department of Agriculture uses a small 9-inch lunch plate, called MyPlate, to promote the concept that most of your daily food intake should come from fruits and vegetables, complemented by grains and proteins. Kids especially need to eat a variety of foods from each food group to get all the calories, protein, vitamins, minerals and fiber that they need.

MEALTIME

Mealtimes provide a unique opportunity for the family to get together and share not only food but companionship. Research shows that family meals have a protective effect on children's health.

Children from families that eat regular meals together consume more-nutritious foods and are less likely to struggle with childhood obesity or eating disorders. They're also more likely to have better behavior, a stronger vocabulary and greater academic success.

As children get older and begin to participate in organized after-school activities, family schedules tend to get a little crazier. But with a little bit of prep, you can make family meals a regular part of your schedule.

Have a plan Having a meal plan makes it easier to stick to healthy, home-cooked meals. Start by planning three or four meals for the week, allowing a night or two for leftovers or a free night.

Rotate in some family favorites with a few new recipes. See page 470 for a sample weekly meal plan with recipes and tips on maximizing your time in the kitchen.

Consider incorporating at least one food you know your child will eat to increase the likelihood that they eat at dinnertime.

Planning your meals ahead of time will help save you time and money. You can look for the best deals while shopping, and you don't have to waste time running to the store to pick up ingredients you don't have.

Remove distractions Cutting out electronic screens at the table allows the family to focus on the meal and on each other. Also, research suggests that watching TV or using phones or tablets while eating can lead to overeating, which can later contribute to childhood obesity. It can also cause a distraction to younger or pickier eaters, who may opt for the television over their meal.

WHAT'S A CHILD-SIZED SERVING?

If visualizing serving sizes in terms of cups and ounces sounds a little overwhelming, you're not alone. It can easily get confusing.

A simple alternative is to use your child's fist as a rough estimate of an appropriate serving size for him or her. For example, for most preschoolers, a fist-size portion is equivalent to about one-half of a cup or one ounce. For kids 9 and older, a fist is more like one cup. A serving of protein is often measured as the size of a child's palm. This works for grown-ups too. A tablespoon can be equated to a woman's thumb, handy for estimating portions of nut butter, for example.

At any one meal, a fist-sized portion of vegetables, fruit, grains and protein should provide roughly a third to a quarter of the daily serving for each food group.

This isn't a hard and fast rule, of course. But you can use these visual cues as tools to help steer you toward a rough estimate of what your child's portions should look like.

WHAT ABOUT FAST FOOD?

Fast food is a big part of American culture and many people enjoy its taste and quick convenience. In general, though, fast food provides more calories and sodium, and fewer beneficial nutrients than food prepared at home. This is true for most restaurants.

Eating fast food too often can result in too many calories and too few nutrients. At the same time, completely prohibiting fast food for your children can be counterproductive. When something's off-limits, kids tend to want it more.

As with most things, moderation is key. An occasional fast-food outing is fine, but don't let burgers and fries replace regular meals at home. Some evidence suggests that eating fast food too often may eventually lead to a preference — an acquired taste — for highly processed or salty foods.

When you do opt for fast food, encourage your son or daughter to make healthy choices. Go for lower-fat milk instead of soda, and yogurt or apples instead of fries. Balance is possible, even when it's a convenience meal, and can help your child learn to organize a nutrient-rich meal whether it's home-cooked or ordered from a menu.

Remember, in the long run, your child's overall pattern of eating matters more than the food eaten on a single day.

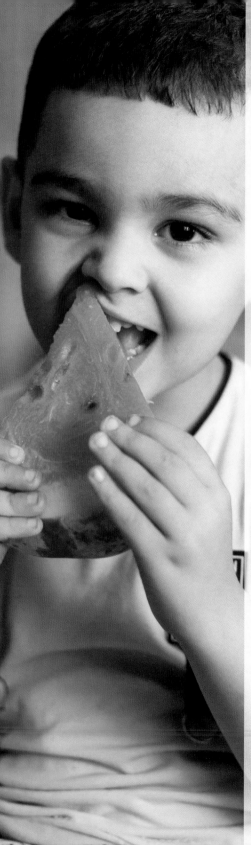

Make it enjoyable Focus on making family meals an enjoyable time. Talk about your day, share funny stories and make plans for good times together.

Expect your child to be a messy eater. Try to overlook spilled milk or dropped food, and avoid being too rigid about table manners. Children will get the hang of where to put their elbows and how to use a fork and knife eventually, especially if they see you behaving in the way you want them to.

Make it easy Just because you eat at home doesn't mean meals have to be complicated or time-consuming. Use healthy shortcuts such as prechopped fresh or frozen veggies, a bagged salad, or a rotisserie chicken or canned tuna to save time. To get the most out of your time in the kitchen, cook extra food one night that you can convert into a second meal the next day. For example, leftover rice from tonight's dinner can be reserved for burrito bowls tomorrow.

SNACK SMARTS

Snacks are fun and can be an important part of your child's diet. Since children have smaller stomachs than adults, a healthy snack between meals is a good way to meet your child's energy and nutrient needs.

Planned snacks help structure your family's eating patterns and discourage grazing. When you plan snacks ahead of time, you have time to strategize a little better and come up with healthier options than you might in the midst of a hungry moment.

To fit snacks into a healthy diet for your child, think about how to space snacks and mealtimes. Also think about the kinds and amounts of foods to offer. Generally, it's OK for kids to eat a healthy meal or snack every three or four hours. Here are some tips for smart snacking.

Include your child Recruit your child's help in planning and preparing snacks. Work with your child to create a snack list and post the list on the refrigerator or cupboard. If your child doesn't read yet, consider cutting out pictures of healthy snacks you have in your cupboards and making a small poster with the pictures on it.

Make it accessible Keep healthy snacks in easily accessible or visible areas. Prep fresh fruits and vegetables — cube a melon or slice up celery sticks — ahead of time so they're easy to grab and go. Place packages of dried fruit or trail mix in a "cookie jar." Set aside special areas of your cupboards and refrigerator so healthy snacks are quickly found.

Time it right Serve snacks at set times rather than anytime throughout the day.

Don't give snacks too close to mealtimes. Plan snacks one to two hours before the next meal and nix snacks directly after a meal. Give your child a chance to get hungry. Being a little hungry helps him or her look forward to the next meal.

Serve child-sized portions Large snacks dull your child's appetite for the next meal. Read labels for serving size information. Remember that prepackaged serving sizes may be too large for preschoolers. Offer a child-sized portion of animal crackers or dry cereal in a snack-sized bowl or bag instead of letting your child eat from the whole package.

Mix it up As much as possible, make an effort to offer whole fruits and veggies as part of a snack, along with a bit of additional carbs or protein. But a taco, a slice of pizza or half of a peanut butter and jelly sandwich can also be a nutritious snack on the way to an afternoon activity. And as long as your child is eating a well-balanced diet, it's OK to occasionally eat a snack high in sugar or fat.

HEALTHY SNACK IDEAS

Examples of healthy snacks include:
- Apple slices or celery sticks with peanut butter
- Pita chips with hummus
- Unsweetened applesauce
- Cucumbers or carrots and yogurt dip
- Pretzels and grapes
- Popcorn
- Small servings of crackers with cheese
- Steamed soybeans (edamame)
- Frozen yogurt or yogurt pops
- Fruit cups, canned in their own juice
- Low-fat pudding

DIY Consider making your own home-made snack mixtures that include items such as whole-grain cereal, raisins or popcorn. Or roast canned chickpeas with your favorite spices. Snacks you make yourself are usually more nutritious and interesting to kids. These homemade mixes often delight younger kids if they have a say in what goes into the mixture.

GETTING YOUR CHILD INVOLVED

As kids get older, they enjoy having a say in the family's decision-making process. Involving your child in meal planning and prepping exposes him or her to lessons in nutrition and increases your child's ownership of home-cooked meals.

You can start by bringing your child to the grocery store with you, or enlist your child's help at home while you're prepping meals. Doing so allows you to teach your child about nutrition in a fun way, while providing a great opportunity for bonding. Getting your child's input while shopping and cooking may even increase your child's willingness to try new foods and recipes.

Go grocery shopping together If your child is just learning about nutrition, take on the role of narrator at the grocery store. Explain to your child why you've made a particular food choice or ask for help in searching for certain ingredients on the shelves. You can even turn it into a fun game of "I spy."

Involving your child in grocery shopping is not only a great way to introduce him or her to different food options, the added conversation can help boost brain development and vocabulary.

Hand over the shopping list If your child is old enough to read — or even recognize a few words — involve him or her in creating the shopping list through writing down or drawing ingredients.

At the grocery store, give your child the shopping list and a pencil. As you put items in the cart, have your child cross them off your list. It will keep you organized while keeping your child engaged in the process.

If your child only makes it through a couple items, don't worry. Your shopping list can also double as a coloring book. Even small doses of learning are beneficial.

Ask for input If the meal you're making gives you latitude on certain ingredients, such as different veggies, fruits or garnishes, ask for your child's opinion on what to choose.

Providing your child with a few choices adds variety you might not have thought of and boosts your child's investment in the meal, making it more likely that he or she will enjoy it.

Get help with your menu Ask for help planning your family's weekly menu. Even if your child chooses only one meal, it can be a fun way to get your child involved and engaged. And if your child insists on hot dogs, complete the overall meal with whole-wheat buns and a veggie.

Plan a dish your child can prepare This might include tossing a salad or washing up fruit for dessert. Set out ingredients beforehand, and if you have more than one child, have your children help each other. Creating a dish for a family meal will give your child a sense of accomplishment and pride, while teaching valuable cooking skills.

Assign a task Older children can learn meal prep skills, such as following a simple recipe or prepping vegetables. Younger children can start with smaller tasks, such as fetching ingredients, dumping in premeasured ingredients or stirring them together in a bowl.

TIPS FOR THE PICKY EATER

Is your child pushing broccoli to the side of his or her plate or not allowing it on the plate at all? Does she turn her nose up at your carefully crafted meals? Will he eat nothing but chicken nuggets or macaroni and cheese?

Young children are often sensitive to the way food looks, tastes and smells. And if your child is rejecting an entire food group, you might start to feel that these picky eating habits are depriving him or her of the benefits of a healthy diet.

Try not to worry. Picky eating is most common in the toddler and preschool years, and it tends to gradually ease with age. It may help to know that you're not responsible for making your child like a certain food. Research indicates that experience is the only real predictor of acceptance and liking. What you can do is provide multiple opportunities for your child to learn about food, whether you're reading about it, shopping for it, preparing it or tasting it.

Here are some additional tips for pulling in picky eaters.

Stay out of food fights Avoid making a big deal of your child's food acceptance – or lack thereof. Resist coercing your child into eating foods he or she doesn't like by offering dessert as a bribe. Try not to force a meal if your son or daughter isn't hungry. This can create a power struggle and cause mealtime to be fraught with stress and anxiety.

Start small Start off with smaller portions along with the option to ask for more. Serving up portions that are too large can be overwhelming. If your child refuses to eat anything at all, ask him or her to stay at the table for the rest of the family meal. Don't cook a separate meal, as this can reinforce picky eating habits.

Be persistent Kids have a better chance of liking a food if you expose them to it regularly. Even if your child doesn't like a food the first time, keep offering it. Research shows that it generally takes eight to 10 times of being offered a certain food, such as a vegetable, before a child is inclined to accept it. Children are usually more willing to try new foods if given one at a time, in small portions, with a meal that includes other familiar foods.

Get creative Sometimes, it's not the food a picky eater objects to necessarily, but the way in which it's presented. Your child might object to mixing foods or having one food touch another on a plate. If this is the case, try changing up the presentation.

For example, offer a buffet of bite-sized portions arranged in small bowls or cupcake liners — maybe try a grouping of pasta shells, cubed ham or tofu, and tiny broccoli florets. It's an easy way for your child to pick and choose from a range of healthy options and to exert some control over his or her eating.

Be patient Don't worry too much about food "jags" or eating patterns that aren't regular. This is common, especially in young children.

Focus on providing healthy options. If your child wants a peanut butter sand-wich every day for lunch that's OK. Occasionally try to mix it up with something different and see how it goes.

Remember that most children consume the right balance of nutrients over the course of the week, so avoid placing too much pressure on yourself, your child or a single meal. A child's pickiness won't change overnight, so take small steps and make note of what works.

If you try these strategies to no avail, or if you're concerned that your child's picky eating is harming his or her health, contact your child's medical provider or a dietitian. He or she can help you create a plan for your child to ensure he or she receives the nutrients needed to support healthy growth.

SPECIALIZED DIETS

There are many reasons a specialized diet could be right for your family, whether based on principle, preference or medical necessity. As with any eating pattern, work to find the right nutritional balance for your child's age, sex and activity level.

Vegetarian and vegan families More families are choosing to raise their children in a vegetarian or vegan household. There are benefits associated with a plant-based diet, including better heart health, a reduced risk of diabetes and a lowered risk of childhood obesity.

With a little planning, a vegetarian or vegan diet can meet the needs of people of all ages. What's important is that your child is receiving all of the vitamins, minerals and nutrients he or she needs to grow and develop. As with any diet, the key is including a variety of foods.

Keep in mind that the more restrictive your child's diet is, the more challenging it can be to get all the nutrients your child needs. A vegan diet, for example, eliminates natural food sources of vitamin B-12, including milk products, which are good sources of calcium.

To be sure that your child's diet is balanced, pay special attention to the following nutrients:

Calcium and vitamin D Calcium helps build and maintain strong teeth and bones. Milk and dairy foods are highest in calcium, but if your child doesn't eat dairy products there are other ways to get the right amount. Dark green vegetables, such as collard greens and broccoli, are good sources of calcium when eaten in sufficient quantities. Calcium-enriched and fortified products — including juices, cereals, soy yogurt and tofu — are other options, along with many plant-based milks such as soy, nut and other milk alternatives.

Vitamin D also plays an important role in bone health. Vitamin D is added to cow's milk, some brands of plant-based

DAILY NUTRITIONAL RECOMMENDATIONS FOR VEGETARIAN KIDS

The following table provides daily nutritional recommendations to ensure your child is receiving the adequate vitamins, minerals and nutrients they need to be healthy.

Calorie Level	1,000	1,200	1,400	1,600	1,800	2,000
Food Group	Daily Amount*					
Vegetables (dark green, red and orange varieties)	1 cup	1½ cups	1½ cups	2 cups	2½ cups	2½ cups
Fruits	1 cup	1 cup	1½ cups	1½ cups	1½ cups	2 cups
Grains (half of daily grains = whole grains)	3 ounces	4 ounces	5 ounces	5½ ounces	6½ ounces	6½ ounces
Dairy	2 cups	2½ cups	2½ cups	3 cups	3 cups	3 cups
Protein (eggs, legumes, soy, nuts)	2 ounces	3 ounces	3 ounces	3 ounces	3 ounces	3 ounces
Oils	15 grams	17 grams	17 grams	22 grams	24 grams	27 grams

Source: U.S. Department of Agriculture

* Cups and ounces are intended as cup-equivalents and ounce-equivalents. For example:

1 cup-equivalent of fruit = a small apple or large banana

1 cup-equivalent of vegetables = 1 cup of raw or cooked vegetables or 2 cups of raw leafy greens

1 ounce-equivalent of grains = 1 slice of bread, 5 whole-wheat crackers or 1 small muffin

1 cup-equivalent of dairy = 1 ½ ounces of cheddar cheese or 8 ounces of fat-free yogurt

1 ounce-equivalent of protein = 1 large egg, 1 tablespoon of peanut butter or 1/4 cup of black beans

For more information on cup- and ounce-equivalents for the different food groups, visit www.choosemyplate.gov.

milk alternatives, and some cereals and margarines. Be sure to check food labels. If your child doesn't eat enough fortified foods, talk to your child's medical provider about giving your child a vitamin D supplement derived from plants.

Vitamin B-12 Vitamin B-12 is necessary to produce red blood cells and prevent anemia. This vitamin is found almost exclusively in animal products, so it can be difficult to get enough B-12 on a vegan diet.

Vitamin B-12 deficiency may go undetected in people who eat a vegan diet. This is because the vegan diet is rich in a vitamin called folate, which may mask a deficiency in vitamin B-12 until severe problems occur. For this reason, it's important for vegans to consider vitamin supplements, vitamin-enriched cereals and fortified soy products.

Protein Protein is important for growth, and it helps maintain healthy skin, bones, muscles and organs. Eggs and dairy products are good sources of protein, and your child doesn't need to eat large amounts to meet his or her protein needs.

Your child can also get sufficient protein from plant-based foods if he or she eats a variety of them throughout the day. Plant sources include nuts and nut butters, beans, legumes, lentils, seeds, and whole grains.

Omega-3 fatty acids Omega-3 fatty acids are important for a healthy heart and eye and brain development. Diets that don't include fish and eggs are generally low in active forms of omega-3 fatty acids.

Canola oil, soy oil, walnuts, ground flaxseed and soybeans are good sources of essential fatty acids. However, because the conversion of the plant-based omega-3 is less efficient than from fish, you may look to additional sources of omega-3 from fortified products, supplements or both.

Iron and zinc Iron is a crucial component of red blood cells. Dried beans and peas, lentils, enriched cereals, whole-grain products, dark leafy green vegetables, and dried fruit are good sources of iron.

Because iron isn't as easily absorbed from plant sources, the recommended intake of iron for vegetarians is almost double that recommended for nonvegetarians. To help your child's body absorb iron, offer foods rich in vitamin C, such as strawberries, citrus fruits, tomatoes, cabbage and broccoli, at the same time as you're offering iron-containing foods — for example, a bowl of cereal with strawberries.

Like iron, zinc isn't as easily absorbed from plant sources as it is from animal products. Cheese is a good option if your child eats dairy products. Plant sources of zinc include whole grains, soy products, legumes, nuts and wheat germ. Zinc is an essential component of many enzymes and plays a role in cell division and in the formation of proteins.

Iodine Iodine is a component in thyroid hormones, which help regulate metabolism, growth and function of key organs. Vegans may not get enough iodine and may be at risk of a deficiency. However, just 1/4 teaspoon of iodized salt a day provides a significant amount of iodine.

Medically restricted diets Sometimes a child's diet needs to be restricted for medical reasons, perhaps because of a food allergy or a condition such as celiac disease, in which the immune system overreacts to a common grain protein called gluten.

FOOD ALLERGIES

Food allergies are fairly common in children. Almost any food can cause an allergic reaction, but most reactions are caused by only a few foods — cow's milk, eggs, nuts (peanut and tree nuts), fish and shellfish, wheat, and soy. Children often outgrow allergies to cow's milk, eggs, soy and wheat. But allergies to nuts, fish and shellfish may be more persistent.

Most food allergies provoke an almost immediate reaction. Symptoms may include itchy skin, hives, swelling and breathing problems. Some kids experience diarrhea and vomiting shortly after the food is ingested.

In a few cases, food allergies can cause life-threatening symptoms in the form of anaphylactic shock (see page 308). Anaphylactic shock requires emergency treatment, including an immediate injection of epinephrine.

If your child shows signs of a possible food allergy, talk to your child's medical provider. He or she may refer you to an allergy specialist who can conduct special tests to identify potential allergens. Having a food allergy typically requires strict avoidance of the food that's causing the problem. If your child has a food allergy, consult with your child's medical provider about carrying an epinephrine autoinjector for emergency use.

Oral allergy syndrome Sometimes, children who have a history of seasonal allergies develop an itchy mouth or throat after eating certain raw fruits or vegetables (oral allergy syndrome). This happens when airborne pollens cross-react with proteins in the raw fruits and vegetables. For example, someone who's sensitive to ragweed may have a reaction to eating fruits such as bananas or melons.

Food intolerance Not every reaction to food is related to the immune system. Food allergies are sometimes confused with a sensitivity or intolerance to certain foods. Intolerance of a certain food usually causes digestive problems — such as a stomachache, gas or diarrhea — but isn't linked to the immune system. For example, some children don't have enough of the enzyme required to digest milk sugar (lactose), making them lactose intolerant.

When a child is diagnosed with a food allergy, food intolerance or a condition such as celiac disease, treatment involves eliminating all foods that contain the offending ingredient. This is typically very effective in relieving symptoms and preventing complications of the condition.

But sticking to a medically restricted diet can present a challenge not just to the child but to the whole family. With some patience and perseverance, though, it can be done.

At home As your child adjusts to life without certain foods, one of the ways you can offer support is by setting up a safe and positive environment at home. Here are steps you can take.

- *Educate your child.* One of the greatest gifts you can give your child is a solid understanding of his or her condition and why it's critical to follow the prescribed diet. Children who are fully educated about their condition and the reasons behind their diet are more likely to adhere to the diet. The opposite is true if they have an incorrect or incomplete understanding of the health effects of consuming the offending ingredient.

- *Transform your kitchen.* Sometimes, bigger changes are necessary. Because gluten is found in so many food products, for instance, it's important to create a kitchen that has separate spaces for foods with gluten and areas that need to remain gluten-free. This might require separate toasters, separate prep areas or closed containers for gluten ingredients. Organizing your kitchen will make it more convenient for the whole family and will make it easier for your child to quickly grab an appropriate snack.

- *Master food labels.* Know what ingredients to watch for and teach these to your child as he or she gets older and is able to read, so that he or she can avoid them.

- *Get your child involved.* Bring your child grocery shopping and let him or her help with food choices. Praise good choices and explain why others aren't safe. At home, involve your child in food preparation. Pass along the skills he or she needs to prepare appropriate snacks and meals. Ask your child to help pack school lunches.

At school and beyond A medically restricted diet may bring up difficulties for your child in social situations — such as making food choices at school or not being able to eat cake at a birthday party.

Rather than focusing on what your child can't have, help your child learn what they can have. Try to anticipate difficulties ahead of time so that you can prepare for them together. To help your child manage social situations:

- *Role play.* Give your child opportunities to practice speaking up for himself or herself. Pretend you're a friend, family member or other adult. Play out a range of situations and help your child come up with the right language to explain why he or she can't eat something.

▶ *Call ahead.* Whether it's a birthday party at a friend's house or a post-game meal at a restaurant, contact the adult in charge in advance. Explain your child's food restrictions and ask what food will be served. Be prepared to explain your child's condition in a simple way, noting that it's a medical indication, not a preference or picky eating. If needed, let the person know that your child will be bringing an alternative treat to eat. As your child gets older, encourage him or her to take on this responsibility.

▶ *Provide safe food alternatives.* If you know that a restricted item will be served at a party, be sure to provide a favorite alternative for your child. Your child is less likely to feel deprived if a similar or more desirable option is available.

▶ *Teach your child to say "No, thank you."* Certain well-meaning children or adults may not fully understand your child's need to avoid all foods containing the offending ingredient. When your child is offered unsafe food, it's important to know how to politely but firmly turn it down.

▶ *Set up a trading system for treats.* Events and holidays such as Halloween can be difficult when your child can't eat some or most of the treats. If your child brings home forbidden goodies, consider having a basket full of safe alternatives. That way, your child can trade in an unsafe treat for an equally desirable safe one.

▶ *Be prepared for post-game snacks.* Many kids' sports teams share a snack or celebratory meal after practices and games. Be sure to inform your child's coach about your child's condition. You may also choose to inform other parents if they're taking turns bringing snacks. Just to be safe, make sure your child always packs a favorite snack in case others bring something he or she can't eat. And have a plan if your child will be eating out.

▶ *Plan ahead for camp.* Call your child's camp well in advance of the start date to determine if the staff can support your child's dietary needs. If you're concerned that the camp won't consistently provide appropriate meals and snacks, provide the food yourself. One suggestion is to fill a large cooler and a suitcase with all of the food your child will need for a stay at an overnight camp. Ask if a cafeteria staff member can be the point person for preparing your child's meals with this food. Or, if your child is able and willing, find out if he or she can help prepare the meals.

▶ *Don't hold your child back.* Encourage your child to take part in all activities that other kids do. It's better for them emotionally and socially. Just follow the extra precautions outlined above.

A note of caution If your child doesn't have celiac disease or hasn't been diagnosed as gluten intolerant by a health professional, it's best not to place your child on a gluten-free diet.

That's because gluten-containing foods — such as whole-grain breads, pasta and crackers — typically contain nutrients such as fiber, vitamins and minerals that help children grow and develop.

Removing key ingredients from your child's diet without consulting a medical provider may lead to malnutrition, along with unnecessary social difficulties that come with a restrictive diet.

VITAMINS AND MINERAL SUPPLEMENTS

You've seen the cute vitamin gummies at the supermarket; your child may have even asked for them. "They're vitamins, Mom, they're good for you!" But when it comes to vitamins and mineral supplements for your child, less is usually more. Most children receive the right amount of nutrients in the foods they eat every day.

Though some multivitamins are OK for kids to consume, many have not been studied or tested for safety or to see how well they work. Large doses of vitamins and minerals can also be toxic to your child, and could interact with medications your child may be taking.

Rather than putting your child at risk, try to get all of the nutrients your child needs from a healthy diet. Supplements can't replicate all of the nutrients and benefits of whole foods, which offer complex micronutrients, dietary fiber and antioxidants.

If your child has a health condition or a specialized diet, your child's medical provider may recommend a multivitamin or supplement to provide nutrients not present in your child's diet. If your child does need a multivitamin or supplement, follow these tips:

▶ Always make sure to choose an age-appropriate multivitamin that doesn't exceed 100 percent of the daily value of vitamins and minerals.
▶ Store multivitamins out of your child's reach.
▶ Teach your child that vitamins are not like candy, even if some of them might look like it.

Vitamin D Some kids have a hard time getting the right amount of vitamin D. Healthy children need 600 international units (IUs) per day.

Responsible for helping to develop strong bones, vitamin D is mainly produced by your skin when it's exposed to the sun. Estimates are that only a few minutes of sun exposure a day are needed for adequate vitamin D production.

Depending on where you live or the time of year, your child may not be getting enough vitamin D production from sun exposure. In these circumstances, your child's medical provider may recommend a supplement.

Fortified foods — such as milk, some brands of orange juice or yogurt, and breakfast cereals — are an important source of vitamin D in the American diet. Salmon, tuna and swordfish also are good sources of vitamin D. If you're concerned that your child isn't getting enough dietary vitamin D, talk to your child's medical provider.

Iron Responsible for transporting oxygen throughout the body, iron is another essential nutrient for children. Healthy children need between 7 and 10 milligrams of iron per day, found in foods such as fortified cereals, lean meats, tofu, lentils, legumes and whole-grain foods.

Cow's milk can inhibit the body's absorption of iron. Children who drink more than 24 ounces a day are at increased risk of iron deficiency anemia. To make sure your child is getting enough iron, serve iron-rich foods and limit the amount of milk he or she drinks.

FOR LIFE

Kids' nutrition can be a stressful topic for parents. Sometimes, it may seem that it's all about numbers and rules and that if you don't get it just right, you'll be failing as a parent. But your child's nutrition is about a lot more than the exact proportions of what he or she eats at any one time. Keep your eye on the long view as you help your child develop healthy eating habits that will last a lifetime. Provide a wide variety of healthy foods. Maintain a regular schedule of family meals and snacks. Set a good example by having good eating habits yourself. Most of all, enjoy eating with your family. Bon appetit!

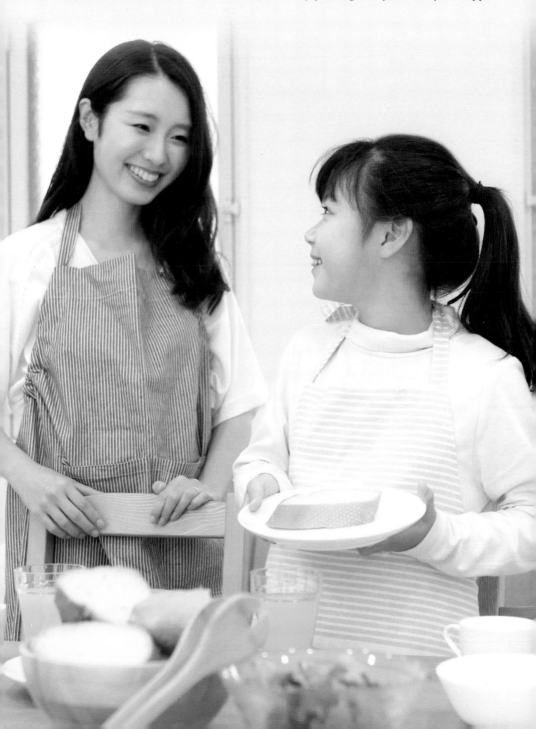

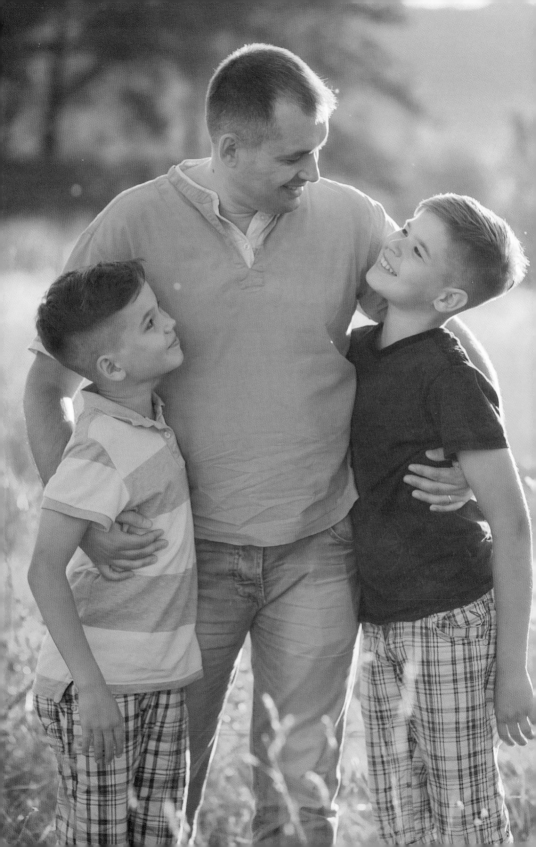

CHAPTER 14

Preventing obesity and eating disorders

For some kids, eating gets complicated by ideas about dieting, body image and what it means to be a "perfect" size. These notions may come from well-meaning parents who want their children to be at a healthy weight, but they can also originate among friends, social media, celebrity news and even doctors. American culture in particular tends to idealize people who are thin and fit, and this is prominently reflected in mass media, popular entertainment and advertising. As a child, it can be difficult to separate what's healthy from what's unhealthy. Without clear direction, kids can fall into unhealthy eating patterns that can have lasting effects.

As a parent, you can protect your child from many of these influences by keeping your attention focused squarely on your child's overall health. This means you don't worry about your child being at exactly the "right" weight or emphasize things such as calories, or "good" and "bad" foods. Doing so has the potential to lead to a child who's al-ways anxious about food and weight control, dissatisfied with his or her body size, and susceptible to unhealthy eating patterns.

Instead, you can actively promote a balanced and accepting view of food and nutrition, one that will help your child form healthy and enjoyable eating habits for life.

PREVENTION IS PARAMOUNT

There's a large and growing body of research on the need to establish measures to prevent both childhood obesity and eating disorders. Concerns about rising obesity rates have led to an increased emphasis on healthy eating and achieving a healthy weight. In general, these messages are important and meant to be helpful, but sometimes they get misinterpreted. In an effort to cut calories and "be healthier," some kids — and grown-ups — resort to unhealthy eating behaviors, such as skipping meals, cutting out entire food groups from their diet, or even doing things such as vomiting or taking laxatives (purging) to lose weight.

To make sure the correct message is getting across, medical experts have come up with some basic recommendations to help parents and children develop healthy concepts of nutrition and body size:

Avoid putting your child 'on a diet' Children shouldn't be "going on a diet" to lose weight. Most forms of dieting, because they're so restrictive, are unsustainable and may be detrimental to a child's growth and development. (Incidentally, most typical diets don't work that well for adults either.)

Research shows that dieting can be counterproductive, ultimately leading to weight gain instead of weight loss. This is because most dieting typically starts and stops. Following a week of feeling deprived, most people naturally want to indulge.

In addition, the way the body adapts to weight loss promotes metabolic shifts toward weight gain. The result is often weighing more than before, which can lead to feelings of disappointment and shame — and another round of dieting ("yo-yo dieting"). This is true for girls and boys. In addition, getting into the habit of dieting can deprive your child of necessary nutrients and increase your child's risk of developing an eating disorder.

So forget about dieting and instead encourage your child to develop good lifestyle habits that include a balanced diet and regular physical activity. By emphasizing what your child can eat and do — and shifting the focus away from food restrictions and weight loss — you'll help your child develop positive, sustainable habits.

Institute regular family meals Frequent and enjoyable family meals decrease the risk of disordered eating patterns in children, especially among girls. The more often families sit down for a meal together, the more likely kids are to consume fruits, vegetables, calcium and fiber, and the less likely they are to consume sugary drinks. In the long term, these habits contribute to achieving and maintaining a healthy weight all the way into adulthood.

Eating together as a family provides kids with healthier options than they might come up with on their own. During family meals, kids also get to interact with their parents and observe their parents make healthy choices. From the parents' perspective, eating together allows for greater awareness of a child's eating patterns and more opportunities to address issues early on.

Avoid weight talk When your child's weight is on your mind, it's hard not to talk about it. But research suggests that talking about body size, dieting or weight loss can be detrimental. Surveys of people recovering from eating disorders show that weight talk at home can have a profoundly negative impact in terms of body image and weight control.

Weight talk at home includes how you talk about not just your child's size but also about your own and everyone else's. Even supposedly positive weight talk, such as saying, "You're so skinny! I'm jealous," indicates to your child that you consider thinness a valuable trait. The implication is that if he or she gains weight, you will see it in a negative light.

When describing yourself or other people, avoid using words such as "awful" or "disgusting." Help your child understand there are many ways to stay healthy, and a healthy weight will look different in different people. Encourage your entire family to use appropriate language about others' appearances, and discourage the use of nicknames when speaking about people who are overweight or obese.

Instead of talking about losing or gaining weight, do more to help your child develop positive habits. Create a home environment that makes it easy to eat healthy foods and participate in physical activity.

Don't tease Teasing is closely related to weight talk. It may be done with affection, but its effects are generally negative. Family teasing about weight often predicts the development of overweight in boys and girls, and binge eating and extreme dieting in girls. Weight-related nicknames or descriptions of a child, such as "fatty" or "tubby," can persist into adolescence and adulthood, as can the hurt these comments cause.

There are plenty of humorous instances in daily life that provide occasions for silliness and laughter. But your child's weight — or anyone else's for that matter — isn't one of them.

Nurture a healthy body image Research shows a clear relationship between being dissatisfied with your appearance and an increased risk of eating disorders. Girls and boys who feel self-conscious about their body size, especially as puberty approaches, are less likely to engage in physical activity and more likely to adopt unhealthy eating behaviors.

When your child asks if he or she looks OK, offer a sincere compliment — let your love shine through your words. Encourage your child to look at his or her body as an amazing gift, one he or she can care for and nurture with healthy, positive choices.

Early on, look for ways to appreciate out loud your child's positive characteristics that go beyond appearances, such as your son's knack for empathy or your daughter's sense of determination.

Also, display a healthy view of your own body. Avoid self-criticism and remind yourself that the ultrafit models or celebrities showcased in magazines and on social media usually don't represent healthy, realistic bodies — quite often, these images have been electronically altered. Focus instead on following healthy habits for yourself and cultivating values beyond appearances.

KIDS AND EATING BEHAVIORS

Full-blown eating disorders typically don't develop until the teen and young adult years, but that doesn't mean troubling or dangerous symptoms don't occur earlier. Girls as young as age 5 or 6 already begin to show a desire for thinness and an awareness of dieting.

According to the American Academy of Pediatrics, eating disorders increasingly are being recognized in children under age 12. And they don't only happen in white girls, as is commonly believed. There are increased prevalence rates among boys and minorities, too, and across socio-economic levels.

Disordered eating Early on, kids may fall into unhealthy patterns called disordered eating. *Disordered eating* is the term used for a wide range of eating behaviors that don't necessarily fall under the category of an eating disorder, such as anorexia or bulimia, but can still be harmful. Signs of disordered eating may include:

◗ Separating foods into "good" and "bad" categories

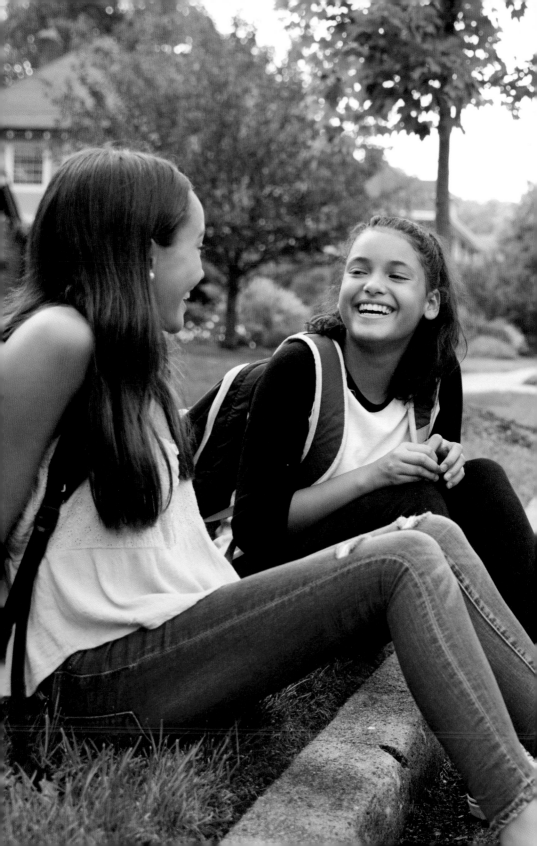

ENCOURAGING A HEALTHY BODY IMAGE

Given the powerful influences of peers and the media, you might notice your child beginning to form a negative or unhealthy view of himself or herself.

As a parent, it's important to get in front of these negative messages early. To help your child develop a healthy body image:

Decode media messages Children today are exposed to plenty of television and digital media, meaning that your child is likely getting input on how to feel about his or her body from TV, movies, music, and his or her favorite streaming video personality.

Get to know what your child is reading and watching. Use these inputs as opportunities for discussion about how society interprets attractiveness. Talk about what makes people attractive in real life, such as empathy or a sunny outlook.

Limit social media access Kids are using technology at a younger age, and this often includes social networking sites. Your child may share pictures or post videos to receive feedback from peers, and you may not always know what your child's peers are saying or what kinds of messages your child is receiving.

Create an open and honest relationship so you know about your child's online behaviors. For young children, you might consider waiting a few years before allowing personal social media accounts. Or consider making social media accounts transparent, where your child can access an account only if a password is shared with you.

Promote body diversity Your child might compare himself or herself to others and may believe a certain body type is superior. Talk with your child to explain that people have different bodies, and that there isn't one type that's better than another. You might point out that every culture over time has created different interpretations of what's considered aesthetically pleasing.

Establish positive role models Exposure to media figures may be inevitable, but you can help influence which people your child is looking up to. Teach him or her about men and women who are notable for their achievements rather than their appearances. When you talk about celebrities or people in the news, avoid bashing them for their body size — whether large or small — or their appearance in general.

Cheer the qualities you value Give your child praise and affirmation for qualities that relate to inner beauty, such as generosity, kindness and courage. Praise these qualities in other people, too. Doing this will help your child understand what you value most.

Encourage healthy friendships In childhood and into adolescence, fewer things are more important to your child than his or her friends. But the influence of your child's friends can have either a positive or a negative effect, so try to get to know your child's friends, their parents and the activities your child is enjoying when spending time with friends.

- Persistent worrying about being fat or talking about losing weight
- Sudden changes to eating habits, such as skipping meals or an excessive focus on eating "healthy"
- Sudden desire to follow an overly restrictive but not medically necessary diet, such as a low-carb or gluten-free diet
- Withdrawing from friends and favorite activities
- Rigid preoccupation with eating and exercise regimens, such as skipping a pizza party to exercise or avoiding "bad" foods
- Chronic dieting

Often, kids with disordered eating patterns don't understand the full impact their choices have on their health.

Consequences of disordered eating may include an increased risk of obesity and eating disorders, bone loss, digestive problems, electrolyte and fluid imbalances, heart and blood pressure irregularities, anxiety, depression, and isolation.

Kids with disordered eating patterns may be under considerable physical, emotional and mental stress.

If your child starts to exhibit these behaviors, gently but firmly guide him or her back toward the principles of flexible eating, where foods themselves aren't good or bad but moderation is key (see Chapter 13).

Eating disorders Some kids with disordered eating habits go on to develop eating disorders. Eating disorders are serious, complex illnesses that can deprive the body of needed nutrition.

Eating disorders can harm the heart, digestive system, bones, teeth and mouth, stunt growth and development, and lead to other diseases. They can be life-threatening.

There are several types of eating disorders. Some of the most common are anorexia, bulimia and binge-eating disorder. These disorders are typically associated with deep-seated feelings of guilt and shame in relation to food and a distorted body image. Extreme measures — such as fasting, excessive exercising, vomiting or using laxatives after eating — may be taken to compensate for calorie consumption.

Avoidant/restrictive food intake disorder (ARFID) is a type of eating disorder that's not as well-known but can also have damaging effects. It's more likely to occur in younger children and involves extreme pickiness in eating — to the point of significant weight loss or failure to gain weight in childhood. Food is avoided because of lack of interest; concern about its color, texture, smell or taste; or fear of hazards such as choking. Fear of gaining weight usually isn't a factor.

A full recovery from an eating disorder is possible, especially if the condition is recognized and treatment begins early. Treatment for eating disorders associated with drastic reductions in caloric intake consists of getting your child's weight back to the level at which his or her body systems work well. This typically involves planning and following a meal and snack schedule that provides your child an appropriate amount of calories.

If your child shows signs of ARFID and has lost weight, seek help from your child's medical provider or an eating disorder therapist. Experts advise encouraging the child to eat bigger portions of favorite foods. Once body weight has increased to an appropriate level, parents can focus on introducing a wider variety of foods. Remember to keep mealtime positive. Offer consistently healthy options, but avoid battling over food choices.

Psychotherapy, which may involve the whole family, is another important part of treatment, especially for a condition such as binge-eating disorder. Your child's care team may include doctors, dietitians, psychologists and therapists trained in managing eating disorders. Parents must be closely involved in treating eating disorders in children, as it isn't appropriate for kids, or even teenagers, to make their own health decisions when the potential consequences are so serious.

Preventing eating disorders is easier than treating them. If you can help your child develop a balanced relationship with food and a healthy body image at a young age, many of these problems can be prevented.

SHOW THE WAY

Image is a big deal in society. As a parent, it's important to help your child form a healthy view of his or her body. You can do this by focusing as a family on healthy eating and physical activity, avoiding dieting, not teasing or talking about body size, and fostering a balanced view of the physical human shape. Perhaps even more important than what you say to your child is your ability to sincerely model these precepts in your own life. Your child is worth it, and so are you.

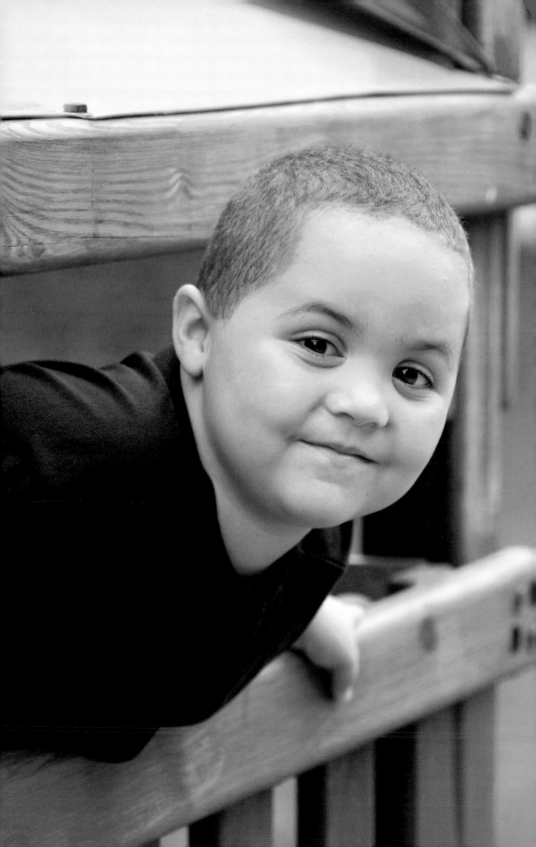

CHAPTER 15

Childhood obesity

What causes a child to become overweight? Is it just a matter of eating too much and not exercising enough? There are many factors that put a child at risk of obesity, including genetics and individual biological make-up and metabolism. Diet and inactivity are important factors in the equation, but scientists also are beginning to discover that excess weight is much more complicated than simply calories consumed versus calories burned. Some people, including children, just seem to gain weight more easily than others.

It's no secret that carrying excess weight can lead to problems, even for kids. Extra pounds early in life often put children on the path to health problems that were once considered adult problems — diabetes, high blood pressure, high cholesterol, bone and joint issues, sleep issues, and liver disease.

Add to these health concerns a cultural bias against being overweight and the social and emotional implications this brings, and a lot of alarm bells may go off in a parent's head when it comes to a son's or daughter's weight.

So what can be done? Reality is, you can't do much about your child's DNA or his or her internal metabolic programming. What's more, an ideal weight for a child is a moving target as he or she grows.

For kids who are overweight or obese, the immediate goal generally isn't to lose weight. Instead, the goal is to develop healthy habits — eating more nutritious foods and spending more time being physically active. Establishing these habits now will help your child carry them over into adolescence and adulthood.

As a family, you can make lifestyle choices that promote healthier habits. The idea is that these habits will gradually become ingrained and automatic — your child reaches for an apple instead of a cookie without even thinking about it. The attention is focused on making positive changes and not solely on the numbers — how much he or she weighs.

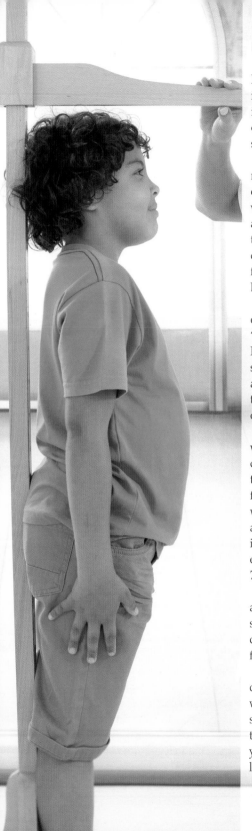

DETERMINING OBESITY

How do you know if your child's weight is a problem? A commonly used screening tool for assessing overweight and obesity in children and adults is a measurement called body mass index (BMI).

BMI measures your child's weight in relation to his or her height and is typically performed during annual checkups with your child's medical provider. There are also various online tools and calculators that you can use to calculate your child's BMI on your own, such as the one from the National Heart, Lung, and Blood Institute.

In children and young adults, BMI is expressed in percentiles (also called "BMI-for-age") based on age and sex. Percentiles allow for more flexibility than standard BMI measurements, taking into account growth over time and the fact that children will carry varying amounts of body fat as they develop.

A healthy weight generally falls within the 5th percentile to 84th percentile range. A child who falls between the 85th percentile and 95th percentile for age and sex may be considered overweight, depending on other factors such as muscle mass and body frame. Obesity is generally defined as a BMI at or greater than the 95th percentile (see pages 75, 77 and 78).

Keep in mind that not all children who are overweight according to BMI measures are considered unhealthy. Some children have larger than average body frames or more muscle mass.

Before you become stressed or concerned about your child's weight, talk with your child's medical provider. He or she can review your child's growth patterns since birth and talk with you about your child's eating habits and your child's level of activity.

THE CHILDHOOD OBESITY EPIDEMIC

Childhood obesity is often referred to as a modern epidemic and an important public health problem. About a third of children and adolescents in the U.S. are currently considered overweight or obese, as defined by BMI measurements. Indeed, children are heavier today than they were a few decades ago. National health data collected between 1976 and 2014 indicate that the prevalence of obesity in school-age children grew from approximately 6.5 percent to 20 percent in that time frame.

There are signs that the trend may be reversing. In preschoolers, obesity rates peaked at approximately 14 percent in 2004 and then fell to just over 9 percent by 2014. Even among school-age children, obesity rates leveled out around 2008 and remained stable through 2014. The prevalence of severe obesity in children and adolescents, however, continues to increase. And the more severe the obesity, the more likely it is to persist into adulthood.

The reasons for this trend are the subject of a lot of research. Often-cited contributors to childhood obesity include increased calorie intake — through greater availability of food, larger portions, and an abundance of high-calorie snacks and beverages — and a less active lifestyle, due at least in part to greater opportunities for sedentary electronic entertainment.

Genetics and individual metabolism also play a large role but are less understood and not as easily changed as lifestyle factors. In addition, the rapid rise in obesity suggests that genetics doesn't play the only role. It's likely that there's a complex interplay between genetic and environmental influences.

Family and lifestyle are important factors, too. Having one parent with obesity increases the risk of a child with obesity two or three times; if both parents have obesity, the risk increases 15-fold.

Because of the potential complications of childhood obesity, there's a sense of urgency in the medical community to fix the problem. But while it's enlightening to look at the big picture, it's also important to remember that each child is unique in his or her own genetic makeup and environment. That's why the focus of treatment is not on short-term weight loss but on helping children — and their families — develop long-term healthy habits that will serve them for life.

In a few cases there may be an underlying medical condition that's contributing to your child's weight. In addition, some medications — such as steroids, antipsychotics or anti-epileptics — can contribute to weight gain. Your child's medical provider may also check for illnesses that may coincide with overweight or obesity, such as sleep apnea or depression. The provider may order lab tests to check your child's level of cholesterol, glucose and liver enzymes.

If an underlying problem is contributing to your child's weight gain, your child's medical provider can help you find ways to manage your child's weight.

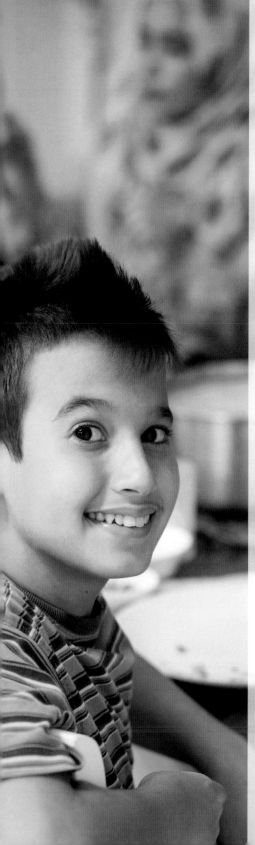

EATING BETTER TOGETHER

The consensus among medical experts is that the best way to address childhood obesity is through a family approach that involves all family members. It can be uncomfortable or embarrassing for a child to be singled out, prohibited from eating certain foods or given a different meal than the rest of the family.

Rather than focusing on just your child — what your child eats and how many calories he or she consumes each day, or how many pounds he or she loses each week — make healthy habits a family affair.

Prepare healthy foods the whole family will enjoy. Follow closely the healthy eating principles outlined in Chapter 13. In addition, plan daily events in which your child is active. Try to make those activities things he or she likes to do.

There's no doubt that all of this is often easier said than done. But here are some practical steps your family can take to adopt a healthier lifestyle while supporting your child in growing into a healthy weight.

Eat at home more often If you notice that your family is eating out a lot or that meals tend to be eaten on the run, start by planning more home-prepared meals.

Childhood obesity is more common in families that eat out more frequently, largely due to excess fat and sugar in restaurant food and the consumption of soft drinks. Also, over the last several decades portion sizes at restaurants have increased for both children and adults. This can influence a child's perception of food servings, which can lead to overeating.

Meals prepared at home are generally healthier, portions are likely to be smaller, and your child is more likely to have milk or water with the meal than a soft drink.

DIETING ISN'T FOR KIDS

Sometimes parents involve kids in popular diets or eating plans that they think will be healthy. Or they think a special diet might help a child who is overweight or struggling with obesity. While achieving a healthy weight is possible for your child, it's important to avoid diets that are meant for adults. These include fad diets or diets that cut out particular food groups, such as a low-carb, paleo or Atkins diet.

For kids in particular, dieting can be dangerous because it can deprive them of nutrients needed for growth and development. Throughout childhood, it's critical that your child receives the appropriate balance of vitamins, minerals and nutrients in the foods he or she consumes. Although restrictive diets may be beneficial for some adults, they're not appropriate for children.

Putting your child on a diet — restricting certain foods or food groups or drastically reducing daily calorie intake — isn't a sustainable solution and can ultimately result in more harm than good. Going "on" a diet inherently requires coming "off" of the diet at some point, which often leads to weight gain. Restrictive eating regimens can fuel a harmful cycle of feeling deprived, craving restricted foods, overeating and weight gain that prompts another round of dieting. Over time, this can lead to unhealthy eating behaviors and eating disorders such as anorexia, bulimia and binge eating (see Chapter 14).

If your child is overweight and you're trying to help him or her grow into a healthy weight, make it about developing healthy habits — not dieting or appearance.

Stock up on healthy foods Take a quick inventory of the foods your family is consuming, from the pantry to the refrigerator. What foods do you eat most often and when? How healthy are these foods? Once you know what you've got, think about ways to make meals and especially snacks healthier and how to add more variety to your family's diet.

Limit the amount of processed foods and high-calorie snacks — such as chips, candy bars and cookies — you keep on hand. It's not that you can't ever have these but place your focus primarily on foods that are rich in nutrients but relatively low in calories. These foods are nutrient dense and include fruits and vegetables, whole grains, lean proteins, and low-fat dairy. You can eat more of these foods — and feel more satisfied — without consuming as many calories.

Cut out sweet drinks Soda and sweetened juices are packed with extra sugar and offer little in terms of nutrients. Essentially, they are "empty calories." Sometimes, it's easiest not to have such beverages around the house. Instead, opt for low-fat or fat-free milk and water throughout the day. Even sports drinks, which are increasingly popular, often contain a lot of sugar and calories. Water is the recommended source of hydration for children and adolescents.

Encourage mindful eating Children struggling with obesity may eat more quickly and take fewer bites than their

THE 5-2-1-0 METHOD

There's so much information out there on nutrition and healthy living that it can get a little overwhelming sometimes to make sense of it. Here's a simple method called the 5-2-1-0, which captures almost everything you need to know about healthy eating and exercise, and is easy to share with kids:

5 servings of fruits and vegetables a day Prepare fresh or frozen fruits and vegetables your child can enjoy for snacks or during meals. Get your child's buy-in on choices and ask for help with preparation. Getting your child involved increases the odds that he or she will adopt this habit.

2 hours or less of screen time a day Technology is everywhere, but that doesn't mean you have to let your child use his or her devices around the clock. Limit screen time to two hours or less per day — one hour or less for children between ages 3 and 5. Swap digital pastimes for other activities such as playing outside or helping preparing meals.

1 hour or more of vigorous physical activity a day Children need to burn off energy to balance the nutrients and calories they consume. Find ways to encourage your child to get up and move. Your child needs to see and understand that there's fun to be had off of the couch.

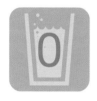

0 sugary drinks a day Keep it simple — stick to low-fat or fat-free milk and water for drinks. If you're going to offer juice, serve only those made of 100% fruit juice and in small portions.

peers. One way to deal with this is to teach mindfulness at the dinner table. First, turn off all distractions such as the television, tablets and cellphones during dinner so that everyone can focus on eating and enjoying each other's company. Next, encourage your family to eat more slowly, enjoying each bite. Teach your child to focus on the smell and texture of the food — to savor it. As your child learns to slow down, he or she will learn to enjoy the meal and to pay attention to hunger and fullness cues.

Watch your own eating behavior
Think about how you eat and the way

you talk about food. If you eat when you're stressed, your child may, too. If you snack throughout the day, your child will do the same.

If you or your partner are struggling with weight issues, developing your own healthy habits will set a positive example for your child. As your child notices your commitment to a healthy diet, he or she will begin to catch on, too.

GETTING EVERYONE MOVING

A big part of being healthy is staying physically active. Physical activity burns energy, strengthens bones and muscles, and helps children sleep well at night and stay alert during the day. Some of the strongest evidence for decreasing childhood obesity lies in increasing physical activity.

National guidelines recommend that all children get approximately one hour of moderate to vigorous physical activity every day (see Chapter 12). The more, the better! Short spurts of movement throughout the day count, too, even if it's only 10 to 15 minutes at a time. To encourage your child to be physically active:

Limit screen time Because of our growing appetite for technology, kids often get stuck in a "screen rut"— watching TV, playing video games or using their tablets. When they're doing this, they're not active. In fact, some research suggests that television viewing is the factor most closely associated with childhood obesity.

You can help your child out by making it harder to sit around and easier to run around. Remove television and other screens from your child's bedroom. Keep electronic devices in a central location where you can monitor their use. Set and enforce limits on screen time — one hour or less for children ages 3 to 5, and two hours or less for children over 5.

Encourage outside time Create regular opportunities for your child to play in the backyard or bike around the neighborhood. Arrange play dates at a playground or city park. Teach your child activities such as jumping rope, hopscotch or a favorite game from when you were a child.

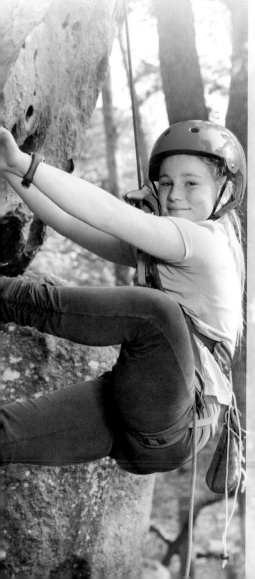

Make it fun It's important to find activities your child likes. For instance, if your child enjoys water, regularly visit a swimming pool or water park. If your child likes to climb, head for the nearest neighborhood jungle gym or climbing wall. If your child likes to read, walk or bike to the neighborhood library to find a new book.

Show more than tell As with eating habits, your child looks to see how you approach physical activity and exercise. While almost every parent has moments where they just want to sit down for a bit, try to find time to be active with your child.

If you view physical activity or exercise as a chore, your child will most likely do the same. But if you approach it as a good thing that will boost your spirits, your child will see similar benefits.

Play catch together, ride bikes, go on a hike or do whatever it is that you both enjoy. Never feel that it's not worth it. When it comes to physical activity, doing something is always better than doing nothing!

MANAGING RESISTANCE

It can sometimes feel like an uphill battle getting your child and family to make healthier lifestyle changes. It's normal to face resistance. Remember that change takes time. Achieving big goals almost never happens overnight.

Instead of letting tensions rise or letting go of your parental authority altogether, try these tips:

Don't police Because you want your child to be at a healthy weight, it can be easy to hover. You might be monitoring what's happening at snack time or checking to see if your child is out playing. While concern about his or her progress is understandable, try not to police your child's every move. Be encouraging but avoid judging or critiquing.

Monitoring your child too closely can make him or her feel singled out, watched or criticized. It can also backfire, leading to unhealthy eating behaviors, such as sneaking food, bingeing or simply giving up on trying to change.

Provide options Instead of asking your child if he or she wants to exercise, provide options, such going on a walk together, playing tag or having an impromptu dance party.

For older children, team sports are a great way to incorporate regular physical activity. Consider giving older children the option of choosing one sport a season. If your child isn't into competitive sports, brainstorm other options — maybe it's joining a dance group or swimming at the community rec center. Even joining a local theater group in which the kids are moving about on stage is better than sitting at home on the couch.

Providing options will help your child practice decision-making skills while feeling a greater sense of control over his or her circumstances. Plus, when given options, your child is more likely to pick something he or she enjoys — which is important if lifestyle changes are going to stick.

Create measurable goals Vague statements such as "I'm going to eat better" or "I'm going to exercise more" are generally ineffective, for children and grownups. Rather than make generalizations, set concrete goals to strive for and achieve.

For example, place a chart with empty check boxes on the fridge that your child marks off each time he or she plays outside. Offer a reward — such as going to see a movie — for biking for 20 minutes four times a week or running the required number of laps in gym class.

Children at this age like to spend extra time with their parents, so take advantage of it. Set goals in which you get to do something fun with your child.

Praise progress Your child will experience challenges. Rather than scolding or criticizing setbacks, praise his or her progress, no matter how small. Support your child's efforts in a way that promotes his or her individual expression and bolsters his or her self-confidence. If your child feels ownership and pride in his or her achievements, it will motivate him or her to continue making healthy choices.

DON'T IGNORE THE PROBLEM

If your child is very overweight and your efforts at home don't seem to be helping, don't give up. You may just need some backup help. Talk to your child's medical provider about it. He or she may recommend enrolling your son or daughter in a pediatric weight management program. These types of programs can often be found at children's hospitals or clinics and they usually involve working with a variety of professionals experienced in treating childhood obesity.

Weight management programs typically include structured dietary and physical activity components that aim to help you and your child learn healthy habits that you can maintain for a lifetime. They can also help your child — and your whole family — develop the necessary confidence to make successful changes.

PART 4

Emotions
and behaviors

CHAPTER 16

Encouraging positive behavior

When you hear the term *discipline*, maybe you think of correcting bad behavior. Or maybe you equate discipline with punishment, as many parents do. But it's actually a much broader concept.

Childhood development experts typically view the practice of discipline as a means of promoting positive behavior and decision-making skills. The focus is on determining how to encourage desired behaviors while minimizing unacceptable behaviors.

When you start thinking this way, use of discipline as a means of correction becomes only a small part of helping a child reach emotional and behavioral maturity.

Encouraging consistently positive behavior in a child involves a lot of patience and hard work — so much for quick fixes! The fact is that positive behavior is developed through hundreds of small exchanges with your child. These daily interactions teach him or her how to exert emotional self-control, make good choices and behave appropriately, even when you're not around.

Although time-intensive, the basic concepts underlying behavioral guidance are relatively simple. Once you grasp them, you'll realize the many possibilities that open up for you to help your child thrive. This stage in your child's life — when you set rules, give directions and provide consistent consequences — will teach your child how to behave for years to come.

WHY DO CHILDREN BEHAVE THE WAY THEY DO?

Most parents want their children to be polite, respect others, show generosity of spirit and be of strong moral character. When a child doesn't behave in this way, it can be disconcerting.

But behavior doesn't occur in a vacuum, and children aren't born knowing the rules. Rather, it's their job to test the limits around them and engage in some trial and error. In this way, they learn as they go and gradually become more independent. It's up to the grown-ups to set up the "bumper lanes" that shape and guide children's behavior.

To know how to set appropriate limits for your child, it helps to understand how behavior works in the first place. In academic terms, this is called functional behavioral analysis. It's often described as the ABCs of behavior:

- *A is for antecedent.* This is what comes before the behavior. It may include your child's past learning patterns, a triggering event or a set of circumstances that precedes the behavior. It's easy to perceive behavior as occurring in isolation or out of the blue. But in most cases, on closer examination, an antecedent can be detected.
- *B is for behavior.* The behavior that flows from the antecedents may be good or bad. The antecedents often have a big influence on the type of behavior that results.
- *C is for consequence.* Generally, behaviors evoke responses, especially from parents or caregivers. These responses may be negative or positive. It's important to note that attention of either kind has the power to reinforce the behavior.

Understanding these three aspects of behavior can make it easier to promote positive behavior in your child. To help your child behave well, you'll want to set the stage for him or her to be successful, clearly spell out your expectations for acceptable behavior, and deliver appropriate and consistent consequences.

You'll probably find yourself taking these steps sometimes simultaneously, sometimes sequentially. But most importantly, you'll want to shift the balance of your energy and attention toward a proactive, positive approach and away from a negative, reactive one.

SETTING UP FOR SUCCESS

Behavior develops over time. In fact, raising a well-behaved child involves a lot of groundwork that rarely produces immediate rewards. But the rewards that do eventually come — in the form of well-grounded relationships and enjoyable time spent with each other and with others — are meaningful and long lasting.

To lay the groundwork for positive behavior, take these steps.

Spend time together Positive behavior is rooted in a warm, secure relationship between parent and child. Parents listen to their children, talk with them and play with them. They observe their children so that they know them well — what motivates them, what frustrates them. Parents are involved and attentive — even in routine, everyday interactions. By being present, parents naturally have the opportunity to sow the seeds of good behavior.

In addition, all children need to spend one-on-one time with their parents. But as every parent knows, other tasks always seem to pop up that limit the time you have to interact with your child. Without realizing it, a child may try to get parental attention by misbehaving or acting out. To the child, negative attention seems better than no attention or not enough attention.

It's important that you work to have a good relationship with your child because it shows that you care and that you're invested in them. And it will help your child improve his or her behavior. To maximize your time with your child:

Guard your calendar Your time is a valuable commodity, and it's best to treat it as such. Modern parents often feel a constant pull to overextend themselves in many different directions, whether it be work, school, volunteering or even leisure activities. Be selective about how you spend precious hours and even minutes. Make your child a regular priority. Use a calendar or other tool to block out time together and don't be shy about protecting that time.

Make it fun When you're spending time with your child, make it enjoyable. Put away distractions. Phone calls, emails, texts and social media can wait. Take time to notice and think about how amazing your child is. Let your child lead the activity and try to avoid giving commands, corrections or directions. Instead, look for ways to commend your child for a bright idea, an empathetic response or a job well-done.

There will be plenty of times where interaction with your child may be less than pleasant. To take the edge off those difficult times, it's important to build up the good times and keep your relationship's goodwill in balance. In general, you want the bulk of your interactions to be positive.

Improvise Most families have a pretty hectic schedule, and finding free time to do fun stuff isn't always possible. But that doesn't mean you can't spend one-on-one time with your child.

Think of all the time you spend together in the car, for example, going to and from school, sports practice, or dental or doctor appointments. Maybe you're just running errands together. Use that time to tell each other funny stories about your day. Take turns being the DJ and sharing or singing your favorite tunes. Or just be quiet together. A kid under stress may find it easier to open up and talk about what's bothering him or her if no one else is around.

Maintain stability at home Tied in with a secure relationship between parent and child is a stable home environment. Regular, predictable routines can help your family stay organized and provide reassurance to your child. It can also help minimize common triggers of poor behavior such as tiredness, hunger and stress.

Some children may need more structure than others, but everyone benefits from some sort of family schedule. Ideally, your family routines should be set up to bring order to your family life but not so inflexible that they end up feeling overly constrictive or controlling.

Daily schedules Try to maintain a predictable schedule for key times of day, such as wake-up times, mealtimes and bedtimes.

---

5 STEPS TO ENCOURAGE GOOD BEHAVIOR IN YOUR CHILD

1. Spend special time together with no distractions.
2. Look for opportunities to praise your child for good behavior.
3. Look for opportunities to give rewards.
4. Give specific, positively worded directions.
5. Follow through with consequences.

HOW TO GIVE GOOD DIRECTIONS

Kids need to know what you expect from them. When you explain your expectations in a way your child understands, and the expectations fit your child's age and development, you make it easier for your child to cooperate. Here's how to give good directions.

Have good body language Be physically close so that you can have a normal conversation (don't shout from another room). Bend down or get on your knees, if needed, so your face is level with your child's face. Have good eye contact. Have a pleasant look on your face and a relaxed body.

Get your child's attention Make sure your child is listening. Turn off the phones, TV and any mobile devices. Use your child's name or a term of affection, and include a gentle physical prompt such as a hand on the shoulder to orient them to you.

Give simple, positive directions Be polite and speak loudly enough to be heard. If you're frustrated, don't show it. Use positive words to tell your child exactly what to do. Typically, the younger the child is, the shorter the directions should be. For example, say, "Kayla, please be gentle with your baby sister" instead of, "Stop being so rough!" which is vague and doesn't really tell the child what to do. If needed, have the child repeat the instructions to avoid confusion. When Kayla is following the rules, say, "Thank you. You're being so careful with your sister. She loves that!"

Wait to mention consequences Focus on the positive aspects of the request and the behavior you want. Don't mention consequences the first time you give directions. Say, for example, "Rocco, please clean your room."

If you must repeat your instructions, include information on consequences. Be specific. For example, say, "Rocco, if you want to go outside, first you need to clean your room." Avoid saying, "Rocco, you can't play outside unless you clean your room."

Don't argue or explain If you repeat the direction over and over or debate with your child about why he or she should listen, your child will be less likely to cooperate. If you must explain a direction, offer that information first. You want your direction to be the last thing he or she hears before taking action.

If you're giving a direction that is reasonable and you expect it to be followed, don't give your child a chance to say no. It may help to offer a choice. For example, don't say, "Lilly, would you like to get into your car seat?" If your child says no or you have to repeat the directions, both you and your child likely will be frustrated. Instead say, "Lilly, would you like to climb into your car seat by yourself, or shall I help you?"

Show your child how to do the task
Kids learn a lot every day. Sometimes they remember what they learned last week, and sometimes they don't. When you give directions for a chore, such as loading a dishwasher, you may need to show your child how to do it.

Give an immediate reaction Only give directions when you're available to watch how your child reacts. If the task is done correctly, smile and give praise right away. For example, smile and say, "Thank you for waiting." Or, "I really like how you cleaned your room so quickly, Kendis." If your child doesn't cooperate, give a timeout or a different consequence.

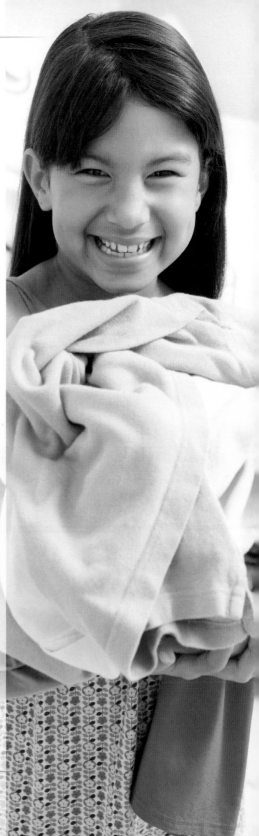

Weekly events If your child's responsible for certain chores, create a weekly schedule so that it's clear when different chores need to be done. For example, your child may be expected to help take out the trash on Tuesday nights and clean his or her room each Saturday.

Family traditions Not all routines have to be practical. Incorporate enjoyable activities into family life. Take a nightly walk around the block, have a weekly movie night, or visit the playground every weekend. Other family routines might be rituals that happen once a year, such as apple picking in the fall or going to a lake in the summer.

Change-ups If an established routine needs to change, try to give your child some advanced warning so there's time to adjust.

Be mindful of your attention Kids respond to parental attention, whether good or bad. Research shows that emphasizing a particular behavior will have the effect of reinforcing that behavior. Often, providing extra attention when your child misbehaves has the unintended effect of promoting that behavior.

On the flip side, kids can also behave well, especially when they know what's expected and they have the skills needed to meet those expectations. All too frequently, though, when behavior improves, parents tend to shift their attention elsewhere. But building a trend of positive behavior requires positive reinforcement.

When you see your child behaving admirably, be purposeful in noticing it and make sure your child knows that you noticed. Try to always be on the lookout for behavior that merits praise. Know what you want to see in your child and promote that.

FAMILY RULES

The expectations you have for your child's behavior must be clearly expressed to your child to avoid confusion and conflict. Family rules allow you to set limits and expectations in a way that enables your child to successfully understand and meet them.

Rules tell your child what's acceptable and what isn't. They help teach your child the values you want to pass on and provide guidelines for you as a parent. Rules that are age-appropriate, consistently enforced, and balanced with warmth and affection help your child navigate life within your family and beyond the walls of your home. Rules vary from family to family, but here are some basic concepts to think about.

Start small If your child's a preschooler, start with two to four key rules. Having a few rules instead of a long list will make it easier for your child to grasp what's expected and give you a better chance to be consistent.

These rules can reflect your family's main priorities, such as showing respect for one another or being safe. Common family rules, for example, are no hitting or name-calling and no jumping on furniture. As your child grows older and masters the rules you've set, add additional, age-appropriate rules to your family's list.

Communicate clearly Your child will be more likely to follow the rules you've established if you've clearly identified and explained them. Break down rules into observable, measurable steps. For example, bedtime rules might consist of specific measures such as brushing teeth, putting on pajamas and getting into bed on time. This allows you to steer your child toward specific activities if he or she acts up at bedtime, rather than reacting to your child's resistance with an emotional outburst of your own. It lets you tell your child what to do, rather than focus on what to stop doing, and helps your child organize a response.

Be prepared to repeat the rules regularly to help your child remember and act on them. Some families find it helpful to post the rules in a place that everyone can see. You could even ask your child to help decorate a rules poster or chart by drawing a picture of each rule.

Explain rewards and consequences
Along with explaining your family rules, make sure your child understands the potential outcomes for following or breaking the rules. Following the rules might earn your child privileges, while breaking them may disallow those privileges.

For example, doing chores in a timely and cheerful way may be rewarded with a half-hour of screen time, whereas not following through with chores may lead to loss of screen time. Establishing these guidelines will help motivate your child to increase positive behavior and help you know how to respond when a rule is broken. You may want to include rewards and consequences on your rules poster or chart.

Follow the rules Family rules work best when they outline expectations for all members of your family. If you've set rules about shouting or screen time limits, be a good role model by following those rules yourself. Children learn a lot from watching how their parents act or react to circumstances.

Enforce the rules consistently All children test limits by breaking a rule now and then. Sometimes, however, they may genuinely forget or not fully understand what's expected of them. In that case, a clear restatement of the rule may be necessary.

Either way, it's important to respond to a broken rule the same way each time. Of course, no parent is perfectly consistent all the time, but the more consistent you can be in your follow-through, the more effective you'll be and the more quickly your child will learn new behaviors.

FOCUSING ON THE POSITIVE

Rewarding positive behavior typically is a more effective teaching tool than punishing negative behavior. To improve your child's behavior, you should feel as if most of your time is spent rewarding positive behavior. Otherwise, you're left chasing negative behaviors.

Recommended rewards for positive behavior generally fall into two categories: social and family rewards, and structured-system rewards. Both work well to reinforce good behaviors. In general, you want about a 4-1 ratio of positive interactions to negative ones.

Social and family rewards Typically, these rewards are a parent's time and attention. Examples include:

Hugs and kisses Expressing physical and emotional warmth through hugs, kisses and pats on the back are great ways to tell your child how happy you are with his or her behavior. The message is easy for children to understand quickly. Young children, especially, respond well to affectionate gestures. Older children might shy away from overt displays of affection but still appreciate a matter-of-fact smile, fist bump or high-five.

Praise Words of appreciation and encouragement are a very useful reward. And they contribute to the development of your child's confidence and self-esteem. Keep an eye out for positive behavior or patterns of behavior change that you can praise. Any genuine praise is appreciated and shows your child that you notice his or her positive behavior.

For example, Dad might say to his son, "CJ, thank you for setting the table while I was making dinner. It made it so much easier to get everyone to the table for our meal." Those two simple sentences praised three of CJ's efforts: noticing a need, making a decision to meet the need and taking action. In addition, when Dad explained how CJ's setting the table helped, it taught CJ about the value of helping others.

Extra time together Many children respond positively to special time with parents as a reward for good behavior. If you catch your child doing something good, offer to spend some time together, maybe an outing to the park or to lunch. This time should be in addition to the usual time you spend with your child. Don't forget to make arrangements for any other children in the family to be occupied during this time.

Structured-system rewards These systems use points, stickers or tokens to reward good behavior. When your child has earned enough points or tokens, he or she can exchange them for activities, privileges, treats or prizes. For preschoolers and children in early elementary school, a sticker chart can be a very effective tool (see next page). Children between ages 4 and 8 often respond to the poker chip system. Older children may respond better to a point system (see page 246).

STICKER CHART

To use a sticker chart:
- ▶ Work with your child to identify two or three behaviors to reward.
- ▶ Make a chart together using words or pictures to explain what's expected.
- ▶ Add a star for each behavior done correctly and offer praise.
- ▶ Point out progress in a positive way at the end of the day. Say, for example, "Julia, look at all you did today — making your bed, getting dressed by yourself and cleaning off the dinner table. You earned three stars today. I want to give you a big hug for that."
- ▶ Set a goal, such as 10 stickers, and work with your child to decide on a reward he or she can receive after meeting that goal.
- ▶ Make sure you have a mix of short- and long-term goals so that it's possible to earn privileges daily while building toward a larger prize.

Maximize your system To get the most out of your reward system:

Decide on rewards together Talk with your child to decide what privileges, rewards or activities he or she enjoys. Helping to make this decision will increase your child's motivation to cooperate. Be prepared to repeat this conversation as your child ages and his or her interests change.

Distribute rewards wisely Give praise and smaller rewards more often instead of a larger reward less often. Children lose motivation when a large reward takes a long time to be earned.

Reward and praise right away Ideally, you want to give a reward as quickly as possible after the positive behavior. Doing this helps the child's brain make a stronger connection between the behavior and the reward. If you need to delay the reward slightly, when you give it, remind your child about the behavior that earned the reward.

Make the reward appropriate and meaningful There are many options for rewards. Choose the best one for each child and be prepared to change it up at times so that it remains meaningful. You might consider restricting access to certain toys or activities for a while to increase your child's motivation for earning them. For example, if you use a favorite TV show as a reward, refrain from allowing your child to watch TV at will. Be specific about why your child is getting the reward, to reinforce the link between the good behavior and the reward.

ALLOWING ROOM FOR CONSEQUENCES

Over time, the positive action of rewarding good behavior typically leads to fewer instances of misbehavior. Still, misbehavior does occur. This is a natural reaction as kids test their limits. But children also need consequences when they misbehave.

POKER CHIP OR POINT SYSTEM

Both systems work the same. Simply substitute points for chips where mentioned here:

▶ Use a set of poker chips. All chips are equal in value. If you have more than one child, use a different color for each child.

▶ Explain to your child that you think he or she hasn't been rewarded enough for doing nice things at home, and you want to change that. Together, set up a reward system so that your child can earn privileges for good behavior.

▶ Find or make a bank to hold the chips. Have your child help decorate a box or plastic jar if needed.

▶ Work with your child to make a list of the privileges that can be earned. This should include special privileges, such as going to events outside the home or buying a toy. It should also include common privileges, such as TV, telephone or computer use, going to a friend's home, or time on the bike. List at least five to 10 items. Decide how many chips each privilege costs.

▶ Make a second list of three to four good behaviors that you would most like to see your child do more often. Choose things your child has difficulty doing. This list is different for each child.

▶ Make it clear to your child that chips are given only for behavior or chores done without directions or after the first request. Chips are not taken away for negative behavior.

▶ Decide how many chips each behavior or chore is worth and record that on the list. Assign one to three chips for most items listed. Assign five chips for bigger items.

▶ Add the number of chips your child can earn in one typical day, such as 10 or 15 chips. Most kids don't earn all of their chips every day.

▶ Try to have your child spend about two-thirds of his or her chips each day on daily privileges like watching TV. This will help your child save about one-third of his or her chips for bigger rewards.

▶ Offer extra chips for behavior or chores done in an especially quick or pleasant manner.

▶ Go out of your way the first week to offer chips for any small, appropriate behavior. Good behaviors not on the list should be rewarded, too.

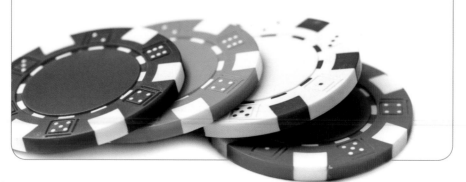

It helps to have a plan for consequences, as well as for rewards. The goal of consequences is never to shame or humiliate your child. Nor is a physically imposed consequence, such as spanking, appropriate.

For consequences to be effective, you and your child must first have a warm and loving relationship. When appropriate consequences occur within the context of a positive environment that recognizes good behavior, provides clear rules and consistently follows through with appropriate outcomes, your child will learn the value of personal responsibility and the benefits of good behavior. Benefits might include less stress at home and at school, and better friendships. There are several ways to match inappropriate behaviors with appropriate consequences.

Ignore misbehavior when you can Sometimes kids act up just to get their parents' attention. This might include doing things like whining, making inappropriate noises or repeatedly asking for things. This type of misbehavior is best ignored — reserve your attention for positive behaviors instead.

If your child's whining or other behavior isn't dangerous or disruptive to others, give your child a single prompt to redirect him or her to a positive choice. If the behavior persists, ignore it. Don't look at or talk to your child. Bury your head in a book or leave the room if you have to. If you're in a public place and you're not comfortable ignoring your child when he or she is being disruptive, it may work best to collect your child and leave.

When you choose to ignore a certain behavior, it may seem like you're not "doing your job" to stop that behavior. Actually, you are. You're refusing to reward the behavior with attention, which would only reinforce the behavior.

When attempting to extinguish an unwanted behavior such as whining, it's natural for the behavior to increase temporarily as the child tests the limits of your new expectation. Be prepared for this "extinction burst" — more whining, louder noises. Don't give in. Continue to completely ignore the misbehavior while watching for opportunities to praise good behavior. When your child realizes his or her efforts are fruitless and that there are better options for getting your attention, he or she will be more likely to give up the annoying behavior. It may occasionally pop up again, but be patient and ignore as needed.

Apply logical consequences This type of consequence closely connects the misbehavior with the results. Once children enter school, they're typically ready to experience and understand logical consequences. Using logical consequences might include:

▶ *Experiencing the natural outcome.* If your child refuses to wear a winter jacket — and there's no danger of frostbite — let him or her experience the natural consequence of being cold. Nature is sometimes the best teacher.

▶ *Losing a privilege.* When a child misbehaves, disallow a privilege — he or she no longer gets to do an activity or have an object that he or she enjoys. For example, when your child doesn't clean up his or her toys, put them away until your child earns them back.

▶ *Making it right.* When it's an option, have your child correct the misbehavior. For example, if your child says something hurtful to a sibling, have him or her give the sibling five sincere compliments or do one of the sibling's chores that day. This consequence addresses the misbehavior and maybe improves the sibling relationship.

Get straight to it If your child pays no attention to your warning, calmly say one time only, "Because you did (name the behavior), you have to have a timeout." Don't repeat the direction or explain it further. Ignore shouting, crying and promises to correct and avoid the behavior in the future.

Don't fuss If your child refuses to go to the timeout, calmly lead him or her by the hand. Be careful not to show any frustration or anger you might feel. Remember that even negative attention from you can reinforce the behavior, so arguing or fighting over the behavior is counterproductive.

Bench your child Find a safe spot to seat your child, such as on a step. Tell him or her to be quiet, and ignore any people or objects that may be nearby. After the child is seated, quickly turn away without saying anything else.

If you're out in public, you can reserve the timeout for when you get home, but don't forget to reinforce it.

Base it on your child's age Use one minute for each year of age. If your child cries, yells or acts out during the timeout, stop the clock. Start it again when the child has been quiet for at least 20 seconds. If this doesn't work, go to your backup plan (read ahead).

If, after the timeout is finished, your child decides to stay in that space for any reason, let it be. He or she may be thinking about his or her behavior and will get up soon.

Set the terms Prior to ending the timeout, your child must agree to follow the instructions he or she ignored earlier and which triggered the timeout. Once the timeout is finished, the child needs to correct the behavior that resulted in the timeout. For example, if toys weren't picked up, they need to be picked up now. If it doesn't happen, give another timeout.

Acknowledge but don't praise When your child cooperates and corrects the behavior, offer a simple acknowledgment but not praise. For example, say, "I'm glad you chose to do what I asked you to do."

Have a backup plan When you put your child in a timeout, warn him or her that an unserved timeout will result in being sent to a backup location to calm down. The backup location should be in a room where your child will be safe — and bored. After he or she has been quiet for 30 seconds in the backup location, the original timeout must be finished.

Get help If your child won't stay in a timeout, make an appointment with your child's medical provider to talk about other options to try.

DON'T GIVE UP

At times it may seem that your child will never learn how to behave well or be able to follow instructions. But don't give up. Raising a well-rounded, well-behaved child takes time, patience and great consistency. It's a challenging job but an important one. And the lessons your child learns now, at an early age, will render benefits over and over again in the years to come.

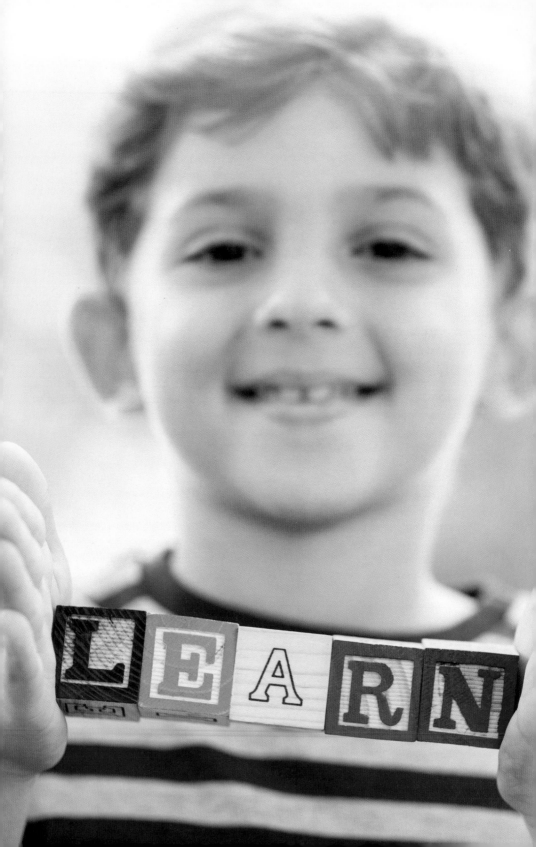

CHAPTER 17

Raising a resilient child

Most parents instinctively recoil when it comes to thoughts of their children facing failure or dealing with a difficult situation. In fact, parents typically think it's part of their job to shelter and protect their children from the storms of life. It's a totally natural assumption. But it's not always the most helpful when it comes to preparing a child for the future.

Ask yourself: Do you want to raise a child who understands the importance of kindness and compassion? Do you want to raise a young adult who knows how to adapt to imperfection, develop new skills, and be confident and independent in the face of adversity?

Research shows that all of these traits are gained through the opportunity to face down tough challenges. Struggles can help your child savor life's best moments and give him or her the rewarding satisfaction of overcoming obstacles — and succeeding.

You can foster your child's ability to seek challenges and bounce back from tough times — to be resilient — from a very young age. This chapter will give you research-backed strategies to resist shielding your child from distress and help him or her learn how to persist through failure.

WHAT IS RESILIENCE?

If you look it up in the dictionary, you might see the term *resilience* explained as having the ability to bounce or spring back into shape after being compressed, stretched or bent. Trees are resilient to wind and storm, for example.

Resilience is also a human quality. A resilient person is someone who recovers his or her strength and spirits after undergoing acute or chronic hardship, someone who triumphs in the face of adversity.

Think of Frederick Douglass, who emerged from slavery as a great orator and intellectual. Or Eleanor Roosevelt, who experienced the early death of her parents but went on to become a noted

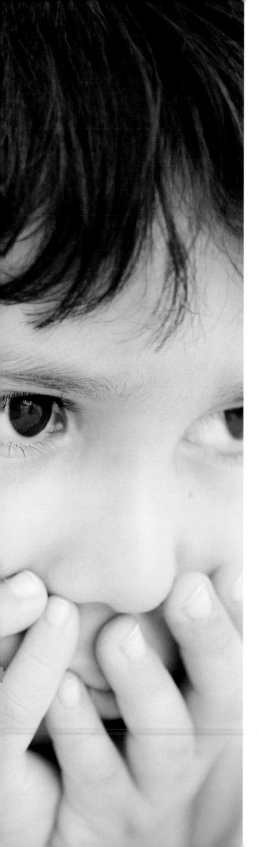

political activist. Frida Kahlo survived a near-fatal accident that ended her dream of becoming a doctor, so she turned to painting. Today she is known worldwide for her art.

But resiliency isn't just found in famous people. It's an important quality for anyone to have because no one can escape life's often unpredictable challenges.

You can gauge your child's current level of resilience by observing his or her ability to cope with everyday stressors, as well as long-term sources of stress. Start by thinking about your child's individual disposition and his or her initial reaction to stress. What's your preschooler's response to being told to put on a seat belt? How does your 9-year-old react to being assigned a big science fair project?

Each child's individual biological response to stress plays a role in his or her level of resilience. Some children show great sensitivity to stress; others are more easygoing in nature. Resiliency isn't just predetermined, though. Your child's ability to adapt and thrive in the face of a challenge also is shaped by experiences and relationships.

Researchers sometimes liken a child's resiliency to a seesaw. Stressful experiences — such as the loss of a parent or having a chronic illness — may pile up on one side of the seesaw, weighing it down in favor of negative outcomes. On the other side, however, are positive relationships and supportive resources. These help make stress tolerable for a child, tipping the seesaw the other way — toward positive outcomes. The stressors don't disappear, but the child is given the necessary tools to achieve a positive balance.

As a parent, you can help your child acquire the skills he or she needs to deal with life's challenges. Resiliency can be built out and developed over time. Here's how to do it.

THE IMPORTANCE OF RELATIONSHIPS

Having the support of a stable, committed grown-up — whether it's a parent, caregiver or teacher — is one of the most important factors in helping a child feel that he or she has what it takes to overcome adversity. This kind of trusted adult-child connection provides young children with a buffer from the stresses of external life, creating a protected space in which to grow and learn.

The supervision and ordered structure provided by a caring adult functions as a supportive scaffold for a child while he or she builds the skills necessary to manage stress. Such skills include the ability to focus, concentrate, plan ahead, problem-solve, exert self-control, and adjust to change. As a child becomes increasingly competent and confident in these areas, the scaffolding can gradually be removed until he or she is able to stand alone.

The more of these stable relationships a child has, the better. Although your own relationship as a parent with your child is of major importance, think about other current trusted relationships your child has in his or her life. This could be a grandparent, aunt or uncle, coach, piano teacher, or family friend. Consider how you might help strengthen these relationships or create others that would benefit your child.

CORE BELIEFS

Resilience is kind of like an emotional muscle. The more you use it, the stronger it gets. To help your child develop this muscle, encourage him or her absorb the following key concepts.

Decisions have consequences Allow your child to experience the outcome of his or her decisions. When parents make all of the decisions, children can get the sense that what they do or feel doesn't matter. They may feel that their parents doubt their abilities to participate in the decision-making process or to make decisions by themselves.

When appropriate, allow your child to make decisions and let the results play out. For example, if your daughter insists on wearing her fancy dress-up shoes to the playground, let her. Soon enough, she'll figure out the best footwear for avoiding hot feet and blisters. If your son is confident that he's studied enough for tomorrow's test, let the test results reveal the rightness or wrongness of his decision. Your child will learn that decisions have consequences, an important life lesson. As your child becomes more experienced in making choices, he or she becomes wiser, more confident and better able to examine the potential outcomes of his or her decisions.

Failure is a part of life It's important for children to learn that failure isn't a deal breaker. If your child sees failure as an opportunity to learn rather than quit, he or she is more likely to try new things and get better at them.

Teach your child that sometimes you win, sometimes you lose, and you don't always come in first. But losing a soccer match or failing an audition shouldn't stop your child from trying again. Emphasize that skills can be learned and developed.

To encourage effort and perseverance, praise your child for working hard at something, even if he or she doesn't win or achieve perfection. Regardless of your child's aptitude for math, for example, focus on the amount of effort he or she puts into learning and practicing math skills. Avoid commenting on your child's innate abilities — this can lead your child to believe that if he or she isn't naturally good at something, then why bother? Instead say, "I really like how you tried a lot of different strategies to figure out that tough math problem." Even if your child isn't able to do everything perfectly or even well, he or she will still learn important skills and grow through the process.

Take a similar approach if your child signs up for a sport or class and wants to stop participating because he or she is bored or doesn't feel good enough at it. Encourage your son or daughter to stick it out until the sport is over or the class is finished. Doing so helps your child learn to see a task or project through and reinforces the idea of not giving up on something too quickly because it's challenging or difficult. If there are legitimate reasons to quit, certainly it's important to do so, but persevering has benefits, too. By the end, your child might even enjoy the activity or decide to pursue it further.

Everyone has strengths Every child has unique abilities. For some kids, conventional areas such as academics or sports may not be their strong suit. But they may have strengths in other areas, such as in creativity or courage.

For example, you might notice that your child, who could really care less about school, has a keen interest in taking things apart to see how they work. Make a visit to the flea market or secondhand shop to purchase an old radio or clock that your child can freely disassemble and rework. Or perhaps your child is fearless when it comes to the outdoors. Find opportunities to safely guide and challenge your child's adventurous spirit, such as joining a scout program or taking a rock climbing class.

Help your child discover and develop his or her character strengths. Be honest about what your child can do — kids know when grownups aren't being sincere — but be positive. Encourage your child to develop his or her strengths and to look for opportunities to use them. Using a skill to help others, for instance, can be a major confidence booster for a child.

A GROWTH MINDSET

Life is rarely a string of continual successes. Most of the time, it's made up of a string of attempts at success.

Think of your child's first steps. Many of those initial efforts to walk likely ended in a tumble. But that didn't stop your son or daughter from getting up again. Soon enough, your child was walking and eventually running. That is how growth works. You try. You fail. You try again.

As your child gets older, you'll help him or her take on bigger and more-complex endeavors — physically, mentally and emotionally. There will be more falls and even some face plants, no doubt. But your job as a parent is to help your child get back up and try again. Cultivating this attitude of resilience helps prepare your child for the many challenges down the road, including high school, college and professional careers.

Make sure your child knows that the process of learning a skill can be as important as the skill itself, and that failure isn't something to be feared or avoided. Help your child see failure as a natural byproduct of learning and experimenting with new things.

When your child loses a hotly contested basketball game, for example, help him or her process what happened. If the

CHORES FOR KIDS

One way you can help your child build resiliency — and keep the household gears moving — is by assigning age-appropriate chores. Doing chores around the house allows your child to not only learn important life skills that promote independence and responsibility but also learn how to stay on task, manage time effectively and gradually get better at something, all within the safety net of the home.

When creating your chore chart, think about essential tasks that need to be done to keep your family's home in working order. Consider your child's developmental level and find a way to include him or her in the daily household operations. Every family has its own priorities, but here are some suggestions to get you started:

Ages 3 to 5	Ages 6 to 8	Ages 9 to 11
• Put away toys • Make bed • Place dirty clothes in hamper • Water houseplants • Set and clear the table	• Put away clean dishes • Fold towels • Match clean socks • Peel vegetables or make a salad • Get backpack ready for school	• Wash dishes • Wipe down table and counters • Clean bathroom • Vacuum • Make lunch

situation stinks, say so. Let your child know that it's OK to be disappointed or upset. Then, when the dust settles a little, encourage your child to think about how to deal with the loss or how to get better at the game.

It can help to share stories about times that you failed and what you learned from the experiences. Even better, let your child see you try new things, even if it's something you're not good at. Try running a 5K race together or taking a pottery class. Find something that challenges you, maybe even scares you a little. You and your child will both learn from the experience. And, you'll be collecting some fun memories.

The three P's Research suggests that three factors, known as the three P's, can diminish a person's ability to recover from a setback and achieve emotional growth:

▶ *Personalization.* What happened is your fault.

▶ *Pervasiveness.* The event will affect all areas of life.

▶ *Permanence.* The effects of the setback will last forever.

HELICOPTER PARENTING

You've probably heard of helicopter parents — it's a term used to describe parents who hover over their children and micromanage their lives. Prime examples of helicopter parenting include following a preschooler around the playground to make sure he or she never falls, calling other parents to sort out your child's relationship issues with their children, and doing or redoing your child's homework. Helicopter parents don't let their kids fail because they want to protect their children from adversity.

Overprotecting your child might feel like the right thing in the moment, but consider the consequences. In doing so, parents prevent children from trying out some very important skills — standing up for themselves, making decisions and learning from mistakes. These skills are important if your child is to eventually become self-sufficient. If you do your child's science poster for him, he will likely get a good grade. But what happens when he has to prepare a presentation in college? How will he do the work then? If he fails the class, will he know how to cope?

Avoid conveying the impression that you doubt your child's abilities, that he or she is too fragile to recover from failure, or that you don't trust him or her. Instead, let your words and actions inspire your child to reach to his or her full potential.

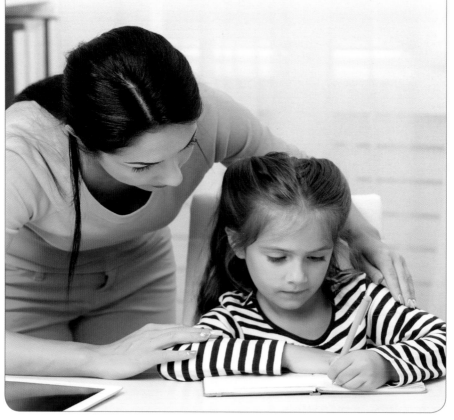

To help your child counter these beliefs, offer these guidelines:

▶ Don't take what happened personally.
▶ Don't let a setback take over your life.
▶ Understand that feelings will pass.

Imagine your daughter is upset about a recent fight with a friend. Caught up in emotions, she says she has no friends, nobody likes her, and she'll never have friends again. First, acknowledge how she's feeling and empathize. Say something like, "Ugh, fighting with friends is such a lonely feeling. It makes a lot of sense that you're feeling this way."

When your child is calm enough to talk and listen, encourage her to test these beliefs. Ask what the fight was about. Gently remind her that friends sometimes argue but that doesn't necessarily spell the end of the friendship. Point out other activities your child is involved in. During these activities, has she been playing with other friends? Were they having fun? Remind her that her social circle can contain multiple friends and that she will likely make other friends in the future.

Remind your child of other positives in her life, too, such as an upcoming science fair, a birthday party or summer break. One lousy event doesn't mean that her whole life is awful or that she'll never be happy again. She can and will move on.

The power of 'yet' Failure can also become a great source of motivation for your child and serve as fuel to get him or her to work a little harder. Explore with your child how a different choice along the way might have led to a different result. If your child expresses feelings of defeat and says, "I can't," ask him or her to add the word "yet" to the end of the sentence. With increased effort, a new strategy or both, your child can try again — possibly with better results.

Assess your expectations Moving forward, think about the role your expectations may play in the development of your child's resilience. Consider your child's abilities and set the bar just high enough to give your child room to stretch and grow. Or let your child set the bar.

Think of it this way: Your child will never fail if you or your child is always setting goals within reach. Plus, your child won't have the chance to understand his or her true capabilities. Instead, set goals that are capable of being attained and that increase your child's skills a little bit more each time.

LETTING YOUR CHILD LEARN

Allowing your child to learn from failure requires you to step back and let your child experience failure in the first place.

If you're like most parents, you might struggle with finding the balance between stepping in and protecting your child versus stepping back and allowing your child to grow — a delicate balance that's continually shifting as your child gets older.

If your child is facing a situation in which his or her safety is at risk, your intervention is appropriate and necessary. But if your child has broken a rule at school or hasn't completed an assignment on time, let him or her face the consequences. This will help your child learn that the rules apply to him or her and to keep better track of assignments and deadlines.

Also, make room for your child to advocate for himself or herself. If your child thinks a teacher is being unfair, encourage him or her to respectfully speak up. If your child experiences bumps in a friendship, avoid interfering. Instead, offer a

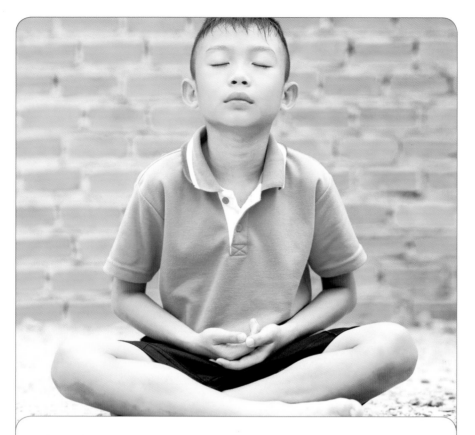

HOW TO RELAX YOUR BREATHING

Relaxed breathing is a technique that your child can use anywhere, anytime to manage stress. It involves slowing and deepening the breath so that mind and body relax. You and your child can practice it together. Here are some kid-friendly instructions you can use:

1. Find a quiet place to sit or lie down.
2. Relax your shoulders.
3. Breathe in through your nose, slowly and evenly. Count to four while you do this, if that helps.
4. Pretend that there's a balloon in your belly. Watch to see if your belly moves out a little when you breathe. If you want to, lie down and put a piece of paper or a small stuffed animal on your belly. See if it moves up when you breathe in. The top part of your chest should stay pretty still.
5. Slowly breathe out through your mouth, as if you're blowing up a big balloon or blowing out a candle. You can count to four while you do this.
6. Let your belly — and the rest of your body — relax for a few seconds. Then start over again. Practice until this is easy and relaxing to do.

listening ear. Work with your child to come up with a solution or discuss what he or she thinks is the best way forward. Offer your support and give advice when asked.

Support your child while letting him or her learn life's lessons. Keep in mind that by allowing your child to face challenges and develop strategies for dealing with them, you're providing important future skills.

MANAGING STRESS

Part of becoming resilient involves the ability to manage stress. Feeling stressed is often uncomfortable. In children, stress can show up in the form of headaches, muscle aches, stomachaches, nausea or disrupted sleep. Your child may be anxious, restless, irritable and lack focus. A visit to your child's medical provider can help rule out underlying problems. But consider the possibility that your child is displaying symptoms of stress.

Even though stress can be distressing, that doesn't mean it's all bad. As with failure, stress is a part of life. If your child learns how to tolerate and manage it, he or she will go through life more content and resilient than otherwise.

Fight-or-flight Stress generally provokes a fight-or-flight response. During this reaction, the brain sets off an alarm system in the body, prompting the adrenal glands to release a surge of hormones, including adrenaline and cortisol. In this mode, the brain thinks there are two possible options: fighting the bad feelings or getting away from them. Rational thinking and problem-solving become difficult. The focus is on quick relief without much thought to long-term outcomes.

To find relief, your child may "fight" by yelling, acting out, talking back or picking a fight for no good reason. Or he or she may opt for "flight" by avoiding the stressful situation. Sometimes, this means literally running away and hiding. Or it might mean getting lost in video games or other hobbies, avoiding friends, or delving into homework or sports. Your child might not even realize what's going on, making it sometimes difficult to discuss.

In the moment As a parent, your first instinct might be to try to eliminate the source of stress on your child. While a loving response, it's unlikely that you can rid your child's life of all stress. Even if you can remove the immediate stressor, you may be denying your child the opportunity to learn healthy coping skills. You might also be sending the message that the best way to deal with stress is to avoid it.

Another option is to help your child put together a toolkit of strategies that he or she can use to cope with stress throughout life. In fact, it's crucial that you expose your child to positive ways to manage and relieve stress so that he or she is able to do so later as an adult, when the stakes are generally higher.

First, help your child become aware of what he or she is feeling. Sometimes just saying, "Whoa, I'm feeling anxious right now" can help reduce the intensity of the emotion. Then, teach your child to calm his or her thoughts by saying, "I am not under attack." In most cases, what's causing your child stress isn't an eminent threat to his or her safety.

Help your child put stressful situations in perspective by reminding him or her that the stressful feelings will subside and that he or she will feel better with time. Also, teach your child to come up with ways of dealing with stress in the moment, such as by telling himself or herself, "I can do this," or by taking deep breaths (see page 258).

Practicing helps There are multiple opportunities in every child's life to learn to manage stress in a positive way.

Stressors can range from something as small and immediate as not being able to find a clean shirt to something larger and more ongoing such as being left out of a group of peers. The resilient child will be able to adapt to different levels of stress over time and ultimately thrive.

As your child continues to develop and mature, his or her coping strategies will change. When stressed, a younger child might cling to a special blanket or stuffed animal, for example, or simply fall asleep. Older children may have already developed more problem-solving skills, but may still need to be reminded that their stress is manageable.

Don't forget that your child is also watching how you cope with stress. This is a good opportunity to assess your stress management skills and maybe learn some new ones. Make healthy coping choices yourself, and your whole family is likely to benefit.

Bear in mind that if a serious event or trauma has occurred, your child will likely need the help of a professional to recover.

Help your child learn ways to adapt to and manage stress by taking steps to:

Address the stressor Encourage your child to identify the problem that's bothering him or her and break it up into smaller, more-manageable pieces.

Sometimes the problem involves less tangible parts, such as stressful feelings or thoughts. Allow your child to describe those feelings and help him or her identify when they come up.

Make sure your child knows that negative emotions, while uncomfortable, aren't necessarily problematic. The goal is to recognize and cope with stressful feelings, not to avoid having them.

Make a plan Once the source of stress and its triggers are identified, it can make it easier for your child to create an action plan. Listen to your child's ideas for solutions first. If necessary, offer some suggestions of your own.

Maybe this involves organizing clothes differently, planning ahead more or practicing harder. Or maybe this means going to a quiet place, even if it's just in the mind, when feelings get overwhelming.

Practice self-care Being active, eating well, getting plenty of sleep, and spending time with family and friends can help your child reduce stress and anxiety. Some kids may be interested in practicing stress-reducing techniques such as deep breathing or mindfulness exercises.

Learn to relax Talk to your child about the power of taking his or her mind off of stress, either by imagining a relaxing place, turning to a hobby, reading a book or listening to music. Ask your child what helps him or her feel relaxed — it may be different than your own list.

Show gratitude Take a moment together each day to share what you're thankful for — perhaps at the dinner table or by placing a slip of paper in a gratitude jar. This can help your child focus on the good things in life.

Be a positive force Did you know your child can relieve stress by helping someone else? Not only will it offer distraction, but he or she will witness that it's OK to give and receive help.

LETTING GO

Building resilience in your child requires a certain amount of letting go from you, the parent and protector. It can be a little scary at times. But it's important to trust your child. It doesn't have to be all at once. You don't want to ask your child to do anything that's inappropriate.

When a parent regards a child with confidence in what he or she can do, that confidence blooms and grows within the child, as well. If you embrace the power of growth and learning, your child will, too. If you believe your child can make it through stressful experiences, your child will believe it, too.

By giving your child the right amount of opportunity to face challenges, learn adaptive skills — even when it involves some trial and error — and thrive in spite of failure, you'll be giving him or her the necessary skills to become an independent, thriving adult.

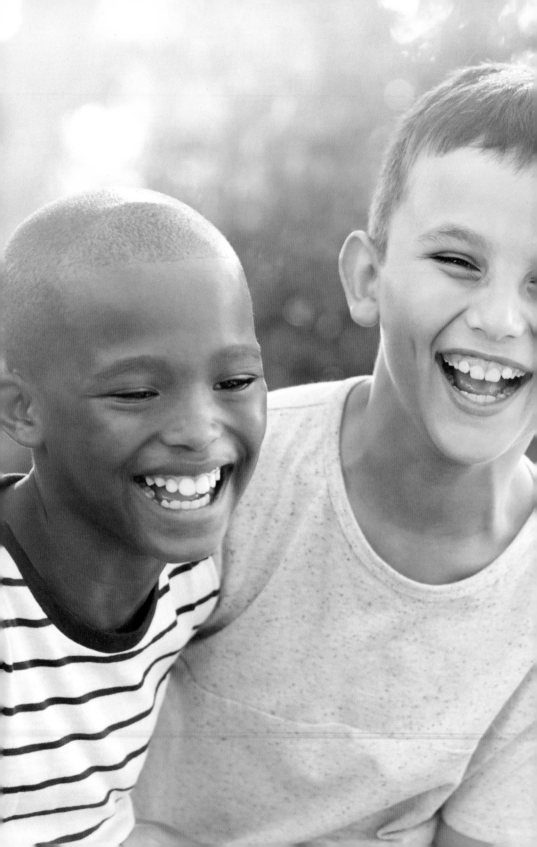

CHAPTER 18

Fostering friendships

When you think about your childhood, some of your favorite memories probably involve good friends. From giggling together under a table to chasing each other wildly at recess, friendships are an important part of being a kid.

Kids need connections with their peers to give them a sense of belonging and support, to broaden their horizons beyond family, and to develop self-worth and an idea of who they are.

Children have different needs when it comes to friendship, but all children can benefit from having friends. While social skills don't come naturally to every child, there's much you can do to help your child make and maintain quality friendships.

HOW KIDS MAKE FRIENDS

Making connections with others is a deeply ingrained human trait, one that's evident from birth. In the infant and toddler years, your child's main connection was you and your family. Now, as your child grows and develops his or her social skills, relationships broaden to others outside the home. Generally, childhood friendships tend to go through specific age-related phases:

- *Ages 3 to 5.* For preschoolers, a friend is a playmate — a fun partner in building a block tower or someone to be silly with on the playground. During this time, children become better able to cooperate with each other, a basic skill that forms the foundation of friendship.
- *Ages 6 to 8.* By the time children enter school, they're able to form more-complex bonds. Your child might consider a friend someone who lives nearby, has cool toys and likes similar activities, such as making crafts or playing with trucks. At this stage, children are less likely to befriend kids who they don't find interesting or who they perceive as difficult to interact with.

WHAT DOES IT MEAN TO BE FRIENDS?

There are many kinds of relationships a child may have, but a true peer-to-peer friendship is meaningful in a special way. A true friendship isn't forced but springs up naturally between two children. A healthy friendship is:

▶ *A two-way street.* Both children like each other and enjoy being together. Sometimes, one child desires a friendship but the other child may not see it in the same light.

▶ *Bound by affection.* Some friendships are based on convenience, because of mutual ties such as classrooms, sports teams or hobbies. Shared talents and interests may lead to friendships and help sustain them. But the basis of friendship itself is mutual affection for each other, regardless of other factors.

▶ *Voluntary.* Both children are friends because they want to be, not because the friendship has been arranged by parents, teachers or others.

Be observant of your child's relationships. If you notice a blossoming friendship that's marked by these characteristics, encourage it. A true friend is a treasure.

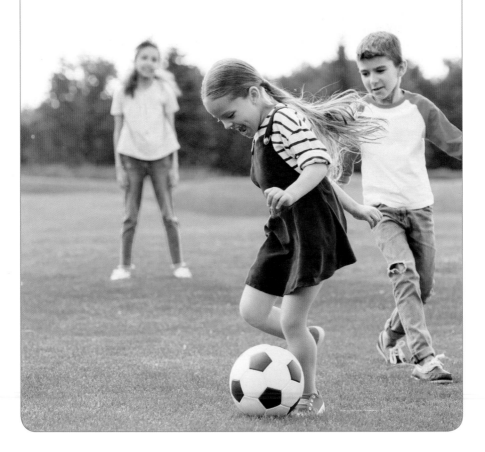

> *Ages 9 to 11.* Children at this age begin relying on peers for support, and strong emotional bonds are more likely to develop. Friends at this age are kids who stick up for and show loyalty to each other. Beyond having similar interests, children also expect a friend to show understanding and share personal thoughts and feelings.

FOSTERING POSITIVE RELATIONSHIPS

What can you do to help your child develop healthy, supportive friendships? You can't make friends for your child, but you can play an important part in helping your child develop quality friendships.

Your own healthy relationships can have a big impact on your child's relationships. When you're supporting and being supported by a partner or spouse, friends, and family members, your child is noticing and absorbing your positive social skills.

Having your own strong bond with your child also shows your child what it feels and looks like to be in a positive, consistent relationship. It enables him or her to trust and enjoy friendships. If your child feels loved and respected at home, he or she is more likely to feel secure and make good choices when it comes to friends.

When your child is younger, you can open the door to friendships by widening your son or daughter's opportunities to meet other kids through activities or classes and connecting with parents of children your child might like to get to know. Listen to your child. Who does he or she talk about a lot? Watch your child interacting with others. Are there some kids your child seems happier around

than others? You might suggest a play date or your child may ask for one. As your child gets older, he or she is likely to become more involved in planning and arranging play dates. Do your best to support his or her efforts.

At the same time, talk to your child about friendship. Discuss what qualities your child appreciates in a friendship and why. Talk also about what qualities your child won't put up with in a friend.

To help support your child's social development:

Make time for friends Modern schedules are hectic, but try to make time each week for your child to hang out with kids he or she likes. Generally, one-on-one play dates are the best ways for kids to develop close friendships. Encourage your child to have fun with friends on the weekends rather than spending time scrolling through electronic media or playing video games.

Teach interactive skills Throw a ball with your child or play board games together. This will give your child a chance to practice social skills by taking turns, following rules, and experiencing winning and losing. Also, it will develop your child's interest in multiplayer activities, so that he or she will want to play with others.

Help your child understand social rules and etiquette If your child wants to join others in play, encourage him or her to look for a group with a similar skill level or with similar interests. He or she can show interest by watching them, making eye contact or complimenting one of them. When there's a pause in the game, your child can ask to join in. If the answer is no, encourage your child to accept it and to not take it too personally.

IS IT OK FOR A CHILD TO FOCUS ON ONE FRIENDSHIP?

Some children concentrate on a single best friend, a person with whom they feel compatible and secure. Sometimes, this can cause parents to worry that their child is too invested in the relationship. As long as the friendship is positive and your child isn't excluding himself or herself from a range of experiences, the situation probably isn't cause for concern.

However, keep in mind that circles of friends frequently shift during childhood. Friends move, kids change and drift apart, and sometimes friendships abruptly end (and start up again). Open the way for your child to have more than one circle of friends. In addition to friends at school, having friends on a sports team, in an after-school activity or within a religious organization can help your child maintain stability if he or she runs into problems with one group.

He or she can look for another group of kids to join or another interesting activity.

When your child has a friend over for a play date, show your child how to be a welcoming host. Remind your child to be considerate of his or her guest's wishes, to avoid criticizing the guest, and to stay with the guest through the whole play date.

Teach good sportsmanship Encourage your child to join in the spirit of the game and to have fun. Discourage pointing out rule violations, criticizing others, or making fun of the game or the players. Encourage high-fives and sincere compliments instead.

Remind your child not to leave in the middle of a game just because he or she is losing or tired. If the activity has become boring, encourage suggesting a new activity, rather than making negative comments.

Offer support As the importance of friendships increases, so do the ups and downs of making friends. As with adult friendships, children can get a lot of emotional support and positive feedback from their circle of friends. But they can also experience sadness, anger and jealousy. They can feel hurt if they think they are being left out.

Offer your love and support during stormy times — be the person in your child's corner. By helping your son or daughter stay true to his or her values, maintain respect for others, and avoid destructive peer pressure, you'll help your child learn important life lessons about navigating social relationships.

WHEN YOU DISAPPROVE OF A FRIENDSHIP

There may be times when your child befriends someone who you perceive as a negative influence or who displays worrying behavior. It can be difficult to hold back on your opinions, but think twice about bad-mouthing the child or demanding that your child end the friend-

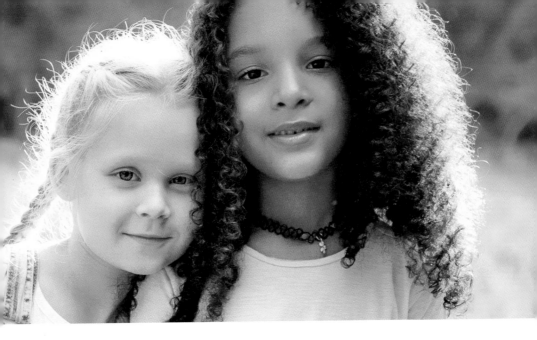

ship. This can sometimes backfire. Your child may feel the need to defend the friend or feel alienated from your trust.

Consider what your child sees in this friend. Sometimes, the other child may fill a gap in your child's perceived sense of self. For example, a child who is typically careful about following the rules might choose a friend who is free-spirited, allowing him or her to explore being more adventurous.

To address your concerns, remind your child of your own family rules and the consequences of adopting unacceptable behavior. Help your child use his or her own mental ruler to determine which friends might be worth investing in versus those who might be better off as acquaintances.

In the meantime, look for situations in which your child might naturally encounter or interact with kids who you feel are a more positive influence. See if relationships develop. Provide the setting for potential friendships to bloom, but allow your child to decide if the connection is right.

HELPING A SHY OR WITHDRAWN CHILD

Some parents become concerned that their child is too shy, and they don't know what to do about it. Being shy or introverted isn't necessarily a problem, as it can just be a natural part of your child's personality.

Children also develop social skills at different rates and they vary in their needs and desires for friends. A child's preferences with regard to friendship may change month to month or year to year.

These changes usually aren't cause for concern. If your child is generally satisfied with his or her social life, there's no need to force friendships. But if your child is being rejected by classmates or seems to have concerns about having no friends, he or she might need some help in strengthening his or her social skills.

Shy children often do just fine in structured settings, such as a classroom, where they know the rules for interacting with others and what's expected of them. It's when they get out on the playground or in the lunchline, where the setting is more ambiguous and expectations more loose, that they have trouble. Because there's no script to follow, they may feel at a loss for what to do or say.

You can help your child get better at handling free play by taking these steps:

Practice skills at home Help your child develop his or her social skills by practicing at home. Don't feel bad — it's no different from practicing reading or language skills. Provide direct instruction and input on ways to handle a situation such as recess. Coach your child on what to say when another child approaches him or her.

For example, when another child stops playing to say hi to your child, your child can say, "Hi. Your game looks kind of fun." This creates an opening for the other child to respond and continue the conversation.

If your child is invited to participate in a game, tell him or her to keep the dialogue simple but positive. Your child can just say, "Sure!" and join in. Providing your child with a social script to follow can give them the basic structure they need to make it through those initial encounters. With time and practice, your child's social skills will become stronger and more adaptable.

Join an interesting club or group Extracurricular activities that align with your child's interests can also provide semistructured environments for your child to practice his or her social skills.

For example, participating in a drama or theater club can provide a good mix of scripted and organic interactions. Or your child might be interested in a robotics or cartoon animation club, where the theme creates a springboard for discussion and interaction.

Take lessons If you feel your child needs additional help, talk to your child's medical provider or a school counselor about joining a social skills group. These groups are led by mental health professionals and are designed to help children overcome gaps in social learning and adaptability. Because of the group setting, kids are able to practice new skills at the same time that they learn them.

PEER PRESSURE

Peer pressure can become an issue during the later elementary years. It's important to talk to your child about what to do if they are pressured to do something they don't want to do or know is wrong. For this age group, the desire to fit in can lead a child to do surprising and unexpected things. This can even include self-destructive things.

You can help your child cope with peer pressure. Talk with your child regularly about friendships and other peer relationships, and about how a friend's actions relate to your family values. When you love, encourage and spend time with your child, you help to develop a strong sense of self-esteem and belonging. Having your unconditional support can help your child stand up to peer pressure.

WHAT TO DO ABOUT BULLYING

Bullying is recurring behavior that intentionally hurts a child, physically or emotionally. It can happen at school, in the community or online. Bullying is different from conflict in that bullying behavior is usually about having power or control over another person. Kids who bully continue with negative behaviors even when they know their words or actions are hurting the other person.

Bullying can have lasting consequences. Children who are bullied may be at increased risk of depression and anxiety, problems at school, and substance abuse. Children who bully others are at increased risk of substance use, school problems and violence later in life. Children who are both bullied and bully others are at the greatest risk of negative outcomes.

Types of bullying In the movies, kids who bully are often big and tough, or mean and popular. In fact, bullying is a behavior. Anyone can bully or be bullied. Some kids who bully are also bullied, as well as the other way around. Bullying can take many forms:

▶ *Verbal bullying.* This is the most common type of bullying. It's quick and direct. Examples include teasing, name-calling, taunting and making inappropriate sexual comments.
▶ *Physical bullying.* This includes doing things such as hitting, tripping or kicking another child, or destroying another child's property. It's easiest to recognize because it's the most visible type of bullying.
▶ *Psychological or social bullying.* This is usually more subtle than verbal or physical bullying. It's often done in groups. It involves spreading rumors about someone, dictating rules of friendship, or embarrassing or excluding a child from a group. It can be more difficult to identify as bullying because kids may feel that the behavior is natural or deserved.
▶ *Electronic bullying (cyberbullying).* This involves using an electronic medium, such as social media, text messages or videos sent through phones, to threaten or harm a child.

If your child is bullied If you suspect your child is being bullied, or your child tells you that he or she is being bullied, it can be upsetting and scary to you as a parent. While it's essential to take the situation seriously, avoid trying to immediately fix the problem or confront the bully yourself. Instead, focus on your child.

Understand your child's feelings Remain calm. Be a good listener. Find out what your child is feeling. Express your own understanding and concern. Avoid attaching any judgment to your child's emotions or reactions to the situation. Reassure your child that telling you about it isn't tattling. When a child is being hurt or harmed, it's important to tell a trusted grownup right away.

Don't spread the blame Remember that bullying isn't about a disagreement between two kids. It's about one child or group of children intentionally hurting another child. Trying to mediate differences or find middle ground isn't an appropriate response. Remind your child that bullying is wrong, that he or she isn't to blame for being bullied, and that your child has your full support.

Learn about the situation Ask your child to describe how and when the bullying occurs and who is involved. Find out what your child may have already

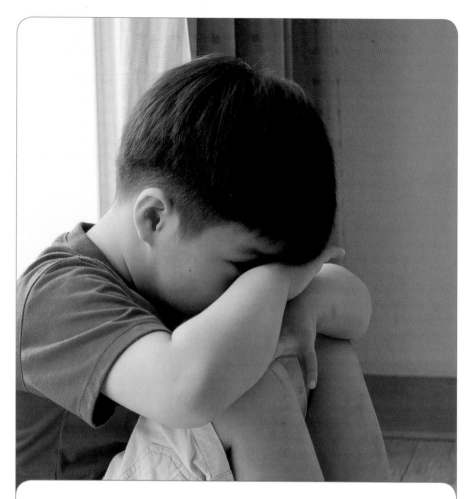

WARNING SIGNS OF BULLYING

If your child is being bullied, he or she might not say anything about it to you or others — often out of fear, shame or embarrassment. Warning signs can be subtle. Be on the lookout for changes such as:

- Lost or destroyed clothing, electronics or other personal belongings
- Abrupt loss of friends or avoidance of social situations
- Not doing well at school or not wanting to go to school
- Headaches, stomachaches or other physical complaints
- Trouble sleeping
- Changes in eating habits
- Regular distress after spending time online or on his or her phone without a reasonable explanation
- Feelings of helplessness or low self-esteem

WHEN YOUR CHILD IS A BYSTANDER

Children who witness bullying have a powerful role to play. They can make the situation worse by joining in the bullying or cheering it on. Or they can make the situation better by discouraging the person doing the bullying, defending the person being bullied, or defusing and redirecting the situation. Bystanders can also rally other kids to stand up against bullying or report bullying behavior to adults.

Kids often know about bullying long before grownups find out about it. According to American Academy of Pediatrics, more than 55 percent of bullying situations end when a peer intervenes.

Encourage your child to take a stand against bullying. As a bystander, your child can support a child who's being bullied by spending time with him or her, being a good listener, reinforcing the idea that bullying is wrong and that no one deserves it, and never encouraging or contributing to bullying. Having friends around is a powerful deterrent to being bullied. Encourage your child to stick up for others who may not have a lot of friends.

done to try to stop the bullying. Ask what has or hasn't worked so far. Ask what you can do to help him or her feel safe.

Come up with a plan Work with your child to come up with a plan to address the bullying. Ask your child what he or she would like to see happen. How can the situation be stopped or prevented? To resolve the situation, who would need to be involved and what could others do? Maybe this includes sticking with friends wherever the bullying seems to happen or asking a teacher, coach or other adult for help.

In addition, think together about your child's strengths and how he or she might use those strengths to counter the bullying. Remind your child that although the situation might seem bleak, there are people who care about your child and don't want to see them bullied.

Be aware of your child's online activity Since so much social interaction today

takes place online, make sure you know how your child is using the internet, social media, or his or her phone to interact with others.

Consider limiting social media use for younger children. For older children, it may be helpful to create a technology contract that lists your family's rules for safe and respectful use of smartphones, gaming devices and tablets. This contract should include the agreement that you reserve the right to look at the content of your child's devices if you have safety concerns, and you will do so in your child's presence, especially for older kids. Sign the contract and post it in a highly visible place in your home.

Avoid isolating your child If your child is being bullied, refrain from removing him or her from social situations or automatically taking away electronic devices or computer access. Children might be reluctant to report bullying for fear of having their online privileges taken away.

LEARNING AND CONSEQUENCES

Parents have a natural tendency to want to rescue their kids from negative consequences. But children learn best when they're allowed to experience the results of their choices. A parent's task is to clearly outline the expectations for a child, equip the child with the skills necessary to meet those expectations, and spell out the potential outcomes that will occur when those expectations are or aren't met. Then comes the hardest part — stepping back and allowing the child to make those choices, including the not-so-good choices, and fully experience the results of those choices.

Constantly altering expectations or accommodating for poor choices creates confusion and ultimately delays a child's learning process. A parent who reinforces some rules sometimes becomes like a slot machine. The child will keep trying to push the limits until he or she hits the "jackpot" and the rules are forgotten.

Allowing your child to experience uncomfortable results not only highlights the value of making a better choice but it also instills in your child the sense that he or she has control over his or her actions and can make things better for himself or herself. In addition, allowing your child to go through discomfort and to realize that he or she still is OK afterward increases your child's resilience and ability to handle stress.

When considering how to change your child's behavior, think about whether you're ready for the task as a parent. It may help to pick a time when you know you'll be able to be strong and support your child, but also refrain from rescuing.

When you decide on a consequence for a particular behavior, tell your child. If the misbehavior happens a lot, tell your child in advance what the consequence will be.

If your child continues to misbehave, calmly follow through with the consequence. If your child complains, don't explain or argue. And don't remove the consequence. If the child refuses the consequence, proceed to a timeout.

Use a timeout Timeouts are best used sparingly to be effective. They generally work well for younger children, up to about age 12.

Timeouts allow a parent to take a child out of the scenario that triggered the misbehavior. They also remove opportunities for the unwanted behavior to be reinforced, and give the child (and parent) a chance to cool off.

Behaviors that might earn a timeout include doing something dangerous or breaking a known safety rule. Timeouts can also be given when a child ignores directions. To institute an effective timeout:

Offer a warning After the misbehavior, give your child a chance to correct the behavior. Wait five to 10 seconds for your child to respond before proceeding to the next step, if necessary. Some behaviors, such as hitting a sibling or intentionally breaking something, may require an immediate timeout.

Assure your child that you will not remove privileges if he or she shares a problem or concern with you.

Take action As a parent, you can take steps to protect your child by saving evidence of bullying and staying connected with your child's teachers, coaches and school staff:

▶ *Record the details.* Write down the date or dates of bullying incidents, who was involved and what specifically happened. Save screenshots, emails and texts. Record the facts as objectively as possible.

▶ *Stay in touch with school staff.* It helps to have a rapport with your child's teachers or coaches from the beginning of the school year so that you feel comfortable asking about your child's social interactions, including bullying situations, in addition to academics and sports. Your child's school guidance counselor or principal also can be helpful in dealing with bullying.

▶ *Explain your concerns in a matter-of-fact way.* Instead of laying blame, ask for help to solve the bullying problem. Bring your own written record of the bullying that's taken place so that you can refer to it. Take notes during these meetings and keep in contact with school officials. If the bullying continues, be persistent.

▶ *Ask for a copy of the school's policy on bullying.* Find out how bullying is addressed in the school's curriculum, as well as how staff members are obligated to respond to known or suspected bullying.

WHAT DOES A PERSON WHO BULLIES LOOK LIKE?

Stereotypes of bullies are plentiful. But it's not appearance that defines someone who bullies, it's their behavior. Because bullying is a behavior, it's important to distinguish between the child and the behavior. No child should be labeled a bully, but any child can engage in bullying behavior. According to PACER's National Bullying Prevention Center, the following characteristics are often associated with bullying behavior:

▶ Unwillingness to accept responsibility for personal behavior
▶ Lack of empathy for or understanding of others' feelings
▶ Being bullied
▶ Lack of social skills
▶ Desire to be in control
▶ Feelings of frustration, anxiety or depression
▶ Trying to fit in with a peer group that's perceived as bullying

If you notice some of these qualities in your child, work to change them. Changing behavior takes time but be patient. Show your child how to respect others' feelings, avoid shielding your child from the consequences of his or her decisions, and help your child learn appropriate social skills. Encourage positive friendships and clarify your family values. If necessary, find a counselor or mental health professional who your child can talk to.

▶ *Make other reports when necessary.* Report cyberbullying to internet and cellphone service providers. If your child has been physically attacked or otherwise threatened with harm, talk to school officials and call the police. Your child may feel hesitant about talking to authorities. While it's important to consider the impact it may have on your child, it's also important to keep your child safe.

If your child is bullying Any child can bully, and it can be surprising and distressing to find out that your child is the one doing it. But it's important to step back and take a deep breath before taking action. Careful thought and consideration is more likely to lead to a positive outcome.

Kids who bully often experience difficulties with school, depression, violence and other problems. Bullying behavior shouldn't be taken lightly. To address bullying behavior:

Take the time to find out why Children bully for many reasons. They might think it makes them cool, they may not realize the impact they're having or they may be bullied themselves. They may bully to deal with cooped up feelings of anger or frustration. To effectively address the bullying behavior, it helps to understand what's triggering the behavior.

Clarify expectations and consequences Your child needs to know from you that bullying is unacceptable behavior. You also need to explain what the consequences will be for engaging in bullying behavior. Be sure to follow through immediately and consistently on the expectations and consequences you've set. Chapter 16 has more information on encouraging positive behavior.

Make a plan Once you understand the situation, brainstorm with your child ways to make things better. Come up with a doable plan for next steps to change the bullying behavior. Think about who might be involved to help your child accomplish these goals. When your child shows positive changes, be sure to praise him or her.

Teach empathy and respect Help your child understand that everyone has feelings and that these feelings matter. Model this by treating your own child's feelings with compassion, as well as those of others. Help your child learn to think from another person's perspective to gain empathy. It may help to say, "Isaac, think about how you might feel if you were in Thad's situation." In addition, teach your child the importance of respecting another child's physical person and property. Boundaries will continue to be important throughout life.

Help your child cope with negative feelings If your child is struggling with negative emotions of his or her own — and people who bully often do — look for ways to help your child develop better ways of handling them. This may involve talking to a school counselor, teacher or religious leader in your community. Your child's medical provider or a mental health professional also can help your child learn how to understand and redirect emotions or internal struggles that may be behind the bullying behavior.

Just because bullying is common doesn't make it a natural or acceptable part of childhood. It's important to address it whenever it occurs. Both adults and children can help stop bullying from happening.

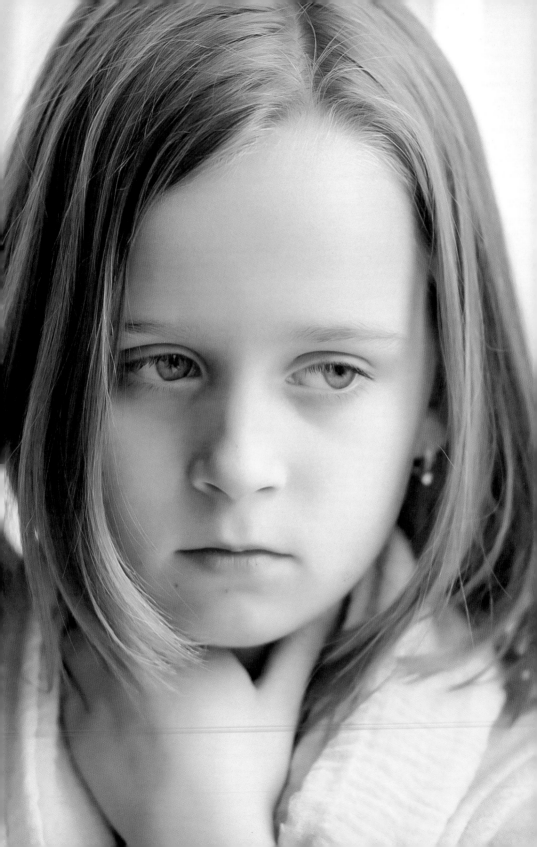

CHAPTER 19

Coping with tough times

Life has a way of throwing curveballs, often when you least expect it. Whether it's a move, divorce, job loss, illness or the death of a loved one, tough times can happen to anyone.

It can be particularly rough to see your child go through difficult circumstances. Many parents' fervent wish is to never have to see their children go through sadness, grief or anxiety. But that's a luxury rarely afforded.

While you can't prevent or eliminate hardship for your child, you can provide comfort and reassurance. You can give your child the mental and emotional tools he or she needs to transition through these experiences and emerge stronger on the other side. It's not unusual for families to report that times of adversity have made their family relationships closer and more meaningful. Positive outcomes are possible.

This chapter offers suggestions for responding to a child's needs when a family is faced with some of life's more difficult challenges.

MOVING

Relocation, whether by choice or because of unexpected circumstances, is a common experience for many families. While the idea of a move can be exciting, it can also create worry and stress for your child. If your family's planning to move, your son or daughter may be focused on what he or she is about to lose — close friends, a sense of belonging at school, and extracurricular activities that he or she is involved in. Your child might worry about finding new friends, what his or her new school will be like, and how he or she will fit in. These are pretty common concerns for any child.

Preparing your child During this time of transition, it's important to acknowledge and empathize with your child's feelings. But stay optimistic. Talk about the experiences you'll have living in a new place. Explain how meeting and getting to know new kids can be fun. Brainstorm on new traditions that you

WHEN A PARENT LOSES A JOB

The loss of a job can be devastating for a parent and create a financial strain on the family. To protect a child from this difficult reality, some parents instinctively want to hide the bad news. Kids, though, can quickly sense when something's wrong or different.

If a job loss in your family is going to affect your financial situation, tell your child the basics of what's going on. You don't need to share all the details. You might say, "Mom's not working right now, so we'll have to cut back on extras for a while." Your son or daughter might still grumble about being denied certain clothes or toys, but at least he or she will understand why now's not a good time to buy those things. If you don't explain what's going on, your child might sense the tension and think he or she has done something wrong.

While it's important to share the job loss with your child, it's also important that you make the communication a two-way street. Allow your child to express his or her feelings about what your family is going through and encourage him or her to share fears or concerns. Provide reassurance that you'll make it through the experience as a family.

can develop. Remind your child that he or she can still maintain old friendships while making new friends.

If your son or daughter has had academic or social problems in his or her current school, a move could provide a fresh start. Be positive, but avoid unreasonable expectations that might invite disappointment. Your child's personality will still be the same in a new town.

To help ease your child's worries, take time out from packing and planning every so often to play with your child or do something fun together. Have your child read books that involve families moving. Or seek out your child's help in picking the color for his or her new room.

If possible, before you make the move, visit your new home and community with your child. To help increase excitement about the move, scout out new places or restaurants you might want to

visit once you've moved. Or sign your child up for activities or events that he or she enjoys or would look forward to.

Keeping up old connections After you've settled, help your child stay in touch with old friends. If possible, visit your old neighborhood from time to time or host old friends at your new home. Help your child reach out to friends by phone, video chat, letters and email. As your child adjusts to the changes a move can bring, make sure he or she feels your support.

DIVORCE

When parents decide to divorce, it can feel to a child like his or her world has turned upside down. Yet thousands of

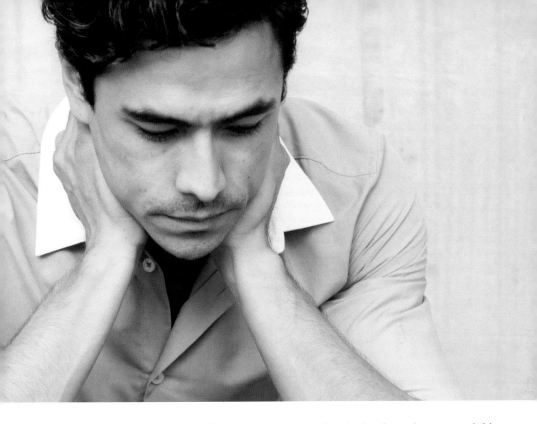

American kids go through a divorce each year and still grow up loved and supported.

An important way that you can support your child's adjustment is by interacting responsibly with your spouse. Sometimes, that may mean placing your child's needs ahead of your own wishes or desires.

Breaking the news Find a time when you and your spouse can sit down together with your child. Speaking honestly and simply, explain that you're getting a divorce. You can skip the details, but be sure to acknowledge that the experience will be sad. Encourage your child to share his or her feelings, worries and questions.

Make sure your child understands that divorce is only between adults. Remind your child — repeatedly — that he or she did nothing to cause the divorce

and that both of you love your child as much as ever. Consider telling your child's teacher, school counselor and medical provider about the divorce. They can observe your child, keep you updated on any concerns and offer guidance.

Easing the transition As you work out custody arrangements and other details, try to always keep in mind that your child needs both parents. Strive to avoid a long custody battle, which might affect your child's well-being and mental health. Instead, help your child maintain a strong, loving relationship with both parents as you and your former spouse work toward meeting common parenting goals.

During divorce proceedings, your child might be worried about a number of immediate concerns. Where will I live? Do I need to change schools? Who will take me to swimming lessons? As much as possible, keep up your child's regular routine. Knowing what to expect will help your child feel more secure.

As the reality of the divorce settles in, you might expect a variety of reactions, depending on your child's age. A pre-school-age child might need extra help understanding that he or she didn't cause the divorce and that nothing he or she does can bring you and your former spouse back together. School-age children might express more anger. They might worry about what will happen to your family, assign blame, and fantasize about you and your former spouse getting back together.

Smoothing the way after divorce
How your child adjusts after your divorce largely depends on how you and your former spouse communicate and cooperate with each other as co-parents. To show respect for your child's relationship with your former spouse:

- Don't speak badly about your former spouse in front of your child.
- Don't expect your child to choose sides.
- Don't argue or discuss child support issues in front of your child.
- Don't pump your child for information about your former spouse.
- Don't use your child as a pawn to hurt your former spouse.
- Don't interrupt your child's time with your former spouse.

It might be tempting to ease up on family rules while your child grieves the divorce, but this may inadvertently create more insecurity for your child. Children thrive on consistency, structure and routine — even if they insist on testing boundaries and limits.

If your child shares time between two households, try to maintain similar rules and routines in both homes. Ideally,
school and extracurricular schedules, daily chores and responsibilities, and family and friend connections should all remain as unchanged as possible.

If you notice that your child is having trouble coping, consider that he or she may benefit from talking with a mental health professional.

SERIOUS ILLNESS

When a family member develops a life-threatening or terminal illness, it can create a deep sense of uncertainty and insecurity in a child. By offering reassurance, stability and age-appropriate information, you and other trusted adults can provide vital support during this challenging time and ensure that your child continues to thrive.

Sharing the diagnosis Telling a child about a family member's illness can be one of the hardest hurdles to face. You want to protect your child from hurt and pain, and it's difficult to know where to even begin sometimes.

Start by setting aside some quiet, un-interrupted time to talk with your child. Be honest about the diagnosis, how the illness will be treated and how it will affect your child's life.

Keep in mind that children, particularly younger children, don't understand illness and death in the same way adults do, so typically they don't experience the shock, anxiety or fear that adults do.

On the other hand, they may see themselves as the cause of the illness. Make sure that your child understands that nothing he or she did or thought caused the illness, and that your child will continue to be loved and cared for no matter what happens.

Encouraging open communication

Encourage your child to ask questions and talk about his or her worries and fears. You may find that your child has misconceptions about the illness or needs help coping with specific concerns. Your child should also be encouraged to share what he or she has heard or learned from others about the illness so that you can help sort out what's true and what's not.

Questions about death can be especially difficult for both parent and child. It may help to admit that this is a time of uncertainty and that uncertainty can be hard to deal with. Ask your child if he or she has specific concerns about what would happen if the person who is sick were to die. Reassure your child that he or she will still be loved and cared for regardless of any possible outcome.

If your child wants to visit the loved one in a hospital, encourage a visit. Your partner or another adult can help you prepare your child beforehand by describing what your son or daughter will see, such as what the person may look like and whether he or she will be attached to things such as IV tubes or oxygen. Let your child stay as long or as little as he or she wants. Afterward, be sure to find out whether your child has any questions about the visit.

Maintaining stability As much as possible, carry on with your child's normal schedule. Let your child know that it's OK to keep up with his or her regular activities and lean on other trusted adults for help. Alert your child's teachers, counselors, coaches and clergy members about what's going on. The goal is to maintain as much stability in your child's life as possible. If you and your partner are feeling overwhelmed, ask other family members to bridge the gap for your child. Don't hesitate to seek professional help if needed.

Understanding anticipatory grief

Children who endure a loved one's extended illness may experience what's called anticipatory grief — living with the loss of qualities and anticipated death of a loved one who's still alive but has undergone significant changes or may be psychologically absent. This can go on for weeks, months and even years.

Anticipatory grief often involves four phases: feeling intensely sad, feeling extreme concern for the dying person, preparing for death and adjusting to changes caused by the death. But not every child experiences all of these phases or goes through them in the same way.

To help your child through this journey, find ways to help him or her identify and process his or her feelings. Your child might benefit from drawing pictures, painting, or illustrating his or her story.

Reading a book or story about someone going through a similar experience can be helpful to some. Reading aloud to young children creates an opportunity to spend time together and opens up room for a discussion of feelings. There are many suitable books for different ages. *Charlotte's Web,* by E.B. White, is an example of a story about moving through the cycle of life. Ask your local librarian for a reference list or search online for the National Association of School Psychologists' list of books recommended for children coping with loss or trauma.

LOSS AND GRIEF

Losing a loved one in childhood is one of life's toughest challenges, whether it's the loss of a family member, a friend or even a beloved pet. For a parent, it can be tempting to intervene or help your child avoid feeling pain. But it's important to

HOW CHILDREN GRIEVE

Among the many factors that influence how your child will grieve, age and development play a critical role in the symptoms you might observe.

Age	Understanding of death	Signs and symptoms
3 to 6 years old	Children in this age range have a hard time grasping that death is final and not temporary. They may talk about the loved one as coming back or sleeping.	• Tantrums • Irritable behavior • Feelings of guilt and shame, thinking that their past actions were a potential cause of death • Difficulty sleeping • Loss of appetite • Poor bladder and bowel control
6 to 9 years old	At this age, children may view death as final, but they're often frightened by it. They may worry that you or other people close to them will die too.	• Fears about going to school • Aggression • Fear of getting sick • Fear of abandonment
9 years and older	Children ages 9 and above start to understand and accept that death is final and can't be changed. Eventually, they'll understand that death is a normal part of life.	• Fear of rejection • Changes in appetite or eating habits • Trouble sleeping • Loss of interest in activities or hobbies • Increased impulsivity • Survival guilt

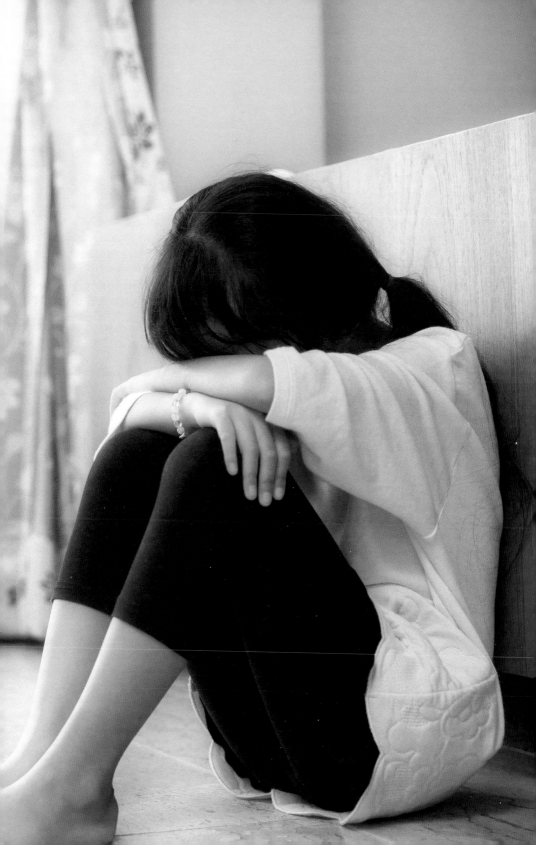

respect the unique way your child experiences the loss and give him or her plenty of time to move through grief.

Being honest Talk to your child about what's happened in an honest way that avoids euphemisms such as "passing away." While this kind of language may seem easier to use, indirect expressions of death can be confusing to children.

Instead, be direct yet kind. Allow your child to talk about feelings such as anger, shock, helplessness or sadness. And don't be afraid to show that you're sad too. Exposing some of your pain might make it easier for your child to open up about his or her grief.

Losing someone close The death of a parent or sibling can be especially traumatic. Losing a parent can make a child revert to younger behaviors. It can bring about feelings of anxiety, anger and depression. The loss of a sibling can cause a child to feel guilty for the times they didn't get along. A child might also experience survival guilt, wondering why he or she is still alive and the sibling isn't. Unanticipated deaths can be harder to cope with, since your child might not have had the chance to say goodbye.

If your child's having trouble coping with the loss, struggling with fears of separation from a surviving parent or showing excessive sadness, talk to your child's medical provider. Your child might need help from a mental health professional to deal with his or her grief.

Parents often have questions about whether a child should attend the funeral or memorial service for a loved one. If the child wants to go, that's OK — it may help him or her process the loss. But there's also no need to force a child to go. Instead, you might look for an alternate way to memorialize the loved one, such

as lighting a candle, saying a prayer or looking over photographs.

Handling grief Children tend to experience grief somewhat differently than adults. Instead of going through grief as a constant or step-by-step process, children tend to have reactions to death based on their age and other factors, including their personality and maturity level, the circumstances of the death, and the family dynamics during grief.

If your child shows symptoms of grief one moment and appears normal the next, don't worry — this is a pretty normal pattern of grief in children. If it seems as if your child doesn't care, doesn't understand what happened or is avoiding grief altogether, bear in mind that a child's grief will ebb and flow — a sign of his or her age and coping abilities.

MASS TRAGEDIES AND OTHER EVENTS

When a mass tragedy — such as a natural disaster, mass shooting or terrorist attack — comes to the attention of your child, you can help your child comprehend what's happened, feel safe, and cope with his or her emotions by taking the following steps. Keep in mind that if your child doesn't know about an event or hasn't heard anything about it, it's not always necessary to tell him or her.

Discussing what's happened It can be difficult to find the right words to address an event that may have left you feeling shocked even as a grown-up. But talking about it can help children process and cope with upsetting information. You might want to start by asking what your child already knows about the event —

and what questions or concerns he or she might have. Let your child's response guide your discussion. Be a good listener.

When you talk, tell the truth and remain calm. Focus on the basics, giving your child accurate, age-appropriate information. Share your own thoughts, and remind your son or daughter that you're there for him or her. Reassure your child that what happened isn't his or her fault.

Some children don't want to talk about a traumatic event, and that's OK. Avoid pressuring them to do so. Let them come to terms with the event on their own, but monitor for any signs of distress.

If your child experiences persistent anxiety, sadness or difficulty engaging in everyday life, get help from your child's medical provider or a mental health professional.

Offering comfort A child's age will affect how he or she processes information about a tragic event and handles the stress.

Preschool children might become clingy or mimic your emotions. Some children might also revert to wetting the bed or sucking their thumbs. Avoid criticizing your child for this behavior. To talk to a preschool child about a disturbing event, get down to his or her eye level. Speak in a calm and gentle voice using words your child understands. Explain what happened and how it might affect your child. Share steps that are being taken to keep your child safe, and give plenty of hugs.

School-age children might fear going to school, have trouble paying attention in class or become aggressive for no clear reason. They might also have nightmares or other sleep problems. Consider letting your child sleep with a light on or sleep in your room for a short time. Extra cuddles might help too. When talking to your school-age child, help him or her separate fiction from reality. Reassure your child that he or she is safe.

Helping your child move forward
Regardless of your child's age, you can help your child process what's happened by doing the following:

▶ Limiting your child's exposure to media coverage of the event.
▶ Maintaining your child's routines.
▶ Encouraging your child to talk about what he or she is feeling.
▶ Doing something for those affected by the tragedy.

Feeling sad, scared and confused after a mass tragedy is normal. However, if your child continues to be distressed for more than two to four weeks or if your child has experienced previous trauma, he or she may need more help coping. Talk to your child's medical provider about your concerns, or seek the help of a mental health professional.

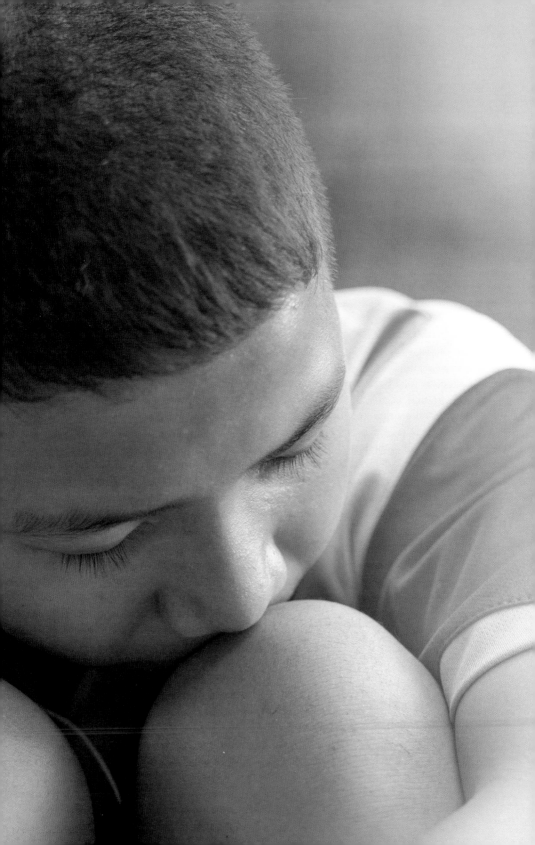

CHAPTER 20

Mental health concerns

Sometimes parents become concerned that there's more to a child's worries or irritable moods than just a bad day. Mental and emotional health concerns can arise throughout early childhood and into adolescence, and it's not always easy to tell what exactly is going on.

Sometimes issues come up around specific life events, such as a move to a different city or the loss of a loved one. Other times, a child may experience ongoing emotional or behavioral challenges, such as chronic depression, anxiety or outbursts of anger.

If your child is struggling with an emotional or behavioral health concern — or even if you suspect that something isn't exactly right — it's important to address it and seek help early on. Being aware of your child's emotional state and knowing when to seek help is a big part of being an effective parent. It's never a sign of parental failure to get help for emotional concerns — you would do the same if your child had a condition such as asthma or diabetes.

Treatment is available from professionals who are trained to help children and adolescents learn how to handle their thoughts, feelings and behaviors. In addition, at-home remedies and supportive routines can offer the stabilizing environment that encourages emotional health in growing children. In some circumstances, medication can be helpful in addition to therapy.

Seeking help when your son or daughter needs it can equip your child to be stronger and more resilient now, as well as later in life. Not only that, it can help make your family life stronger and more functional.

ANXIETY

Every child has worries and fears. In fact, children's fears often follow a developmental pattern. During the preschool years, children may fear many things, including separation from their parents,

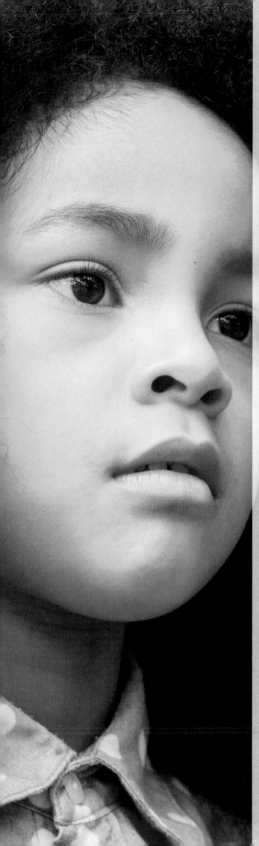

loud noises, monsters or the dark. As children move into the school-age years, fears tend to become more abstract, such as the death of a parent, intruders in the home or growing up. As children get older, they may be more reluctant to share these fears. During adolescence, children often have fears related to their social abilities, such as being rejected by peers or talking to a member of another sex. Failing at school and getting injured are also common fears.

A certain level of anxiety is normal and healthy. Every child becomes anxious from time to time. Anxiety becomes a problem when it persists or interferes with your child's ability to participate in daily life — to do well at home and at school, and to make friends. In this situation, your child may need help understanding that he or she is experiencing a lot of "false alarm" fear reactions to situations other children would consider non-threatening. He or she may also need help learning how to work through these emotions.

Symptoms of anxiety Anxiety in children can take different forms. If your child has generalized anxiety, you might notice that he or she worries a lot, often about unlikely problems. Your child might feel tense or nervous, or as if something bad is going to happen — such as someone in the family getting sick or someone breaking into the house — even when there are few reasons to feel this way.

Other children may have social anxiety, where they feel distressed being around other people or strangers. For these kids, going to school can be a challenge. For other kids, separation anxiety remains an issue beyond the normal separation anxiety of early childhood. Less commonly, a child may have a panic disorder or a specific fear (phobia).

Children with anxiety often have a hard time sleeping. Your child may talk about lying in bed a long time without falling asleep or not being able to "turn her brain off." Some children may have difficulty falling asleep without a parent nearby.

Feeling overly fearful, stressed or worried may lead children to hold back from favorite activities. In addition, children who are feeling distressed will often report headaches or stomachaches, which can also be signs of an anxiety disorder. A school nurse or teacher might observe these signs before you do.

When to seek help If anxious feelings last longer than you think is normal, are distressing to you or your child, or get in the way of daily life, talk to your child's medical provider. The provider may want to rule out any physical health issues that may be contributing to your child's anxiety. If there is an underlying problem, treating it may help ease some of your child's symptoms.

Your child's medical provider may also conduct an evaluation for childhood anxiety. This evaluation is based on questionnaires you or your child fill out and face-to-face interviews the provider has with you, your child, and your spouse or partner. The provider will ask about your child's symptoms and how they've affected your child and your family.

In some cases, the provider may refer you to a specialist in mental health conditions, such as a licensed counselor, psychologist or psychiatrist.

Treatment options Research shows that cognitive behavioral therapy (CBT) is one of the most effective treatments for anxiety in children (see page 288). Particularly helpful is a form of CBT known as exposure therapy. The goal of this kind of therapy is for your child to learn through guided experience that his or her fears are unlikely to happen and that he or she can handle feeling uncomfortable. For some children, an anti-anxiety medication may be recommended in addition to therapy.

Exposure therapy During exposure therapy, a therapist guides your child through a process of exposure to triggers that typically induce anxiety in your child, over time helping him or her to respond in a healthier way.

For example, if your child is afraid of dogs, a therapist might begin by showing your child a picture of a dog. After a gradual progression, your child may practice petting live dogs. Or if your child has a social phobia, he or she might go through a progression of talking to acquaintances, then strangers.

The goal of exposure therapy is not only to reduce excessive feelings of anxiety but also to help the child learn to tolerate anxiety or discomfort. Exposure therapy may be done in an individual or a group setting.

Medication Exposure therapy is generally considered the most effective treatment for anxiety in children. But if it's not enough, an anti-anxiety medication, such as a selective serotonin reuptake inhibitor (SSRI), may help ease symptoms. SSRIs are associated with more side effects than CBT.

Helping your child manage anxiety
Therapy can be very effective in helping kids with anxiety disorders. But you also can help your child at home:

Let your child work through it As a parent, it's important to provide information and support in situations that would

WHAT IS COGNITIVE BEHAVIORAL THERAPY?

Cognitive behavioral therapy (CBT) is a specific type of psychotherapy that's used to treat many mental health conditions, including anxiety and depression. Adults, adolescents and children can benefit from CBT. Young children — under age 7, for example — may not have developed the thinking and reasoning (cognitive) skills yet that CBT requires. Nonetheless, CBT often can be adapted for younger kids to be used with the help of their parents.

Cognitive behavioral therapy is based on the principle that your thoughts, feelings and actions have a powerful effect on one another. In particular, negative thoughts or patterns of self-talk can promote feelings of fear, hopelessness and helplessness. These feelings in turn can make you behave in ways that reinforce negative thoughts and subsequent feelings, creating a harmful distress cycle.

For example, your child may be anxious at lunchtime at school. She may enter the lunchroom believing that no one will want talk to her and that no one will like her. As a result, she moves to sit by herself. Others assume she wants to be left alone, and the cycle continues.

Some kids get stuck in these distress cycles and are unable to break out of them, so they become chronically anxious or depressed. CBT can help break the cycle by helping a child learn how to actively handle fears. CBT can help a child:

- Identify situations (triggers) that lead to distress
- Recognize when negative thoughts pop up
- Actively change his or her behavior to boost confidence and feel better
- Use newfound knowledge and experience to challenge and replace negative thoughts

For some conditions such as anxiety or obsessive-compulsive disorder, CBT also includes exposure therapy. Exposure therapy gradually brings a child closer to an anxiety-producing trigger, such as insects or large groups of people. Through repeated exposure and readjusting negative thought processes, the child becomes increasingly confident in his or her ability to handle the trigger.

LUNCH BAG

cause any child to be anxious — such as moving to a new school or dealing with friendship problems. But avoid trying to remove all anxiety triggers or offering continuous reassurance about commonplace issues. If you do, you'll deprive your child of opportunities to face and deal with uncomfortable feelings — things your child will get better at over time.

Test the hypothesis Encourage your child to test the reasoning behind his or her fear. For example, have your child ask, what's the worst that can happen if I order directly from the server at a restaurant rather than asking mom or dad to do it? Or together, role-play buying lunch in the school cafeteria. Help your child gain the confidence to effectively deal with anxiety, rather than always working to avoid it.

Offer plenty of warm support When your child is trying to face his or her fears, give lots of warm support. Let your child express his or her feelings without judgment or criticism. Offer to help your child come up with a plan to address his or her worries, such as breaking down a task into smaller, more manageable steps. Help your child see that most problems, though seemingly huge, are temporary or solvable.

Maintain the basics Adding stability to daily life can minimize worries about what's happening next and help your child feel greater control over his or her circumstances. Make sure your child gets enough sleep, eats regular nutritious meals, and has enough time for homework, chores and playtime. Treatment approaches will have a better chance of success when your child is supported with consistency and stability at home and at school.

OBSESSIVE-COMPULSIVE DISORDER

Kids often develop specific habits and routines for doing things and form their own unique beliefs about the world and themselves. This is a normal part of childhood development. But if you notice behaviors or beliefs that start to become repetitive or intrusive, it could be a sign of obsessive-compulsive disorder (OCD).

What does OCD look like? Symptoms of OCD often start with repeated, upsetting thoughts or mental images (obsessions). These can range from worrying about germs to having thoughts that may be disturbing or inappropriate. As a result, children with OCD may feel ashamed or that something is wrong with them. To try to get rid of these obsessions, children may perform certain behaviors, such as:

◗ Washing their hands or cleaning themselves to alleviate a fear of germs or sickness
◗ Repeatedly checking locks or doors if they're afraid of danger or intruders
◗ Excessively arranging or organizing items to meet the need for symmetry or perfection
◗ Counting or repeating certain things
◗ Repeatedly asking parents or others for reassurance

The ritual makes the child feel better, so the ritual is repeated whenever the thought comes up. But the relief provided by the ritual is temporary and precludes the child from learning that he or she can manage the distressing thoughts without the ritual, leading to a perpetual cycle.

Even though obsessions and compulsions are typically linked, there could be compulsions your child acts out that won't make sense to you, such as tapping, arranging items in precise patterns or avoiding certain numbers. People with OCD often feel a strong need to perform a compulsive action to prevent something bad from happening. They also may do it as a way to feel "just right."

If you notice such behaviors in your child or suspect that your child is struggling with obsessive thoughts, it's important to make an appointment with your child's medical provider for an evaluation. Understand that while these intrusive thoughts and images can be very disturbing to your child, they don't mean that your child is deviant or that he or she wants to do these things. On the contrary, a child with OCD performs compulsive rituals and behaviors to try to get rid of the thoughts. OCD can be disabling, but it also responds well to treatment.

Diagnosing OCD As many as half of all people with OCD are first diagnosed in childhood. While symptoms of OCD can crop up in younger children, most symptoms begin around age 10. Boys are most commonly diagnosed between ages 7 and 12; girls in adolescence.

The first step to getting help is to schedule an appointment with your child's medical provider, who may refer you to a mental health expert. An evaluation for OCD may include:

▶ Discussions with the parent and child
▶ Age-appropriate questionnaires
▶ Testing for co-occurring disorders, such as anxiety or depression

It's common for two or more mental health conditions to occur alongside each other, and each should be treated separately.

Treating OCD A variation of exposure therapy called exposure and response prevention therapy (ERP) is usually the first line of treatment for symptoms of OCD in children.

Exposure and response prevention therapy ERP allows a therapist to guide your child through a process of exposure to situations that trigger fears or obsessive thoughts. Studies show that repeated exposure to anxiety-provoking scenarios result in decreased anxiety over time. Similar therapy is used to treat anxiety disorders.

With OCD, the second component of ERP — response prevention — seeks to break the connection between the obsession and the compulsive response. It involves guiding your child away from performing rituals. For example, if your child is worried about germs, the therapist may gradually help your child go from being near something your child considers germy, such as a coin or a door knob, to eventually handling it. The response prevention part of the equation would involve not washing or sanitizing hands afterward. The therapist might stand with your child near the perceived germ source until the compulsion has passed. As this process is repeated over time, your child will learn to feel less anxious about passing thoughts and more in control of his or her actions.

Medication Most children do well with ERP. But if behavioral therapy isn't providing adequate relief or if symptoms interfere with behavioral therapy, medications — such as a SSRI — may be recommended in addition to ERP.

Parenting a child with OCD Coping with childhood OCD can be a challenge not just for your child but for the whole family. Although the condition may feel all-consuming, it may help to remember that your child is more than his or her OCD. Even small steps to support your child's progress toward mental and emotional wholeness can help.

WHAT ARE TICS?

Some children make sounds or body movements without meaning to. These involuntary actions are called tics. They can happen one at a time or all at once, and can be difficult for a child to stop or control.

Tics appear in many forms, but can look like:

▶ Rapid eye blinking
▶ Throat clearing
▶ Movement of the face, hands or legs
▶ Jumping
▶ Shaking the head

Tics may be triggered by a number of factors, including caffeine consumption, seizure disorders and stress, to name a few. While tics can be embarrassing or uncomfortable in social situations, most tics are not harmful and get better over time, with many going away completely by adulthood.

A specific type of tic disorder is Tourette syndrome — a chronic condition that causes both movement-oriented (motor) and vocal tics that are beyond the child's control. Tourette syndrome is believed to be caused by multiple factors, including genetic and environmental factors. Signs and symptoms typically develop around age 6 and usually before age 11. Tourette syndrome is more common in boys than in girls. It often occurs along with other conditions such as OCD or ADHD.

What to do If you notice that your child has a persistent tic, consider reviewing symptoms with your child's medical provider. The provider can help your family understand the condition and guide you to treatment options, if needed.

If tics aren't bothersome, your child may not need any treatment other than support and understanding of the disorder. But if he or she is having problems at school or making friends, treatment such as comprehensive behavioral intervention for tics (CBIT) may help. CBIT teaches your child to recognize an oncoming tic and perform a separate, more appropriate action until the tic urge passes. For example, a throat-clearing tic may be countered with slow, rhythmic breathing.

Certain medications can minimize severe tics. If a tic involves a single body area, onabotulinumtoxinA (Botox) injections can calm or block nerve signals to the affected muscles.

Support for your child As a parent, you can help your child by:

▶ Not getting angry or shaming your child for the behavior or vocal expression
▶ Not giving tics a lot of attention
▶ Expecting your child to continue meeting his or her responsibilities, such as chores and schoolwork, despite tics
▶ Talking with your child's school about learning options that may be available, such as support staff for your child or an individualized education program (IEP) (see page 470)

MENTAL HEALTH PROFESSIONALS

When looking for someone to help your child with an emotional or a behavioral concern, seek out a qualified professional who has training and experience in caring specifically for children. Most of the time, psychotherapy is preferred over medicine as a first step in treating children. Mental health experts generally include:

Psychologists A psychologist has a doctoral degree in psychology or counseling and is trained in psychotherapy. All states license psychologists, who may also be certified by the American Board of Professional Psychology. Psychologists use testing and other methods to help diagnose, evaluate and treat individuals with psychological problems. They use various forms of psychotherapy, but in most states they can't prescribe medications. Child psychologists specialize in helping children and adolescents with mental health concerns.

Psychiatrists A psychiatrist is a medical doctor who has had at least four years of specialty training after earning a doctor of medicine (M.D.) degree. Psychiatrists must be licensed to practice medicine in the state in which they work, and most are certified by the American Board of Psychiatry and Neurology. Psychiatrists are qualified to carry out many aspects of treatment, including prescribing medication. They also lead treatment teams in hospitals. Child and adolescent psychiatrists have extra training in child and adolescent mental health and behaviors.

Social workers A clinical social worker must have a master's degree in social work and be licensed or certified by the state in which he or she practices. To be designated a licensed clinical social worker (L.C.S.W.) or a licensed independent clinical social worker (L.I.C.S.W.), candidates usually undergo supervised training in psychotherapy. Licensed clinical social workers can provide therapy, although they can't prescribe medications. They may also help coordinate your child's care and make sure you and your child have access to available resources. Your child's school may employ a licensed clinical social worker as a counselor.

Advanced practice prescribers Advanced practice prescribers include individuals such as nurses and physician assistants who have advanced training in medical care. A psychiatric nurse has a degree in nursing, is licensed as a registered nurse (R.N.) and has additional experience in psychiatry. A clinical nurse specialist (C.N.S.) has a bachelor's degree in nursing, is licensed as an R.N., and holds a master's degree in psychiatric and mental health nursing or a related field. A nurse practitioner (N.P.) or a physician assistant (P.A.) also may work in psychiatry. They both have advanced training in physical assessment, physiology, pharmacology and physical diagnosis. They may prescribe medications.

Simplify Because OCD can demand a lot of energy and treatment can be time-consuming, some parents find it helpful to simplify things at home. Whether this means putting extra activities temporarily on hold or saying yes to fewer commitments, simplifying your routine can help reduce the stress you feel while coping with an already difficult disorder. However, it's also important to avoid putting your family's life on hold just to accommodate the disorder.

Help your child overcome compulsions Consistency is key. If your child is in exposure therapy and is working to overcome compulsions, you can help your son or daughter at home by reinforcing the same practices learned in therapy.

Model healthy behavior As your child works to find new, healthier ways of handling frequent intrusive thoughts or worries, it can help your child to see you respond with a calm and loving reaction. It will help reinforce new thinking patterns and may even help your child reduce compulsions by seeing a new way of responding.

DEPRESSION

Maybe you've noticed your child has been feeling particularly sad or out of sorts for a few weeks. It's certainly normal for any child to feel down from time to time. And every child has his or her own unique temperament and demeanor — there's no universal ideal of a "happy kid." But if you notice that sad feelings or isolating behaviors linger for more than a couple of weeks or are hampering your child's ability to function, it may be that your child is experiencing depression.

DEPRESSION AND SUICIDE

As your child gets older, depression becomes a risk factor for suicide. It can be hard to acknowledge that your child might be having thoughts tied to suicide, but it's important to face it head on. A healthy conversation between you and your child can help you assess what's really going on in your child's mind and can be an important step to getting your child the help he or she needs.

Despite some beliefs, talking about suicide will not bring up or promote an idea that a child hasn't thought of before. If you're having a hard time with the conversation, simply ask your child this: "Have you ever had thoughts about harming yourself?" or "Have you ever had thoughts about ending your life?"

Take your child's response seriously. If your child reports having these thoughts or feelings, talk to your child's care provider or counselor promptly. If your child is actively contemplating suicide, this is an emergency. Call 911 or emergency help, or take your child to the emergency department.

Although depression doesn't occur as often in children as it does in adults or even adolescents, it can still have a big impact. A child with depression may find it increasingly difficult to function at school and at home, and may become disconnected from important relationships. If left untreated, depression can continue or worsen, and may be associated with school and social difficulties, substance use, and suicide.

On the other hand, children with depression can get better with the right treatment and support. This usually includes psychotherapy and sometimes medicine. Parent or family counseling also can be part of treatment, to help parents understand how best to help and support a child experiencing depression.

Recognizing depression One of the biggest symptoms of depression is feeling sad or irritable most or all of the time. But other signs and symptoms often are present. Signs and symptoms to watch for in your child include:

▶ *Withdrawal from family or friends.* Children with depression may begin to feel as if it's too much effort to play with friends or hang out with family. They may spend a lot of time in their rooms, away from others.

▶ *Loss of interest in favorite activities.* This includes uncharacteristic behaviors such as quitting a sport or after-school activity your child previously enjoyed or avoiding play dates or sleepovers with good friends.

▶ *Physical complaints.* Children may not have reached an emotional maturity level that allows them to tell the difference between emotional and physical pain. Instead of talking about feeling sad, they may complain of feeling sick or having a headache.

▶ *Changes in appetite or weight.* Your child may not show much interest in eating, or conversely, may snack more than usual. Some kids with depression lose weight; others gain weight. Or some fail to gain weight and grow as expected for their age.

FAMILY THERAPY

Often, it's hard for just one family member to make changes, especially when certain patterns of behavior — in both children and parents — have become ingrained in family life. Family therapy may be used in treating a variety of diagnoses, including depression, anxiety, behavior problems and eating disorders.

The therapist works with the family to take a fresh look at how family members interact and to change patterns that are causing problems. Therapy sessions might include learning to communicate better with each other through active listening and regulating emotional reactions.

Therapists also help family members learn to problem-solve together by understanding the problem, setting achievable goals, brainstorming solutions, developing and implementing an action plan, and evaluating how well that plan is working. Evidence suggests that, for a number of conditions, family therapy helps kids recover faster and stay in remission longer.

▶ *Sleep problems.* You might observe changes in your child's sleep patterns, such as sleeping during the day, feeling restless, waking up in the middle of the night or having difficulty falling asleep. Children with depression often say they feel tired. You might notice it's harder to wake your child in the morning.

▶ *Lack of energy.* Children with depression may feel aimless, weighed down or low in energy.

▶ *Feelings of worthlessness.* Children with depression are often overly critical of themselves and express feelings of guilt, shame or worthlessness. They may compare themselves negatively with their friends, or even blame themselves for circumstances beyond their control.

▶ *Difficulty concentrating.* You might notice your child has trouble focusing and remembering, or processes information more slowly than before. This can often impact a child's school performance or learning ability.

▶ *Restlessness.* An increase in fidgety or hyperactive behavior may be a sign of internal agitation or distress when a child is depressed.

Sometimes, depression runs in families, meaning that some children are born with a genetic vulnerability to a condition such as depression. Life events — such as a divorce in the family, moving to a new city, or the loss of a friend or family member — also can trigger bouts of sadness that may become chronic and lead to depression in children. If your child continues showing signs of depression beyond a two-week period, talk to your child's medical provider.

Diagnosing depression If you suspect your child is dealing with depression, bring it up with your child's medical provider, who may make a referral to or work along with a mental health professional, such as a child psychiatrist or psychologist, counselor, or social worker.

An evaluation for childhood depression typically includes written and verbal assessments filled out by both you and your child, as well as in-person interviews with you, your child and close family members.

Treating childhood depression
Most kids with depression, as well as their families, benefit from some form of psychotherapy. This might include:

Cognitive behavioral therapy One of the most common forms of therapy for depression is cognitive behavioral therapy, or CBT (see page 288). CBT is also used for anxiety and other mental health conditions. The therapist helps your child identify and challenge negative or distorted thoughts and beliefs — such as unrealistic self-standards (perfectionism) or catastrophic thinking that consistently pictures bad outcomes to ordinary events — and replace them with more-positive and realistic perceptions. Your child also learns to cope and behave differently in response to redirected thoughts.

Interpersonal therapy Interpersonal therapy is another common form of psychotherapy. It involves learning communication and problem-solving skills to improve relationships. It can help your child learn to function in social situations with adults and other children. Interpersonal therapy can be especially helpful for dealing with unresolved grief or loss, conflicts with others, and transitions between different home settings.

Behavioral activation therapy Both adults and children with depression often avoid doing things they once enjoyed because of loss of interest. Behavioral activation therapy is a newer type of treatment that specifically targets this avoidant aspect of depression. There's evidence that it may be helpful in treating childhood depression and may have a positive effect on sleep. The therapy uses scheduled activities, along with positive reinforcement, to re-engage the child, reduce avoidant behaviors and improve mood. Parents help out by supporting the child in his or her chosen activities and problem-solving together to overcome obstacles to re-engagement.

Family therapy This option focuses on helping the whole family and is used for a range of mental health concerns in children, including depression. It may involve teaching the parents and other family members how to help the child with depression. It can also include ways to improve family dynamics (see page 295).

Medications If your child's symptoms are moderate to severe, your child's doctor or psychiatrist may prescribe an antidepressant such as fluoxetine (Prozac, Sarafem, others), which has been shown to improve symptoms in children between ages 7 and 17. Fluoxetine is a SSRI, a common drug used for depression, OCD and other mental health concerns. It can help improve mood and emotional regulation.

Combined therapy Sometimes a combination of psychotherapy and medications is used. Medications can be useful in the short term, while psychotherapy can teach your child and your family life-long skills for managing depressive thoughts and tendencies.

Periodically over the first few months of treatment, your child's medical provider will schedule visits to see how well the treatment is working and make adjustments as needed.

Treatment for depression typically involves long-term follow-up with your child's mental health team to watch for relapses and to provide "booster" therapy sessions as necessary.

Helping your child at home No matter what treatment option works best for your child, there are things you can do at home to help him or her start to feel better:

Keep a regular schedule As much as possible, maintain your child's normal schedule at home and at school. Stay on track with regular, nutritious meals. Have your child keep up with chores, homework and other family routines. This will give your child something concrete to do and help shift his or her focus away from negative thoughts and emotions.

Encourage physical playtime Not only is plenty of free playtime an important

BIPOLAR DISORDER

Bipolar disorder is a complex disease that many people don't understand well. It's known for extreme mood swings — high periods characterized by markedly elevated levels of excitement and activity, little need for sleep, and an exaggerated sense of self, interspersed with deep lows filled with feelings of sadness, hopelessness and apathy. These highs and lows, called episodes, may last for days or weeks.

Diagnosis of bipolar disorder in children can be challenging for several reasons. The disorder tends to unfold in a less standard way than it does in adults, so it's a little less predictable. Children may fluctuate more rapidly between moods during an episode, and it can be difficult to tell if symptoms are related to bipolar disorder or to another condition, such as depression or attention-deficit/hyperactivity disorder (ADHD). It's not uncommon for these conditions to occur together.

Add to that the difficulty children may have in describing their symptoms and the variable nature of childhood development in general, and you can start to see how it might be tough to make a firm diagnosis. Typically, bipolar disorder is diagnosed more often in the late teen years than in middle childhood.

Having a thorough assessment by a qualified professional is important, though, because an accurate diagnosis and appropriate treatment contribute to a better outcome. Treatment for bipolar disorder usually involves taking a mood-stabilizing medication, such as lithium (Lithobid). Although these medications are associated with increased risks and side effects, they can be appropriate in children when mood symptoms are severe.

Following recovery from bipolar episodes, children commonly continue medication maintenance treatment for another one to two years to prevent relapses. Many children and families also receive psychotherapy — which may include learning about bipolar disorder, how it's treated and how to manage symptoms — and family therapy to improve communication and problem-solving among family members.

factor in healthy growth and development, physical activity releases natural endorphins and serotonin, two chemicals in the brain that are known mood boosters. Encourage your child to play, especially with friends.

Uphold the importance of sleep Because sleep problems often accompany depression, finding a balanced sleep routine is critical. Try improving your child's sleep hygiene — turning off screens well ahead of bedtime, removing electronics from the bedroom, and adding books, cozy pajamas, a white noise machine or a new blanket. See Chapter 8 for more information on sleep.

Develop your child's support system While your relationship with your child remains a cornerstone of your child's social network, having other healthy adults in his or her life can be helpful, whether this is an aunt, an uncle or grandparent.

Promote fun with friends Social involvement is important to healthy growth and brain development in children. As depression symptoms improve, promote typical childhood activities that will help your child spend time with other kids, such as playing sports, trying a new hobby or having a play date with a close friend.

OPPOSITIONAL DEFIANT DISORDER

Even the best-behaved children can be difficult and challenging at times. But some kids may show a frequent and persistent pattern of anger, irritability, arguing, defiance or vindictiveness toward parents and other authority figures. If such patterns persist over a period of six months or longer, they may be part of a conditon called oppositional defiant disorder (ODD).

Oppositional defiant disorder is a complex problem. Multiple factors likely contribute to ODD, including genetics and a child temperament marked by difficulty regulating emotions. Sometimes, there's a home environment that's inconsistent, harsh, or characterized by parental difficulties with mental health or substance abuse. Attention from peers at school or inconsistent discipline from other authority figures in the child's life can reinforce negative behaviors.

Treatment of ODD usually involves helping parents learn skills to build positive family interactions and to manage problematic behaviors.

Symptoms of ODD Sometimes it's difficult to recognize the difference between a strong-willed or emotional child and one with oppositional defiant disorder. It's normal for a child to exhibit op-positional behavior at certain stages of development.

Signs of ODD generally begin during preschool years. Sometimes ODD may develop later, but almost always before the early teen years. These behaviors cause significant impairment of family life, social activities and school work.

A child with ODD displays some or most of these characteristics frequently over several months:

- Loses his or her temper
- Is easily annoyed by others
- Argues with adults or authority figures
- Deliberately annoys or upsets people
- Blames others for his or her mistakes
- Is spiteful or vindictive

Many children with ODD have other conditions, such as attention-deficit/hyperactivity disorder (ADHD), depression, anxiety or a learning disorder. Although it can be hard to distinguish symptoms of ODD from those of other conditions at times, it's important to recognize and treat each condition separately.

Finding help If your child shows behaviors that may indicate ODD or if you're concerned about your ability to parent a challenging child, seek help from a psychologist or a psychiatrist with expertise in disruptive behavior problems in children. Ask your child's medical provider to refer you to the appropriate professional.

Your child's evaluation will likely include an assessment of:

- Overall health
- Frequency and intensity of behaviors
- Emotions and behaviors across multiple settings and relationships
- Family life and interactions
- Strategies that have been helpful — or not helpful — in managing problem behaviors
- Presence of other mental health, learning or communication disorders

Treatment Treatment for ODD primarily involves parent-based interventions, but it may include other types of psychotherapy and training. Treatment often lasts for several months or longer.

It's also important to treat any other existing problems your child may have, such as anxiety or ADHD. Left untreated, these conditions can contribute to or aggravate symptoms of ODD.

Medications generally aren't used for ODD unless your child also has another condition. If your child has coexisting disorders, such as ADHD or depression, medications may help improve symptoms related to those conditions.

The cornerstones of treatment for ODD usually include:

Parent training A mental health professional with experience treating ODD can help you strengthen your parenting skills so that they're more consistent and positive and less frustrating for you and your child.

In some instances, your child may participate in this training with you, so everyone in your family develops shared goals for how to handle problems. Involving other authority figures, such as teachers, in the training may be an important part of treatment.

Parent-child interaction therapy (PCIT) is considered the gold standard of parent training. During PCIT, a therapist coaches parents while they interact with their child. In one approach, the therapist sits behind a one-way mirror and, using an "ear bug" audio device, guides parents through strategies that reinforce their child's positive behavior.

The desired result of PCIT is that parents learn more-effective parenting techniques, the quality of the parent-child relationship improves, and problem behaviors decrease.

Individual and family therapy Individual therapy for your child may help him or her learn to manage anger and express feelings in a healthier way. Family therapy may help family members learn better ways to communicate and interact (see page 295).

Problem-solving training This type of therapy is aimed at helping your child identify and change thought patterns that lead to behavior problems. Collaborative problem-solving — in which you and your child work together to come up with solutions that work for both of you — can help improve ODD-related problems.

Social skills training Your child also may benefit from therapy that will help him or her be more flexible and learn how to interact more positively and effectively with peers. It can be done individually or in a group setting. A group setting can be helpful because it allows your child to practice new skills and receive feedback.

Hang in there Although some parenting techniques may seem like common sense, learning to use them consistently in the face of opposition isn't easy, especially if there are other stressors at home. Learning these skills will require routine practice and patience.

Most important in treatment is for you to show consistent, unconditional love and acceptance of your child — even during difficult and disruptive situations. Don't be too hard on yourself. This process can be tough for even the most patient parents.

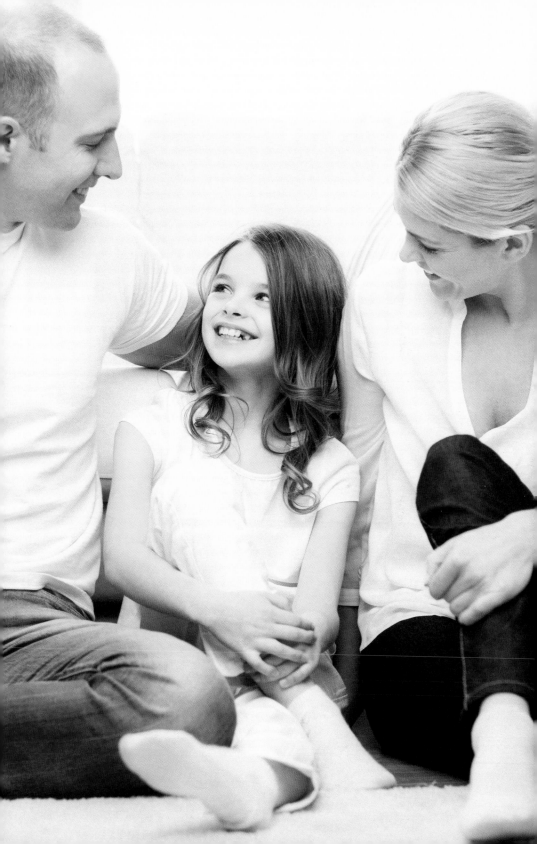

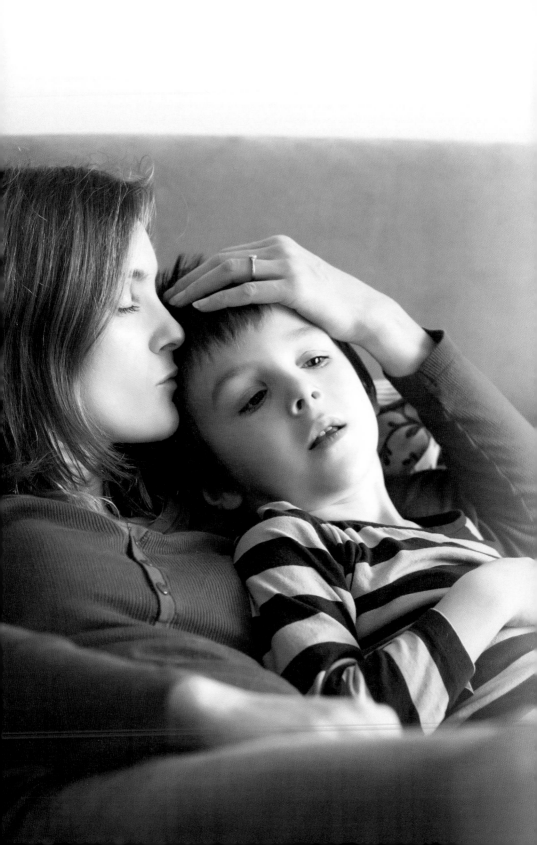

PART 5

Common illnesses and concerns

Colds, earaches, stomach bugs — these are all part of being a kid. The good news is that as children grow and develop, the frequency with which they get sick tends to decrease overall.

To be sure, there are some months of the year — especially with a preschooler — where you feel as if a stop at the doctor's office is a routine part of your week. But as your child continues to mature, his or her immune system becomes stronger and better adapted to the environment. By the time your child is in elementary school, you're likely to see your child's medical provider much less often for most common illnesses.

Even if your child does seem to fall prey to every virus that hits the block, don't let it worry you too much. If your child is active and growing, he or she is likely doing just fine. Your child's immune system will be exposed to many viruses before it develops its own immunity. In addition, following the recommended vaccination schedule for your child's age will help prevent infections.

Although serious disorders can occur in childhood, most common illnesses in preschool and school-age children don't have lasting consequences. At this age, children are extraordinarily resilient and their young bodies easily recover from most common conditions.

This part of the book contains helpful information on some of the more common illnesses and concerns that affect children. Sections on each condition tell you how serious an illness is, when to call for help and what you can do to care for your child at home.

Remember that you know your child best — including details about his or her current and previous illnesses and how he or she behaves when sick. You can tell when your child is feeling under the weather or not being his or her usual self. Trust your instincts. Parents' instincts about sick children are usually very good. When in doubt, reach out to your child's medical provider. Together, you can address most problems that come your child's way.

GIVING MEDICINE TO YOUR CHILD

When it comes to medications, whether for adults or children, the benefits of the medication must always be weighed against the risks. While some medications certainly can play a role in helping children feel better, many others do not. Plus, almost all drugs have potential side effects. So it's important to choose wisely when and what type of medication to give.

The general approach to over-the-counter medications in an otherwise healthy child is that they're rarely needed. If you do use nonprescription medications, use only those that are designed for children. Use them only when necessary and as indicated by your child's medical provider.

When giving your child medicine, follow these precautions:

Give the right dose Children's medicines usually come in liquid form but in different strengths based on the individual medicine. Use only the dispenser that came with the medication, and follow the directions on the label carefully so that you give your child the right dose. Avoid using cooking utensils, such as teaspoons, to measure out doses. If you know your child's weight, use that as a guide. See the dosage charts for acetaminophen (Tylenol, others) and ibuprofen (Advil, Motrin, others) on pages 478 and 479.

Avoid overdosing Avoid giving your child multiple medicines with the same active ingredient at the same time, such as a pain reliever and a decongestant, which can lead to an accidental overdose. Some parents alternate between pain relievers such as acetaminophen and ibuprofen, but this generally isn't recommended. Each medicine requires a specific interval between doses. Trying to keep the two straight may become confusing, and you may unintentionally overdose your child.

Avoid aspirin Aspirin is not recommended for children under age 18 because of its association with a serious illness called Reye's syndrome, which can damage the brain and liver. The risk is mostly associated with using aspirin to treat symptoms of a viral illness, such as the flu or chickenpox. But since it's not always easy to accurately distinguish between a viral illness and a nonviral illness, experts recommend avoiding aspirin altogether in children under 18, unless specifically prescribed by a medical provider.

If you have any questions about giving your child a medication, call your child's medical provider. If your child vomits or develops a rash after taking a medicine, call the provider promptly.

SINGLE USE ONLY

CARING FOR A SICK CHILD

Many common childhood illnesses can be treated at home. If you have any questions, seek the advice of your child's medical provider. When you have a sick child at home, a little extra loving care is always in order. To help your child recover quickly and fully, there are some simple steps you can follow.

Encourage rest Make sure your child has plenty of opportunity to rest. Getting enough sleep will help ease crankiness and smooth over irritability and discomfort. Take the opportunity to snuggle up and relax together. A mild illness is often just the excuse you need to pause the family's hectic schedule and spend quality time with your child.

Offer plenty of fluids One of the biggest risks associated with infections and other common childhood illnesses is dehydration. Dehydration occurs when your child loses more fluids than he or she is taking in — because of vomiting, diarrhea, difficulty eating and drinking, or just the increased demands on your child's metabolism (see page 321). If your child is having difficulty eating or keeping fluids down, offer small, frequent sips of water or an oral rehydration solution, such as Pedialyte. Kids often enjoy sucking on an ice pop or crushed ice.

Make your child comfortable If your child is congested, adding extra moisture to the air by running a cool-mist humidifier or vaporizer may help. Or have your child breathe the moist air in a steamy bathroom. Saline drops into the nose can help with congestion. If your child's room feels hot and stuffy, circulate the air with a fan. Make sure your child isn't dressed too warmly.

Use medications wisely If your child has a fever but is eating and sleeping well and playing normally, medication may not be necessary. But if your son or daughter is in pain, it's fine to give him or her acetaminophen (Tylenol, others) or ibuprofen (Advil, Motrin, others) to relieve the discomfort. Follow the directions on the label or the advice of your child's medical provider. Be sure to wait the appropriate amount of time before giving your child another dose. If the provider has prescribed antibiotics or another medication, follow the instructions exactly and take the complete course as prescribed to maximize the drug's benefits and reduce possible risks.

Call your child's medical provider When caring for a sick child, trust your intuition as a parent. If you feel like you should call your child's medical provider — call. Describe what's worrying you and what you've tried so far. A phone call to a provider often solves a lot of problems and gives you reassurance that the steps you've already taken are the right ones. If you feel like you should have your child seen in either the doctor's office or the emergency department — go in.

Prevent the spread of germs Take commonsense steps to keep germs from spreading around the house and to others. Sneeze or cough into a clean tissue or into your elbow if tissues are unavailable. Toss used tissues promptly. Don't share eating and drinking utensils. Keep high-use surfaces clean, including on toys and play areas. If needed, stay home to prevent spreading an infection. Above all, wash your hands frequently and thoroughly and make sure your child and other family members do the same. You may want to keep bottles of hand sanitizer in various places around the house.

A TO Z ILLNESS GUIDE

Following are some of the illnesses most common to preschoolers and school-age children. Learn how to recognize signs and symptoms, when things might be serious and when to call for help, and get tips on home treatment.

ALLERGIES (ENVIRONMENTAL)

Allergies occur when your child's immune system reacts to a substance — such as pollen, bee venom, pet dander, or a certain food or medication — as if it's harmful, when for most people it isn't.

Some children are genetically predisposed to developing allergies. Allergic conditions — such as asthma, eczema or food allergies — tend to run in families. Children don't usually develop seasonal airborne allergies until after their immune systems have had multiple seasons of pollen exposure.

Although there are no cures for allergies, treatment can relieve some of the bothersome symptoms they cause, especially those produced by airborne allergies, asthma and eczema. For other allergic conditions, avoiding allergy triggers is key to preventing an allergic reaction.

How to recognize it Symptoms vary based on what's causing the allergy. Generally, symptoms are mild or manageable. But in some cases, exposure to certain allergens can lead to a severe reaction (anaphylaxis), which requires emergency treatment. Signs and symptoms of anaphylaxis typically develop soon after exposure to the allergen and may include difficulty breathing, swelling, hives, vomiting, diarrhea, accelerated heart rate and dizziness or fainting (see page 308).

Airborne allergies Airborne allergies — also called allergic rhinitis or hay fever — may occur seasonally as allergens, such as pollen, are transported through the air. Airborne allergies typically cause signs and symptoms such as:

▶ A runny nose with a thin, clear discharge
▶ Sneezing
▶ Itchy, watery or mildly swollen eyes
▶ Itchy skin or rash
▶ Cough (postnasal drainage)
▶ Worsening of asthma symptoms, such as wheezing or shortness of breath

Food allergies A food allergy can cause:

▶ Swelling of the lips, tongue, face or throat
▶ Hives
▶ Anaphylaxis

Allergies to stings and bites An allergic reaction to an insect sting may include:

▶ Hives all over the body
▶ Coughing, chest tightness, wheezing or shortness of breath
▶ Anaphylaxis

Allergies to drugs An allergic reaction to a drug may include:

▶ Hives
▶ Swelling of the face, extremities or throat
▶ Wheezing or trouble breathing
▶ Anaphylaxis

How serious is it? Environmental allergies can make your child miserable but usually aren't serious. Treating symptoms and avoiding allergens are key to reducing your child's discomfort.

Some children have severe, anaphylactic reactions to a certain food, insect venom or medication. If your child is allergic to peanuts or bee stings, for example, your child's medical provider will

WHEN TO CALL RIGHT AWAY

Parents often wonder when signs and symptoms in their children signal something more serious than a simple runny nose or a skin rash. If you're ever unsure, a quick to call your child's medical provider can provide reassurance and guidance on next steps.

Keep in mind that common infections can quickly become serious in kids who have a chronic illness, especially one that impairs the immune system's ability to fight infection. The same goes for kids who aren't current with their vaccinations.

The following signs and symptoms require prompt evaluation either by your child's medical provider or in the emergency department. If you're not sure it's an emergency, call your child's provider first.

- *Persistent or high fever.* A fever that lasts more than three days or a fever that reaches 103 F or higher.
- *Rash with fever.* A red or purple rash with fever that doesn't disappear or become lighter (blanch) when pressure is applied (petechial rash or purpura).
- *Difficulty breathing.* Shortness of breath, inability to complete a sentence without taking a breath, or having trouble eating or drinking. Other signs include flaring of the nostrils and drawing in of the skin above or below the rib cage or between the ribs (retractions).
- *Changes in alertness.* Disorientation, confusion, unresponsiveness, inability to stay awake or persistent drowsiness that prevents eating and drinking.
- *Stiff neck.* Inability to move the neck, especially when accompanied by fever and sensitivity to light.
- *Seizure.* Loss of awareness or sudden, uncontrollable jerking movements.
- *Feeling faint.* Inability to see or hear clearly or stand upright.
- *Weakness.* Inability to walk, self-feed or get dressed.
- *Dehydration.* No urination in the last eight hours, dry or cotton mouth, sunken eyes.
- *Intense abdominal pain.* Severe and persistent belly pain.
- *Acting very sick with fever.* Lack of improvement one hour after being given a fever-reducing medication.
- *Extreme irritability.* Difficult to comfort or calm.
- *Severe sore throat.* Inability to swallow foods, drooling.

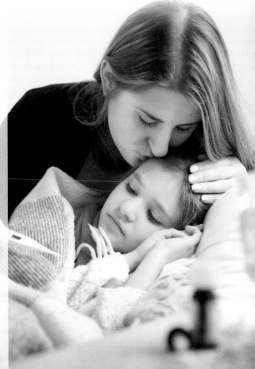

SEVERE ALLERGIC REACTION (ANAPHYLAXIS)

Sometimes, exposure to an allergen can lead to a severe, potentially life-threatening allergic reaction (anaphylaxis). This kind of severe reaction can occur within seconds or minutes of exposure to something your child is allergic to, such as peanuts or bee stings. The most common anaphylaxis triggers in children are food allergies.

Anaphylaxis requires immediate injection of epinephrine and a follow-up trip to an emergency room. If you don't have epinephrine, you need to go to an emergency room right away. If anaphylaxis isn't treated promptly, it can be fatal.

Symptoms Anaphylaxis causes the immune system to release a flood of chemicals that can lead to shock — blood pressure drops suddenly and airways narrow, blocking breathing. Although anaphylaxis usually occurs immediately, sometimes it can occur a half-hour or longer after exposure. Signs and symptoms of anaphylaxis include:

▶ Severe shortness of breath, coughing or wheezing
▶ Swelling of the lips, tongue or throat or a funny feeling in the mouth
▶ Hives or itching
▶ Pale, cool or clammy skin
▶ Fainting or loss of consciousness
▶ Sudden onset of abdominal pain, nausea or vomiting
▶ Fast or pounding heart rate
▶ Low blood pressure

What to do in an emergency If your child is having an allergic reaction and shows signs of anaphylaxis, act fast. Do the following immediately and seek urgent medical care.

▶ Use an epinephrine autoinjector, if available, by pressing it into your child's thigh. This is the only lifesaving medication for anaphylaxis.
▶ Make sure your child is lying down.
▶ Check your child's pulse and breathing and, if necessary, administer CPR or other first-aid measures.
▶ Call 911 or emergency medical help.

Even if symptoms improve after administering the epinephrine autoinjector, you still need to take your child to an emergency room. In some cases, some children may need additional medical intervention or more than one epinephrine autoinjector administration.

Schedule a follow-up appointment If your child has had an allergic reaction or anaphylaxis, schedule an appointment with your child's medical provider or an allergy specialist to discuss triggers for the reaction and long-term management. The provider will give you epinephrine autoinjectors to keep with your child and show you how to use them, if you don't already have them.

MEDICATIONS FOR AIRBORNE ALLERGIES

Airborne allergies — such as to pollen, mold or pet dander — make lots of people, including children, miserable. In many cases, avoiding the outdoors or a friend's house with pets isn't always feasible or even desirable. As a result, many families turn to allergy medications for control and relief of symptoms. But which allergy medications are best for kids?

Several allergy medications are approved for use in children. Although allergy medications can be taken as needed to ease mild symptoms, they're most effective when taken regularly.

Several types of nonprescription and prescription medications can help ease allergy symptoms. They include:

▶ *Oral antihistamines.* Antihistamines can help relieve sneezing, itching, a runny nose and watery eyes. They typically come in the form of a nonprescription syrup or a tablet, some of which are chewable. Diphenhydramine (Benadryl), though a popular medication, isn't generally recommended because it can cause drowsiness. Recommended nonsedating antihistamines include loratadine (Claritin), cetirizine (Zyrtec) and fexofenadine (Allegra). Your child's medical provider may advise taking one of these antihistamines regularly throughout the allergy season.

▶ *Glucocorticoid nasal sprays.* These may be recommended alone or in combination with other allergy medications depending on the severity of allergies. These are available over-the-counter and by prescription. Examples of glucocorticoid nasal sprays approved for children include fluticasone (Flonase), triamcinolone acetonide (Nasacort) and mometasone (Nasonex). These medications are considered generally safe and don't have the systemic side effects associated with oral steroid medications.

▶ *Montelukast (Singulair).* This is an oral medication that can be helpful for allergy symptoms and has the added benefit of improving asthma symptoms. This medication, available as a chewable tablet, may be used alone or in combination with other allergy medications. In some children, there's a small but possible risk of mood disturbance as a side effect. It's considered generally safe for long-term use in children.

▶ *Antihistamine nasal sprays.* Some antihistamines also come as prescription nasal sprays. These medications include azelastine (Astepro) and olopatadine (Patanase).

likely recommend that your child have emergency treatment in the form of an epinephrine autoinjector with him or her at all times.

When to call If your child has symptoms of anaphylaxis, don't wait to see if symptoms go away. Call 911 or your local emergency services, or go to the nearest emergency department. Meanwhile, administer an epinephrine autoinjector, if you have one, to your child right away.

After emergency treatment, see your child's medical provider to determine what caused the reaction and to figure out how to avoid another one. Your child's provider may refer you to an allergy specialist (allergist).

For food allergies, doctors will prescribe an epinephrine autoinjector that you can keep with your child at all times. This medication is the only lifesaving medication for anaphylaxis. Make sure the medication is available for use wherever your child goes. All adults caring for your child should be aware of your child's allergy and know how and when to administer the emergency medication.

If your child has a constant runny nose, chronic cough or dry, itchy skin, make an appointment with his or her medical provider to discuss the possible causes and options for treatment.

What you can do The best way to prevent an allergic reaction is to avoid the trigger behind it, such as avoiding certain drugs or offending foods and taking precautions against insect stings.

But it's not always feasible to completely avoid some allergens, especially airborne ones. Here are some steps that may help with airborne allergies:

▶ *Rinse out nasal passages.* Saline nasal irrigation — rinsing out the sinuses with a salt and water solution — may help flush out allergens and irritants from your child's nose. Saline solutions in specially designed squeeze bottles are inexpensive and readily available over-the-counter at drugstores and supermarkets.

▶ *Reduce household airborne allergens.* For dust mite allergies, reduce your child's exposure by washing bedsheets once weekly and getting dust mite encasements for the pillows, mattress and box spring. Use of high-efficiency particulate air (HEPA) filters is helpful for cat allergies. Turning on air-conditioning in the car and home, if possible, can help with reducing exposure to pollen allergies.

▶ *Use medications.* A number of allergy medications have been approved to ease symptoms in children over age 2 (see page 309).

ASTHMA

In children with asthma, the lungs' airways (bronchial tubes) become easily inflamed and constricted, making it hard to breathe.

Inflammation, swelling and an increased production of mucus narrow the bronchial tubes and reduce airflow. In addition, the airways of a child with asthma are much more sensitive to certain conditions (triggers).

When a child with asthma is exposed to a trigger — such as cold air or exercise — the muscles surrounding the bronchial tubes tighten up or constrict (bronchospasm). This is commonly referred to as an asthma attack, where breathing becomes difficult, sometimes severely.

In young children, the first sign of asthma may be wheezing that's triggered by a cold, goes away and then recurs with

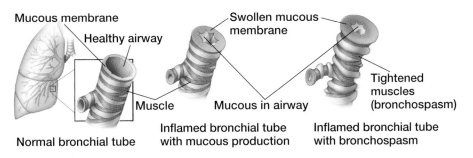

Mucous membrane
Healthy airway
Swollen mucous membrane
Tightened muscles (bronchospasm)
Muscle
Mucous in airway
Normal bronchial tube
Inflamed bronchial tube with mucous production
Inflamed bronchial tube with bronchospasm

An asthma flare is typically caused by inflammation and constriction of the bronchial tubes.

the next cold. It can be a challenge to diagnose asthma at a young age because about 20 percent of those who wheeze outgrow it by the time they're 6 years old.

A number of childhood conditions — bronchiolitis and pneumonia are examples — can have symptoms similar to those caused by asthma. As a child gets older, it becomes easier to get accurate results on lung function tests that help confirm an asthma diagnosis.

Asthma is more common in children who have a family history of allergic diseases, such as asthma, allergies or eczema (atopic dermatitis).

How to recognize it Wheezing — a high-pitched whistling sound produced when your child breathes out (exhales) — is a common sign of asthma. Other signs and symptoms include a cough that worsens at night, tightness in the chest and shortness of breath. With asthma, wheezing or coughing episodes tend to recur. Signs and symptoms are typically triggered or worsened by a cold or other upper respiratory infection or exercise. Exposure to cold air, tobacco smoke or allergens, such as pollens or mold, are also common triggers.

While wheezing is most commonly associated with asthma, not all children with asthma wheeze. Some kids with asthma may have only one sign or symptom, such as a lingering daytime cough, a nighttime cough that persists even without illness, or continued chest congestion.

Conversely, not all children who wheeze have asthma. Wheezing can also be caused by a cold or other respiratory infection that blocks your child's airways.

How serious is it? Asthma signs and symptoms vary from child to child and may get worse or better over time. Some preschoolers who experience wheezing outgrow it by the time they reach school age. For others, asthma symptoms may stop and then recur again later in life. Still others have chronic, persistent symptoms that require daily management.

If your child has symptoms of asthma, your child's medical provider will prescribe medication, depending on the severity and type of symptoms (see page 312).

If your son's or daughter's wheezing persists throughout the preschool years, his or her medical provider will likely recommend a full evaluation for asthma. Lung function testing can be done typically around age 6 or older. This type of testing provides valuable information about the degree of underlying obstruction and inflammation in your child's lungs and how reversible these factors are after administering medication such

ASTHMA MEDICATIONS

Medication is the primary form of treatment for asthma. When used correctly, it can greatly reduce your child's symptoms and help prevent asthma attacks.

Asthma medication is typically given through an inhaler, but it can also be given in pill, capsule or nebulizer forms. The inhaled medication comes in two main forms: quick-relief (rescue) and controller (maintenance) medication.

Quick-relief medication All children with asthma should be prescribed a quick-relief medication for asthma attacks. The medication helps ease acute signs and symptoms of cough, shortness of breath, wheezing and chest tightness. Albuterol is a commonly used quick-relief medication that acts fast to relax the smooth muscle surrounding the airways, expanding the airways and making it easier to breathe.

Children with asthma should carry quick-relief medication with them at all times, as well as a spacer device to ensure proper delivery of the medicine to the lungs. This includes at child care, school, sporting events and other activities. Caregivers, teachers, coaches, and other school or child care staff should be aware that your child has asthma and ideally know how to help your child if an attack occurs. Asthma symptoms or attacks can come on quickly, and albuterol will help improve airflow and relieve symptoms rapidly. If symptoms don't improve promptly, seek medical care right away.

Quick-relief medication such as albuterol is typically prescribed in the form of an inhaler. Sometimes a less preferred method of giving the medication called a nebulizer is prescribed. A nebulizer is a device that vaporizes liquid medication into a fine mist that can be inhaled.

Using a spacer device with an inhaler is important for all children. Spacer devices make delivery of the medication to the small airways more targeted and efficient, so there's less absorption by other parts of the body (systemic absorption) and fewer side effects. The type of spacer used varies depending on the child's age and ability to perform correct technique. In younger children, a mask attached to a plastic tube with a valve makes it easier to breathe in the correct amount of medication. In older children, a plastic tube that goes into the mouth is usually sufficient.

Controller medication Whereas quick-relief medications ease airway muscle spasms during an asthma attack or flare, controller medications work to reduce the underlying inflammation that obstructs and narrows bronchial tubes. Reducing inflammation helps maintain free airflow and reduces the chance that future asthma attacks will occur. Controller medications are prescribed for children who've been diagnosed with persistent asthma based on how much symptoms interfere with their daily life.

Long-term control of asthma symptoms typically involves taking a daily controller medication, such as inhaled corticosteroids and sometimes oral pills or capsules. Forgetting these daily medications is the most common cause of frequent asthma flares. Helping your child take all doses of these medications will improve overall asthma symptoms. When your child isn't having problems, it may not seem necessary to give him or her a medication. But it's very important not to stop the medication. Left untreated or undertreated, childhood asthma can lead to permanent lung changes that can result in poor lung function in adulthood. Because asthma can have a variable course, it's also important to check in with your child's medical provider regularly to assess symptoms and adjust your child's treatment plan as needed.

Asthma medications are very safe. All medications carry risks if used inappropriately, but when asthma medications are used correctly, their benefits far outweigh their small risks. Talk with your child's medical provider if you have concerns about correct use or side effects.

ASTHMA ACTION PLAN

If your child is diagnosed with asthma, you and your child's medical provider can create a comprehensive treatment plan — often called an asthma action plan — to guide home management of day-to-day symptoms. The Centers for Disease Control and Prevention lists several sample asthma action plans.

These plans are typically color-coded into zones of increasing symptom severity:
- **Green.** Symptoms are well-controlled.
- **Yellow.** A call to your child's medical provider is in order.
- **Red.** Seek emergency care.

Periodically, go over your child's asthma action plan with your child's medical provider. This way you can make sure the plan is still meeting your child's needs. If asthma symptoms are severe or become uncontrolled with your current treatment plan, other types of maintenance or controller medications may be added. After control of symptoms has been achieved, medication dosages are usually stepped down to the lowest effective dose for your child.

---

as albuterol. In children over age 6 with asthma, regular lung function testing is recommended to monitor how well treatment is working.

When to call Knowing when to call for help is important in managing your child's asthma. Use the following guidelines:

There's no need to call if your child:
- Has few daytime asthma symptoms
- Isn't troubled with asthma symptoms at night
- Doesn't miss school due to asthma
- Can engage in normal daily activities without being limited by asthma symptoms
- Doesn't have unplanned trips to the doctor or emergency care
- Has few asthma attacks and those flares can be controlled with medicine
This means your child's asthma symptoms are under control. This scenario is reflected by the green zone in an asthma action plan (see above).

Call your child's medical provider when your child:
- Has frequent symptoms (daytime symptoms more than two days in one week or symptoms that affect sleep more than two nights in one month)
- Experiences an asthma flare without any known trigger
- Experiences symptoms during activities that usually don't cause a flare
- Doesn't get full relief from symptoms with quick-relief medication
- Has to use quick-relief medication more than twice in one week (not including preventive use before exercise or active play)
These symptoms are reflected in the yellow zone of an asthma action plan.

Seek emergency care if your child:
- Is still struggling to breathe several minutes after taking quick-relief medication
- Suddenly begins wheezing

- Is unable to speak more than three words in a row without coughing or struggling to breathe
- Experiences increased wheezing, coughing or chest tightness that isn't relieved by quick-relief medications
- Has severe chest pain
- Feels lightheaded or faint
- Has a bluish tint to the lips, face or fingernails
- Has an alarmingly severe or intense asthma flare

These emergency signs and symptoms are reflected in the red zone of an asthma action plan.

What you can do Keep track of your child's asthma symptoms, preferably in a journal if you can. If you notice that certain things tend to trigger your child's symptoms, such as dust or pollen, try your best to avoid them. Clean regularly to eliminate dust and use air conditioning while keeping windows closed during pollen season to keep out airborne allergens.

Avoid tobacco and wood smoke, which are known to trigger symptoms. If your child's symptoms are worsened by cold air, have your child wear a hat and scarf to keep the air around his or her face warm and moist. Not all studies show that allergen-avoidance measures are effective in controlling asthma, though, so don't feel as if you need to surround your child in a protective bubble at all times.

Since colds and other respiratory infections can worsen asthma symptoms, try to limit your child's exposure to people who are sick, when possible. Also, it's important for your child and the rest of your family to receive the flu shot every year, as it reduces your child's risk of getting the flu. Children with asthma are at risk of severe complications from the flu.

If your child has asthma and you suspect he or she has the flu, visit your child's medical provider for a prompt evaluation.

In many kids, asthma symptoms are brought on by exercise. But having asthma doesn't mean your child can't be active. Medication taken before exercise, as prescribed by your child's medical provider, will help your child during activities such as sports and physical education class. Doing a proper warmup and cool-down before and after exercise also may help reduce exercise-related asthma symptoms.

BED-WETTING

If waking up to soggy sheets and pajamas seems to be the norm for your child these days, don't despair. Bed-wetting (sleep enuresis) isn't a sign of toilet training gone bad. Usually, it's just a normal part of a child's development. The way bladder function matures is the result of a complex relationship between different parts of the brain and nervous system. Every child matures at a slightly different rate. Most children outgrow bed-wetting on their own — but some need a little help.

Bed-wetting can happen to any child, but it's more common in boys than girls. It also runs in families, probably due to an inherited pattern of development. If one or both of a child's parents wet the bed as children, their child has a 50 to 75 percent chance of wetting the bed at older ages.

Stressful events — such as becoming a big brother or sister, starting a new school, or sleeping away from home — may trigger bed-wetting in a child who already has been dry for longer than six months. This type of bed-wetting is called secondary enuresis. It usually resolves with time and patience, as well.

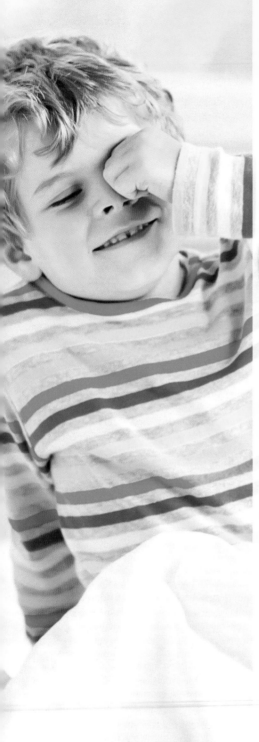

How serious is it? Generally, bed-wetting before age 7 isn't a concern. At this age, your child may still be developing nighttime bladder control. Most kids are fully toilet trained by age 5, but there's really no target date for developing complete bladder control. Between the ages of 5 and 7, bed-wetting remains a problem for some children, but the rates of bed-wetting decrease significantly during this time period. For some kids, it may take a little longer. But even after age 7, about 15 percent of children every year will achieve nighttime dryness without help.

In some cases, bed-wetting may be a sign of an underlying condition that needs medical attention, such as a urinary tract infection, chronic (and often unrecognized) constipation or poor daytime urination habits. An infection can make it difficult for your child to control urination. Also, the same muscles are used to control urine and stool elimination. When constipation is long term, these muscles don't work as well and contribute to bed-wetting at night and dysfunctional urination. Obstructive sleep apnea, a condition in which the child's breathing is interrupted during sleep, may be a cause of secondary enuresis.

Although frustrating, bed-wetting without a physical cause doesn't pose any health risks. In addition, bed-wetting is rarely caused by an emotional or psychological problem. However, bed-wetting can create some issues for your child, including:

- Rashes on the child's bottom and genital area — especially if your child sleeps in wet underwear
- Guilt and embarrassment, which can lead to low self-esteem
- Loss of opportunities for social activities, such as sleepovers and camp

Keep in mind that children don't wet the bed on purpose or because they're lazy or defiant. Nighttime continence is something their bodies are still working on. Try to be patient as you and your child work through the process together.

After eliminating risk factors such as constipation, initial treatment generally includes strategies you can use at home, such as following a bedtime toilet routine and having your child use the toilet regularly during the day.

If these changes aren't helpful, your child's medical provider may recommend the use of an enuresis alarm — a small, battery-operated device that connects to a moisture-sensitive pad on your child's pajamas or bedding. When the pad senses wetness, the alarm goes off, waking your child so that he or she can go to the bathroom. You may need to help your child to the bathroom with every alarm for the first couple of weeks. It may take several weeks to months of use before your child consistently wakes up dry. But the device is readily available and carries a low risk of relapse or side effects.

As a last resort, your child's medical provider may prescribe medication for a short time to slow nighttime urine production or calm an overactive bladder. Medications don't cure the problem, though, and bed-wetting may resume when medication is stopped.

When to call Make an appointment to talk with your child's medical provider if your child still wets the bed after age 7, or he or she starts to wet the bed after six or more months of being dry at night. Also call if you notice your child is experiencing painful urination, unusual thirst, pink or red urine, hard stools, or snoring. These additional signs and symptoms may indicate an underlying problem.

What you can do Here are changes you can make at home that may help:

▶ *Limit fluids in the evening.* It's important to get enough fluids, so there's no need to limit how much your child drinks in a day. However, encourage drinking liquids in the morning and early afternoon, which may reduce thirst in the evening. But don't limit evening fluids if your child participates in sports practice or games in the evenings.

▶ *Avoid beverages and foods with caffeine or high sugar.* Beverages with caffeine or high sugar content are discouraged for children at any time of day. Because caffeine may stimulate the bladder, it's especially discouraged in the evening. Sugary drinks cause the kidneys to produce more urine.

▶ *Hit the bathroom before bed.* Encourage your child to empty his or her bladder just before going to bed. Remind your child that it's OK to use the toilet during the night if needed. Use night lights to light the way between the bedroom and bathroom.

▶ *Encourage regular toilet use throughout the day.* During the day and evening, suggest that your child urinate every two hours or so, or at least often enough to avoid a feeling of urgency.

▶ *Prevent rashes.* To prevent a rash caused by wet underwear, help your child rinse his or her bottom and genital area every morning. It also may help to cover the affected area with a protective moisture barrier ointment or cream at bedtime. Ask your child's medical provider for product recommendations.

▶ *Be sensitive to your child's feelings.* If your child is stressed or anxious, encourage him or her to express those feelings. Offer support and encouragement. When your child feels calm and secure, bed-wetting may become less problematic. If needed, talk to your child's medical provider about strategies for dealing with stress.

▶ *Plan for easy cleanup.* Cover your child's mattress with a plastic cover. Use thick, absorbent underwear at night to help contain the urine. However, avoid the long-term use of diapers or disposable pullup underwear. These may encourage the sensation that it's OK to "let go" without heading to the toilet first. Keep extra bedding and pajamas handy. Sometimes, covering the wet area with a thick towel will do the trick until morning.

▶ *Enlist your child's help.* If age-appropriate, consider asking your child to rinse his or her wet underwear and pajamas or place these items in a specific container for washing. Taking responsibility for bed-wetting may help your child feel more control over the situation.

▶ *Celebrate effort.* Bed-wetting is involuntary, so it doesn't make sense to punish or tease your child for wetting the bed. Also, discourage siblings from teasing the child who wets the bed. Instead, praise your child for following the bedtime routine and helping clean up after accidents. Use a sticker reward system if you think this might help motivate your child.

COLDS AND COUGHS

Preschoolers average about six to eight colds in a year, as many as four times more than the estimated number adults tend to have. Colds can be especially common if a child has older siblings or he or she attends child care or school. Each bout generally lasts a week or two, but occasionally it persists longer. Spread those colds out over a year, and it's no wonder if you think your child constantly seems to have a runny nose.

Viruses account for most colds. Some of the same viruses that cause colds — coronaviruses, influenza viruses and respiratory syncytial virus, for example — also cause other infections such as pneumonia, flu and croup.

Colds are often spread when someone who is sick coughs, sneezes or talks, spraying virus-carrying droplets into the air that others breathe in. Nasal discharge, commonly called snot, is easily spread and, in kids with a cold, is a rich source of viruses. It can quickly go from nose to hand to other objects and surfaces, which are then touched by other kids who in turn touch their eyes, noses and mouths. Some viruses can live on surfaces — including human skin — for a few hours. This makes hands, utensils, toys and school supplies prime vehicles for germ transmission. Washing hands and other surfaces is key to minimizing the spread of germs.

How to recognize it When your child has a cold, he or she will likely develop a stuffy or runny nose. Typically, a child's snot is clear at first, then turns yellow, thicker and even green — a familiar sight to almost every parent. After a few days, the discharge again becomes clear and runny. At this point, your child may sneeze and have a cough, a hoarse voice or red eyes. While infants typically start a cold off with a fever, older children may not have a fever with a cold. Other symptoms might include sore throat, headache and ear pressure.

A common myth, even in the medical world, is that greenish-gray or yellowish snot is a sure sign of a bacterial infection. Both viral and bacterial upper respiratory

IS IT STREP THROAT?

The term *strep throat* is often spoken with a certain amount of dread among parents because strep throat is the kind of sore throat that typically means a trip to the doctor, a course of antibiotics, and staying home from school or child care.

Strep throat is caused by the bacterium group A streptococcus. It's most common among children 5 to 15 years old — an age group that's more susceptible to strep throat than younger or older groups. Most sore throats, however, don't result from bacterial infection but from a viral infection. And if the infection is viral, home care is usually all that's needed.

So how can you tell the difference between a viral sore throat and strep throat? Red eyes, a runny nose, cough and hoarseness accompanying the sore throat are generally signs of a viral infection. But diagnosing strep throat requires testing a swab sample of the infected person's throat. When deciding whether to test, here's what medical providers look for and what you can look for, too:

- Is there an accompanying fever? Group A streptococcus is the most common cause of sore throat with fever in children between ages 3 and 15.
- Is there no cough present? Coughs are typically associated with a viral infection, not strep throat.
- Are lymph nodes near the throat swollen and tender? Swollen lymph nodes may be a sign of strep throat.
- Do tonsils look swollen or full of pus? A throat infected with group A streptococcus often looks inflamed and may have characteristic red dots on the tonsils.

If the answers to these questions are mostly yes, your child's medical provider may recommend testing for strep throat. Even then the likelihood of strep throat is about 50-50. Another factor the provider will consider is whether anyone in your house has been recently diagnosed with strep throat.

Treatment for strep throat is usually with antibiotics. If taken within 48 hours of the start of symptoms, antibiotics reduce the duration and severity of symptoms, as well as the likelihood that the infection will spread to others. Complications aren't common, but antibiotics can help decrease the risk that the infection will spread to other parts of the body. If taken within 10 days, it can decrease the rare risk of rheumatic fever. Rheumatic fever can cause painful and inflamed joints, a rash and sometimes heart valve damage.

infections can cause similar changes to the quality and coloration of snot. The color is likely due to an increase in the number of certain immune system cells, or an increase in the enzymes these cells produce. Over the next few days, the discharge tends to clear up or dry up.

How serious is it? Colds are mostly a nuisance but not much more. If your child has a cold with no complications, it should resolve within a week or two. Sometimes a mild runny nose or a dry cough may linger a bit longer, but should steadily improve over time.

COLD AND COUGH MEDICATIONS

When your child is sick with a cold or cough, your first instinct may be to make a pit stop at the drugstore. But be aware before you buy.

In children under age 6, studies show that over-the-counter cold and cough medications don't really help and may even be harmful due to potentially serious side effects.

The benefits of decongestants and antihistamines in children between 6 and 12 years old is unproved. Also, these medicines do carry risks. Many experts recommend against using them until age 12. If you choose to give these to your child, make sure you supervise the administration of the medicine. Avoid giving multiple medications with the same active ingredient, which could lead to an overdose.

If fever or headache is making your child uncomfortable, acetaminophen (Tylenol, others) or ibuprofen (Advil, Motrin, others) may help. Carefully follow label instructions. **Don't give aspirin.** Aspirin use in children, especially after a viral illness, is associated with Reye's syndrome. This is a rare but serious condition that causes swelling of the brain and liver.

Zinc lozenges, echinacea and vitamin C are often touted as helpful for colds, but unfortunately there's little evidence to support these measures. In small doses, they're unlikely to be harmful. In addition, cough drops or hard candy may help ease a cough or sore throat.

When to call Colds usually don't require a visit to a medical provider. But if symptoms are severe, persist for more than 10 days without getting better, or improve then worsen again — such as a new fever at the end of an illness — it's possible a bacterial infection of the ears or sinuses may have set in and a visit to the doctor is in order. Other signs and symptoms of a secondary infection include persistent fever and ear pain.

What you can do Unfortunately, there's no cure for a cold. Antibiotics kill bacteria but do nothing against viruses, which cause the vast majority of colds. And, overuse of antibiotics can be harmful. It tends to make bacteria more resistant to antibiotics, lessening the effectiveness of treatment for bacterial infections.

Most of the time, the best treatment for colds is time, rest and a little extra love and attention. To make your child feel more comfortable:

Offer plenty of fluids Drinking liquids is important to avoid dehydration. Encourage your child to take in his or her normal amount of fluids. Warm fluids, such as chicken soup or tea, may help ease congestion and soothe inflamed airways.

Milk and dairy products also are fine to give. Although drinking milk may make mucus in the throat (phlegm) thicker, it won't cause the body to produce more phlegm. In fact, frozen dairy products can soothe a sore throat and provide needed calories when your child otherwise may not eat.

TREATING DEHYDRATION

Dehydration occurs when your child uses or loses more fluid than he or she takes in, and his or her body doesn't have enough water and other fluids to carry out its normal functions. If lost fluids aren't replaced, dehydration occurs. The most common cause of dehydration in children is severe diarrhea and vomiting.

Signs and symptoms of dehydration vary based on severity:

Mild dehydration	Moderate dehydration	Severe dehydration
• Decreased urine output (urinating less than three times in 24 hours) • Mildly increased heart rate	• Decreased urine output • Increased heart rate • Dizziness on rising or standing up, due to decrease in blood pressure • Decreased skin elasticity and sunken eyes • Dry mouth • Cold hands and feet	• Moderate dehydration signs and symptoms • Low blood pressure • Mottled appearance to hands and feet • Listlessness, lethargy • Deep, labored breathing • Weak pulse

Mild to moderate dehydration can be treated with ice chips or ice pops or with frequent sips of water, an over-the-counter oral rehydration solution (Pedialyte), or a half-and-half mixture of water and either apple juice or a sports drink.

Start with about a teaspoon every five minutes for a couple of hours, up to three to four hours. It may be easier to use a syringe for young children. Once your child is keeping these liquids down for several hours, you can increase the amount you're offering. If your child starts vomiting again, rest the stomach for 30 minutes to an hour before restarting the process. Allowing your child to drink immediately after vomiting will likely trigger more vomiting episodes. A slow and steady process better allows the stomach to absorb the liquids.

Children who are severely dehydrated need emergency care. Call 911 or your local emergency services, or seek care at a hospital emergency department. Salts and fluids delivered through a vein (intravenously) are absorbed quickly and speed recovery.

Give a spoonful of honey Remember the old advice of giving honey and lemon juice for a cold or cough? Your grandmother may have been onto something. Evidence suggests that taking ½ to 1 teaspoon of honey can help decrease cough frequency, especially at night when taken before bedtime. If your child likes honey, this might be a soothing option. Your child can take it straight from the spoon or you can dilute the honey in tea or juice.

Thin nasal discharge If the discharge from your child's nose is thick, saline nose drops or nasal sprays may help loosen it up. These nose drops and nasal sprays are made with the optimal amount of salt and water. They're inexpensive and available without a prescription. Avoid using home preparations because tap water can contain unwanted germs. Place a couple of drops, or spray once or twice, in each nostril. You can follow up by suctioning the mucus with a nose bulb, if desired.

Moisten the air Running a cool-mist humidifier in your child's room can add moisture to the air and help improve a runny nose and nasal congestion. To prevent mold growth, change the water daily and follow the manufacturer's instructions for cleaning the unit. It might also help to have your child take a warm bath before bedtime. In general, avoid hot steam vaporizers because there have been reports of burns to children from their use.

Stop colds from spreading Use common sense and plenty of soap and water. Emphasize proper hand-washing techniques (see page 359) and refrain from sharing cups and utensils with a sick child. Clean surfaces often. Make sure that all child care and school items are clearly labeled to avoid accidental sharing. Teach everyone in the household to cough or sneeze into a tissue — and then toss it. If you can't reach a tissue in time, cough or sneeze into the crook of your arm.

CONCUSSIONS

Almost all children bump their heads every now and then. This may be upsetting to you or your child, but keep in mind that most head injuries are minor and don't cause problems.

Sometimes, however, a bump, a fall or physical contact during a sporting event can lead to a concussion. A concussion is a traumatic brain injury that affects brain function but doesn't involve bleeding of the brain or a skull fracture. Its effects, which are usually temporary, may include a headache and problems with concentration, memory, balance and coordination.

If you suspect that your child may have a concussion, see a doctor. Most children recover fully from a concussion, but the healing process can take days to weeks.

How to recognize it Signs and symptoms of a concussion can be subtle and may not show up immediately. In addition, concussions can be difficult to recognize in young children because a child may not be able to fully describe how he or she feels.

Signs and symptoms in a child may include headache, loss of balance, dizziness, nausea, sensitivity to light and noise, irritability and change in mood, confusion, problems with memory and concentration, and changes in eating or sleeping patterns.

How serious is it? The human brain, which has the consistency of gelatin, is cushioned from everyday jolts and bumps by the skull and fluid inside the skull. However, a major blow to the head and neck can cause the brain to slide back and forth forcefully against the inner walls of the skull. Sudden acceleration or deceleration of the head, caused by events such as a car crash or being forcefully hit or thrown during a game, also can cause brain injury. These types of injuries affect brain function, usually for a brief period, resulting in signs and symptoms of concussion.

CONCUSSION SIGNS AND SYMPTOMS

Physical	Emotional
• A headache or feeling of pressure in the head • Loss of balance and unsteady walking • Nausea • Sensitivity to noise or light	• Irritability and crankiness • Excessive crying

Mental	Sleep-related
• Confusion • Difficulty concentrating or memory loss	• Listlessness or feeling sleepy • A change in sleeping patterns

The best treatment for a concussion is rest. Most concussions get better on their own. For the first 24 to 48 hours, your child may need to stay home from school, sports or other extracurricular activities. After this initial period, have your child gradually increase his or her activity as tolerated while taking care to eat and sleep well. A recent study published in the medical journal *JAMA* concluded that some activity can be beneficial. The study looked at more than 3,000 children who'd been diagnosed with concussions in emergency rooms. It found that those children who didn't take part in any physical activity the first seven days after injury were more likely to have persistent symptoms a month later than were those who began mild activity a couple of days after the concussion.

There aren't any medications proved to speed recovery from a concussion or prevent long-term effects from injury. However, your child's medical provider may prescribe medication to treat certain symptoms, such as headache or nausea.

Your child may take over-the-counter pain medication, such as acetaminophen (Tylenol, others) or ibuprofen (Advil, Motrin, others) to help with headache pain. Don't give or let your child take as-pirin. If your child's doctor suspects there's a risk of bleeding in the brain, he or she may request a brain-imaging test such as a CT scan to rule out bleeding and ask you to avoid ibuprofen, which can increase the risk of bleeding.

When to call The American Academy of Pediatrics recommends that you contact your child's medical provider for anything more than a light bump on your child's head.

If your child doesn't have signs of a serious head injury, remains alert, moves normally and responds to you in a normal fashion, the injury is probably mild and no further evaluation may be needed. If symptoms are present, additional evaluation may be necessary.

In some cases, a forceful head injury can lead to more-serious problems such as a skull fracture or bleeding in or around the brain, which can be fatal. That's why a child who experiences a head injury should be monitored after the incident. If your child is experiencing the following after a head injury seek emergency care:

- Repeated vomiting
- A loss of consciousness lasting longer than 30 seconds

RETURNING TO SPORTS

If your child is involved in athletics and experiences a concussion, he or she should be evaluated by a medical provider, preferably someone trained in pediatric concussions. Child and adolescent athletes with a concussion should not return to play on the same day as the injury.

Ask the provider when your child can play sports or do usual activities again. The timing will depend on your child's injury and symptoms, ability to tolerate activity, previous concussion history, and the type of sport your child plays. In the U.S., individual states generally have certain requirements a child must meet before returning to sports after a concussion. Most children are symptom-free and able to return to full activity within a month.

Don't rush it, though. Your child's brain needs to heal completely after a concussion. If your child gets another concussion before his or her brain has healed, it could lead to more-serious problems.

When your child does return to his or her usual activities, he or she might need to slowly ease into them. A doctor may recommend starting with light activity, gradually increasing to moderate activity and eventually regular activity. Your child has recovered when he or she is able to engage in regular activities without experiencing any symptoms.

- A constant headache, especially one that gets worse
- Noticeable changes in his or her behavior
- Changes in physical coordination, such as stumbling or clumsiness
- Confusion or disorientation, such as difficulty recognizing people or places
- Slurred speech or other changes in speech
- Seizures
- Vision or eye disturbances, such as dilated pupils or pupils of unequal sizes

What you can do During the healing period, monitor your child to make sure he or she doesn't do too much and symptoms are improving. Rest includes limiting activities that require thinking and mental concentration, such as playing video games, watching TV, doing schoolwork, reading, texting or using a computer, especially if these activities trigger symptoms or worsen them.

Generally, kids need a couple of days of full rest before returning to school and other activities. Depending on how your child is doing, his or her medical provider may recommend shortened school days initially or reduced school workloads or work assignments.

Once all signs and symptoms of concussion have resolved, discuss with your child's medical provider what steps should be taken to safely play sports again. Resuming sports too soon increases the risk of a second concussion and a more serious brain injury (see left).

CONSTIPATION

Almost everyone becomes constipated at some point in in life. Being constipated can be uncomfortable and frustrating. When your child is constipated, particularly when it happens often, it can be especially difficult.

Bowel habits vary from child to child just as they do in adults. Babies generally poop several times a day. As kids get older, the amount of time food spends going through the gastrointestinal tract increases. Preschoolers and school age children have a bowel movement once or twice a day, or every other day, on average.

In kids, constipation may occur when a child ignores the urge to poop or doesn't take enough time on the toilet. This can happen when he or she is transitioning to a new phase, such as during toilet training or when starting child care or school. If poop builds up in the rectum and colon, it can become dry and hard, and lead to constipation. Stress, lack of exercise, inadequate water intake or a poor sitting position on the toilet also can contribute to constipation, as can eating a lot of dairy or not enough fiber.

How to recognize it It's not always easy to tell if your child is constipated, especially if you don't see him or her during the day. And once your child is older, "How's your poop?" isn't always at the top of the list of conversation starters. But here are some ways you can tell whether your child is constipated:
- Your child does not have a bowel movement very often (three times a week or less).
- Your child tells you often that his or her tummy hurts.
- Your child tells you that his or her bottom is itchy or you notice your child scratching his or her rear end.
- Your child has streaky poop marks in his or her underwear.
- Your child leaks very loose stool, a result of chronic constipation and dysfunctional pelvic muscles.

- Your child's bowel movements are very large, firm and painful to pass, and may plug the toilet.
- Your child has daytime pee or poop accidents or bed-wetting accidents or both.
- Your child has repeated urinary tract infections (UTIs).
- Your child has to pee often or has to run to make it to the bathroom in time.
- You are having trouble toilet training your child by 4 to 5 years of age or kindergarten.

There's not a lot of space in your child's abdomen and pelvis. If poop fills up the rectum and colon, it presses on or even blocks the bladder. Then the bladder can't completely empty or hold as much pee as it should. Or, the poop pushes on the bladder, causing it to squeeze and leak. This is not something your child can control or stop if he or she is constipated. If the bladder isn't completely emptied or poop has been sitting in the rectum for too long, bacteria can grow in the urinary tract and cause urinary tract infections.

How serious is it? Although occasional constipation can be uncomfortable, it usually isn't serious. If constipation becomes chronic, however, bowel movements can become painful or difficult, and your child may become afraid to go to the bathroom. As a result, your

FIBER-RICH FOODS TO TRY

A serving of ...	Has approximately this much fiber ...
Cereals, beans and seeds	
Bran cereal (⅓ cup)	9 grams
Chickpeas* (½ cup)	8 grams
Black or pinto beans* (½ cup)	7 to 8 grams
Shredded wheat cereal (1 cup)	5 grams
Roasted pumpkin seeds (1 ounce)	5 grams
Fruits	
Medium pear with skin	5 to 6 grams
Medium apple with skin	4 to 5 grams
Raspberries (½ cup)	4 grams
Vegetables	
Artichoke* (½ cup)	7 grams
Avocado (½ cup)	5 grams
Mixed vegetables* (½ cup)	4 grams
Collard greens* (½ cup)	4 grams
Green peas* (½ cup)	3 to 4 grams
Winter squash* (½ cup)	3 grams

*Cooked

Source: U.S. Department of Agriculture

child may hide when he or she feels like pooping or try to hold back pooping. Doing these things can then cause your child to become even more constipated and the cycle continues. In some cases, small, painful tears in the skin around the anus (anal fissures) may develop.

When to call Take your child to his or her medical provider if the constipation lasts longer than two weeks or is accompanied by:

▶ Fever
▶ Vomiting
▶ Red streaks or signs of blood in the poop
▶ A swollen or bloated belly
▶ Weight loss

What you can do A few changes in your child's diet and daily routine may be all that's needed to get your child back to having soft, squishy bowel movements on a regular basis. Chronic constipation will take some time to improve — often months and sometimes up to a year. But stick with it, and you'll be setting your child up for a lifetime of good habits.

▶ *Emphasize a balanced diet.* Offer your child plenty of fruits, vegetables, beans, and whole-grain cereals and breads. These foods are rich in fiber, which helps poop stay soft. If your child isn't used to eating these foods, start by adding them in gradually to prevent gas and bloating. If your child drinks a lot of milk or eats a lot of dairy products, you might consider minimizing them for a while to see if it helps.

▶ *Encourage your child to drink plenty of fluids.* Water is often the best. Avoid drinks with caffeine or high sugar content. One way to tell whether your child is getting enough fluid is to look at his or her urine. It should be clear or light yellow by the middle to end of the day.

▶ *Promote physical activity.* Regular physical activity helps stimulate normal bowel function. Limit screen time and encourage your child to move.

▶ *Create a toilet routine.* Regularly set aside time after meals for your child to use the toilet. Generally, the colon becomes more active about 15 minutes after eating a larger meal, which makes this the best time for having a bowel movement. If you're still toilet training, consider taking a break in training until your child's constipation is resolved.

▶ *Position for success.* If necessary, provide a footstool so that your child is comfortable sitting on the toilet and has enough leverage to release the poop. If your child is still small, consider adding a toilet seat ring to allow your child to relax his or her body and bottom muscles.

▶ *Remind your child to heed nature's call.* Some children get so wrapped up in play that they ignore the urge to go to the bathroom. Ask your child's teachers or care providers to encourage your child to use the bathroom every two to three hours, even if he or she doesn't feel the urge to go.

▶ *Take care of chapped skin.* For young children, during routine bathing, rinse the skin around the child's anus with water only and gently pat it dry. Skip the soap. If your child's skin is irritated, do this daily. If your child is older, encourage him or her to do these steps independently. A waterproof cream or ointment also can help protect skin from moisture. Review proper wiping techniques with your child.

- *Review medications.* If your child is taking a medication that causes constipation, ask his or her medical provider about other options.

If these measures don't work, your child's medical provider can recommend additional treatment such as a laxative. Sometimes this starts with treatment to clean out the bowels and then continues with maintenance therapy. Don't give laxatives or enemas to your child without the provider's OK.

EARACHE

Most often, ear pain is due to an ear infection. Middle ear infections (otitis media) usually result when another illness — cold, flu or allergy — causes congestion and swelling of the nasal passages, throat and eustachian tubes. The eustachian tubes are a pair of narrow tubes that run from each middle ear to high in the back of the throat, behind the nasal passages. Swelling, inflammation and mucus in the eustachian tubes from an upper respiratory infection or allergy can block them, causing the accumulation of fluids in the middle ear (see right). A bacterial or viral infection of this fluid is usually what produces the symptoms of a middle ear infection.

The outer ear canal also can become infected (otitis externa), causing itching and discomfort. An outer ear infection is sometimes known as swimmer's ear because it tends to occur after frequent swimming. Water gets stuck in the outer ear canal and becomes infected.

A buildup of earwax can sometimes block the ear canal, putting pressure on the eardrum and causing discomfort. Objects stuck in the ear or injury to structures in the ear — caused by attempts to clean the ear, for example, or a more blunt force, such as being hit on or around the ear by a soccer ball — also can cause ear pain.

Earache sometimes occurs not because of something in the ear itself but because of a condition in a nearby structure, such as a sinus infection or a dental cavity.

How to recognize it Kids with an ear infection usually develop the infection after a cold or other upper respiratory tract infection. Most likely, your child will be able to tell you which ear is hurting and a recent history of events may help you pinpoint the cause, such as spending days at the pool or using a cotton swab in the ear. Other signs and symptoms to look for include:
- Ear pain, especially when lying down
- Difficulty hearing or responding to sounds
- Drainage of fluid from the ear
- A feeling of fullness in the ear
- Itching or redness of the outer ear canal
- Fever
- Ringing in the ear
- Problems with balance

A sudden drainage of fluid from the ear followed by a decrease in pain is a possible sign that the eardrum has ruptured.

How serious is it? Most of the time, earache is caused by an ear infection and doesn't present a serious problem. Most ear infections clear up on their own within one to two weeks.

On occasion, buildup of pus and fluid in the middle ear can create enough pressure to tear (rupture) the eardrum. The resulting pressure relief frequently leads to pain relief, as well. However, large ruptures may cause recurring infections. Since you can't tell whether a rupture is large or small by looking at the ear, visit your child's medical provider promptly if you think a rupture has occurred.

Rarely, an ear infection may spread to nearby structures such as the mastoid bone behind the ear (mastoiditis). This can present a more serious problem and needs prompt evaluation and treatment.

Excess earwax and objects stuck in the ear generally don't cause long-term problems when removed properly.

When to call If you know your child has experienced blunt force or trauma to the ear region, see your child's medical provider right away for an evaluation.

Also call your child's medical provider if:

▶ Earache lasts for more than a day or two
▶ Fever is present
▶ Ear pain is severe
▶ A discharge of fluid, pus or blood is released from the ear
▶ Redness or prominent swelling develops behind the ear, which could be a sign of mastoiditis

If your child's medical provider suspects a middle ear infection and your child's symptoms are mild, the provider may wait to see if the condition improves on its own before prescribing antibiotics.

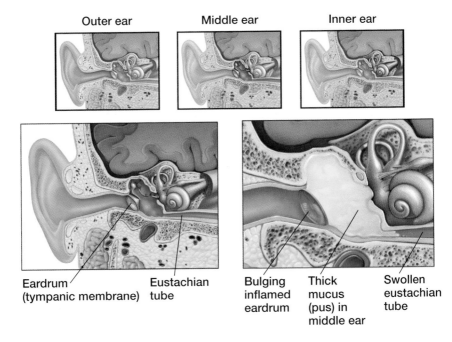

Outer ear   Middle ear   Inner ear

Eardrum / Eustachian
(tympanic membrane) tube

Bulging   Thick   Swollen
inflamed   mucus   eustachian
eardrum   (pus) in   tube
            middle ear

In babies and young children, the passages between the middle ear and throat (eustachian tubes) are narrower and shorter and have a more horizontal angle than in grown-ups. These factors promote the accumulation of fluids in the middle ear. A bacterial or viral infection of this fluid is usually what produces the symptoms of an ear infection.

As your child matures, though, the eustachian tubes become wider and more angled, making it easier for secretions and fluid to drain out of the ear. Although ear infections may still occur, they probably won't develop as often as during the first few years of life. In addition, ear infections in older children are more likely to be viral and go away on their own.

Although antibiotics are more frequently recommended for children under age 2, middle ear infections in older children usually improve without them. About 80 percent of the time, middle ear infections get better without antibiotics. But antibiotics may be appropriate if your child's symptoms are severe or recurrent.

Outer ear infections are often treated with topical antibiotic drops. These drops may also contain steroids to reduce inflammation.

Eardrum perforations often heal up on their own, but antibiotics may be prescribed. If the eardrum hasn't healed within a couple of months, a minor surgical procedure can repair the tear.

What you can do Placing a warm — not hot — moist washcloth over the affected ear may help lessen the pain. An over-the-counter pain reliever such as acetaminophen (Tylenol, others) or ibuprofen (Advil, Motrin, others) also can help. Follow instructions on the label carefully.

To reduce your child's risk of ear infections, practice good infection prevention skills by washing hands frequently, not sharing eating and drinking utensils, and avoiding contact with others who are sick. Avoid secondhand smoke, which also can contribute to frequent ear infections. Stay current on your child's immunizations. Vaccines such as the flu shot

---

EARWAX

Earwax is a helpful and natural part of the body's defenses. It protects the ear canal by trapping dirt and slowing the growth of bacteria. Normally, it will dry up and tumble out of the ear on its own. But occasionally, wax buildup occurs, perhaps because of a narrower than usual ear canal, an excess production of earwax or even well-meaning attempts to clean out the ear, which can push the earwax farther into the ear and cause a blockage.

A buildup of earwax is unlikely to cause serious problems, unless you try to dig it out yourself. Trying to remove earwax with a cotton swab or other instrument may push the earwax farther into your child's ear and cause serious damage to the lining of the ear canal or eardrum.

The best thing to do is to call your child's medical provider if you see a lot of waxy discharge coming out of your child's ears or if you notice hearing problems.

If your child frequently experiences earwax buildup — and he or she doesn't have an ear tube in place or a ruptured eardrum — you can try using earwax softening drops, available over-the-counter at drugstores, to help clear the earwax out. Follow the package instructions carefully.

Alternatively, you can mix equal parts of hydrogen peroxide and water and place a few drops in the affected ear twice a day for up to five days. A drop or two of mineral oil may be helpful in softening the earwax, as well. As the earwax softens, it should drain out on its own. Avoid the temptation to use a cotton swab to get it out, as the swab usually pushes the earwax in farther and creates a greater obstruction.

and pneumococcal vaccine can help prevent upper respiratory infections and reduce the risk of ear infections.

Germs thrive in moist environments. Keeping your child's ears dry can help heal and prevent swimmer's ear. This typically means no swimming until an outer ear infection has cleared. To prevent infection, have your child tip his or her head to the side to get the water out and dry the ear opening carefully. Use a hair dryer on a cool setting to gently dry the ear canal after bathing or swimming.

You can also rinse your child's ear canals with a few drops of rubbing alcohol or a solution of half rubbing alcohol and half white vinegar after swimming or bathing to help dry the ear canals dry and kill germs. The vinegar restores the normal acid balance to the ear canal.

Unless you can see and remove an object stuck in your child's ear without probing or digging, wait for your child's medical provider to remove it. The same goes for earwax. Otherwise you risk pushing the object or earwax in farther and possibly injuring the ear.

ECZEMA

Eczema is a common skin condition in young children that produces dry, itchy skin with red bumps and patches. Also known as atopic dermatitis, eczema tends to run in families and it can affect both children and adults. In children, symptoms usually start before age 5.

Symptoms of eczema often come and go (flare). Your child may have a flare that lasts for a few weeks or months, then he or she may go for a long time without symptoms. Flare-ups tend to occur when your child's skin is dry, such as in the winter, or when the skin gets infected.

Many kids who have eczema also have asthma or allergies, which can worsen symptoms of eczema.

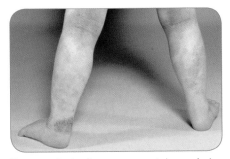

Eczema typically causes patches of dry, rough, reddish-brown skin.

How to recognize it Eczema typically produces red to brown patches of dry, bumpy skin. These itchy patches often occur where the skin flexes — inside the elbows and around the knees. Other common areas include the hands, wrists and ankles. You may find that your child tends to scratch these areas more at night. Repeated scratching can make the skin raw, swollen and more prone to infection. Over time, the skin may become thickened, cracked and scaly.

How serious is it? Eczema isn't contagious or life-threatening. But it can make your child uncomfortable, and sometimes it can be severe enough that it gets in the way of a good night's sleep. Keeping your child's skin moisturized and using medicated ointments when necessary will help ease the itching and discomfort.

When to call Make an appointment with your child's medical provider if your child:

▶ Is so uncomfortable that his or her sleep or activities are affected

- Continues to experience symptoms even after you've tried caring for the condition at home
- Has a skin infection (red streaks, pus, yellow scabs)

If your child has a skin infection that's accompanied by a fever, seek urgent care.

What you can do Be sure to always keep your child's skin moisturized, whether symptoms are present or not. Use fragrance-free, hypoallergenic lotions, creams or ointments at least twice a day. For example, you might use an ointment before bedtime and a cream before school.

It's especially important to moisturize immediately after bathing, to keep the skin from drying out. When bathing, have your child use lukewarm water and a hypoallergenic, fragrance-free soap that won't strip the skin of its natural oils. After a bath or shower, teach your child to pat dry and moisturize quickly — within three minutes.

Other measures that might help include avoiding secondhand smoke, products with perfumes or fragrances, and irritating nonbreathable clothing.

If a flare occurs:

- *Apply an anti-itch cream to the affected area.* A nonprescription hydrocortisone ointment or cream, containing at least 1 percent hydrocortisone, can temporarily relieve the itch. Apply it no more than twice a day to the affected area, after moisturizing. Using the moisturizer first helps the medicated cream penetrate the skin better. Once the skin has improved, you may use this type of cream less often to prevent flare-ups. If symptoms don't improve, ask your child's medical provider about a prescription cream or ointment. There are different ones the provider can try.

- *Take an oral allergy or anti-itch medication.* Taking a nonprescription antihistamine — such as cetirizine (Zyrtec) or fexofenadine (Allegra) — may help control the itching. Also, diphenhydramine (Benadryl, others) may be helpful if the itching is severe. But diphenhydramine causes drowsiness, so it's best taken at bedtime.

- *Prevent scratching.* For some kids, it may help to try pressing on the skin rather than scratching it. But it can be hard for a child to resist the urge to scratch. In this case, cover the itchy area with a bandage or gauze and tape. Keeping your child's nails trimmed and wearing gloves at night also can help protect sensitive areas.

- *Use a humidifier.* Hot, dry indoor air can parch sensitive skin and worsen itching and flaking. A portable home humidifier or one attached to your furnace adds moisture to the air inside your home.

- *Wear soft clothing.* Avoid clothing that's rough, tight or scratchy. Instead, have your child wear soft, smooth clothing that breathes well, such as cotton. Also, wear appropriate clothing in hot weather or during exercise to prevent excessive sweating.

EYE INJURIES

Eye injuries are often accidental. Sometimes shampoo or a household cleaner gets in the eye, or a foreign object enters the eye. During sports, an eye might get hit by a ball or a bat. An eye can get scratched during roughhousing.

Some eye injuries can be serious. When there's trauma to the eye or something gets stuck in the eye and can't be easily removed, urgent care is a priority.

How to recognize it If an eyelash or a speck of dust gets caught in an eye, it might cause tearing or redness, as can soap or shampoo in the eye. In such cases, the discomfort is usually temporary. Other times, an eye injury may be obvious and serious. The following signs and symptoms require immediate medical care:

- Obvious injury to the eye itself
- Obvious pain, trouble opening the eye or trouble seeing
- A cut or torn eyelid
- One eye not moving as well as the other eye
- One eye sticking out farther or seeming more prominent than the other
- An unusual pupil size or shape
- Blood in the white part of the eye
- An object on the eye or under the eyelid that can't easily be removed

How serious is it? Eye injuries are generally treated with caution, even if the injury seems minor. Trauma to inner parts of the eye may not always be readily apparent. Delaying care could lead to permanent vision loss or blindness. Because of the potential complications, eye injuries almost always require the care of a medical provider.

When to call When an eye injury occurs — and it's not a simple matter of blinking away dust or rinsing out shampoo — seek medical help as soon as possible, preferably from an eye doctor.

What you can do Eye injuries are generally treated by a medical provider. But there are things you can do at home.

Prevent further damage To prevent any further damage to the eye, follow these do's and don'ts:

- *Don't* touch, rub or apply pressure to the eye.

- *Do* flush out any chemicals the eye has been exposed to with plenty of clean water.
- *Don't* try to remove an object that appears stuck on the surface of the eye or an object that appears to have penetrated the eye.
- *Don't* apply ointment or medication to the eye.
- *Do* gently place a shield or gauze patch over the eye until you can get medical attention.

Examine the eye To examine your child's eye for a small foreign object:

- Wash your hands. Seat your child in a well-lighted area.
- Gently pull the lower lid of the eye down and ask your child to look up. Then hold the upper lid while the child looks down.
- If the object is floating in the tear film or on the surface of the eye, try flushing it out with clean, lukewarm water or saline solution. Put water or solution in a clean cup. A small paper cup or shot glass will work. Position the glass with its rim resting on the bone at the base of the eye socket. Gently tilt your child's head back, keeping the eye open, and pour the fluid in.
- If the object doesn't come out, seek emergency care.

Put safety first To prevent eye injuries:

- Don't allow your child to play with nonpowder rifles, such as pellet guns or BB guns. Avoid projectile toys, such as darts, bows and arrows, and missile-firing toys. Don't allow your child to play with fireworks, including firecrackers, rockets and sparklers.
- Don't allow your children to use laser pointers. Laser pointers, especially those with short wave lengths such as green laser pointers, can permanently

damage the retina and cause visual loss with exposures as short as a few seconds. As an adult, be cautious when using laser pointers. Avoid directing the beam toward anyone's eyes.

▶ Wear protective eyewear during sports. Any sport featuring a ball, puck, stick, bat, racket or flying object carries a potential risk of eye injury. Choose sports protective eyewear labeled as ASTM F803 approved. Eyewear that hasn't been tested for sports use, such as sunglasses, can cause more harm than no eyewear at all.

▶ Keep small children safe around dogs. When young children are bitten by dogs, eye injuries frequently occur.

FEVER

A fever is a sign that your body is working to fight off an infection. Viral infections, strep throat and ear infections are the most common causes of fever in children. More-serious illnesses also can cause fever, but fortunately they aren't common, especially in fully vaccinated children.

Fever is one of the most common reasons parents call their children's medical providers. A fever in and of itself doesn't need to be treated. But if it persists for more than a few days, or it's accompanied by other signs or symptoms of illness, it makes sense to have it evaluated.

How to recognize it A "core" temperature of more than 100.4 degrees F is generally considered a fever. Often, a child's temperature is a little higher or lower than the average body temperature of 98.6 F during different parts of the day. A temporary rise in temperature can sometimes result from exercise, hot weather, being overdressed or drinking hot liquid.

Some parents swear they can tell if their child has a fever by feeling his or her forehead and cheeks. This method may be helpful in ruling out a fever. But it can't tell you your child's temperature.

To do that, you'll need a thermometer. The American Academy of Pediatrics recommends taking rectal measurements up until 4 years of age. A reading taken under the tongue, in the armpit or near the temples also can give you a good idea of your child's temperature. There's no need to add or subtract a degree. Just be sure to tell your child's medical provider what method you used. What's generally more important than the actual number is how your child is behaving.

How serious is it Although children tolerate most fevers quite well, high temperatures often provoke a great deal of anxiety for parents. But even high fevers aren't always a sign that there's a serious problem.

It's more important to take note of how your child is acting. If your child is responsive, continues to drink fluids and wants to play, there's probably nothing to worry about. Usually, your child's temperature will return to normal in one to three days.

Vaccinations help to protect your child against many serious illnesses. If your child hasn't been fully vaccinated and develops a fever, check in with your child's medical provider since your child will be at greater risk of serious illness. Tell your child's provider if your child's vaccinations aren't up to date.

When to call Call your child's medical provider promptly if your child has:
▶ A fever that persists for more than three days without a known cause or that reaches 103 F or higher

- A fever that returns after having gone away for 24 or more hours
- Burning or pain with urination
- Ear pain or ear pulling
- A cough and seems to be working harder to breathe
- A sore throat with fever

Seek urgent care if your child is acting very sick or your child's fever is accompanied by considerable listlessness, dehydration, difficulty breathing, a rash, stiff neck, severe headache, seizures, joint pain or swelling, or persistent vomiting or stomachache.

What you can do These suggestions may help your child feel better:

- Make sure your child is taking in plenty of fluids. Fever causes children to lose more fluids than usual. Water, ice chips, frozen juice bars or soup broth can provide extra fluid. Drinking plenty of fluids replaces those lost while sweating.
- Let your child decide how much he or she feels like eating.
- Avoid overdressing or bundling your child. This can make your child feel even warmer.
- Encourage extra rest and quiet play for two to three days.
- It's not necessary to give your child a cool bath. The benefits don't last long, and it may increase discomfort.

Most kids can return to school or child care after 24 hours of no fever without fever-reducing medications.

If you think your child will be more comfortable if you lower the fever, you can use acetaminophen (Tylenol, others) or ibuprofen (Advil, Motrin, others) to help reduce it. However, fever medications will not make the illness go away faster.

Follow the label instructions carefully. It's preferable to dose according to your child's weight rather than his or her age.

FEBRILE SEIZURES

Sometimes kids with a high fever react by having a seizure (febrile seizure). Although febrile seizures can be alarming, most are harmless and don't indicate an ongoing problem in a fully vaccinated child. In a child whose vaccinations aren't current, a fever and seizure could point to a more serious problem, such as meningitis or encephalomeningitis.

Febrile seizures are most common in younger children between the ages of 6 months and 3 years. The fever is often caused by either a bacterial or viral infection of the ears, nose and throat, or the stomach and intestines.

More than half of children who have a febrile seizure never have another one. But some kids may have repeated febrile seizures in early childhood. Febrile seizures sometimes run in families. The majority of children — whether they have one or more febrile seizures — stop having them by the time they are 4 or 5 years old.

What does a febrile seizure look like? Symptoms may include staring into space, shaking or involuntary tightening of the muscles. Sometimes, loss of consciousness occurs.

There are two types of febrile seizures — simple and complex. Most are simple. Simple febrile seizures involve both sides of the body and usually last less than 15 minutes. Complex febrile seizures may last longer than 15 minutes, involve one side of the body more than the other or occur more than once within 24 hours.

What should I do if my child has a seizure? You can't make the seizure stop, but you can help your child remain safe during the seizure. Gently help your child to a reclining position and turn your child on his or her side to prevent the tongue from falling backward and blocking the air passage. Don't put anything in your child's mouth and avoid restraining your child.

Most seizures aren't life-threatening, and they usually stop on their own within five minutes. If the seizure goes on for more than five minutes, if there's vomiting or difficulty breathing, or if the area around your child's lips turns a dusky or bluish color during the seizure, call an ambulance.

It's normal for children to sleep or feel especially groggy after having a febrile seizure. They may sleep heavily and may be difficult to arouse for 10 to 20 minutes. They may not remember the seizure happening and that's OK. If your child doesn't recover completely after an hour, seek emergency care.

After the seizure is over and your child is able to drink and swallow, you can give your child medication, such as acetaminophen (Tylenol, others) or ibuprofen (Advil, Motrin, others), to reduce the immediate fever and discomfort. Fever-reducing medications don't seem to be able to prevent recurrent febrile seizures, however.

Should I seek medical care for my child after he or she has a febrile seizure? Yes. Although febrile seizures rarely require treatment, a physician needs to determine the reason for the seizure and the fever to make sure they're not being caused by a more serious infection.

In some cases — such as a complex seizure, or if meningitis or another infection of the nervous system is suspected — your child may undergo a spinal tap (lumbar puncture). Certain blood tests also may be done. Less frequently, an electroencephalogram (EEG) or imaging of the brain such as a CT or MRI is done. The EEG measures brain function and is helpful to the medical provider in deciding how to treat your child. Generally, these tests aren't necessary, however.

Avoid giving both fever reducers and cough and cold medications, as the latter often contain fever reducers, too, and can increase the risk of overdose. Fever-reducing medications typically decrease core temperature by 1 to 3 degrees, regardless of the cause of fever. Don't use aspirin to reduce a fever in a child. Aspirin use in children has been linked to Reye's syndrome — a potentially life-threatening illness.

FLU (INFLUENZA)

Influenza, routinely known as the flu, is a common fall and wintertime viral illness that affects the upper respiratory system. It's often confused with the common cold, although the flu usually leaves your child feeling more achy and miserable than does a cold.

Several types of viruses can cause influenza (A and B are the most common), with each type having several strains. Influenza viruses are constantly changing, with new strains appearing regularly. This is why it's important to receive an annual flu vaccine — each year's vaccine is developed to prevent the three or four strains most likely to appear that year. The Centers for Disease Control and Prevention (CDC) recommends annual flu vaccination for all Americans over the age of 6 months. It's typically available as an injection in the inactivated form. Sometimes it's offered as a nasal spray. Always check the CDC's current recommendations to find out which form provides the best protection for the year.

How to recognize it The flu typically starts off with a sudden fever along with chills and shaking (unlike a cold, which usually develops slowly). Other flu symptoms may include headache, loss of energy, body aches and a dry, nonproductive cough. A runny or congested nose may follow. Young children occasionally experience nausea, vomiting or diarrhea. While a common cold can be a nuisance, the flu usually makes you feel much worse.

How serious is it? Most kids recover from the flu in about a week or so without any major problems. Some symptoms may persist a bit longer, such as a cough in younger children or weakness and tiredness in older kids. Influenza infections are contagious a day or so before your child becomes sick and while he or she is sick. The virus can still be spread after the fever has resolved.

Influenza can cause serious complications including death for some children, particularly those with an underlying health problem, such as asthma, diabetes or another chronic illness. Children with a condition that weakens the immune system, or who are taking a medication that suppresses the immune system, also are at high risk for flu-related complications. In addition, children younger than 5, and especially those under 2, are more susceptible to the dangers of the flu.

The most common complications of influenza are ear infections and pneumonia; bacterial pneumonia can get serious very quickly in some cases. Influenza can also worsen symptoms of asthma or another underlying respiratory condition.

When to call If your child is at high risk of complications of the flu, call your child's medical provider at the first sign of flu symptoms. Also call if your child is generally healthy but symptoms are severe. Severe symptoms include working hard to breathe, dehydration, persistent drowsiness or lethargy, inability to see or hear clearly, extreme weakness, and a severe sore throat making it hard to swallow.

For children at high risk of complications or with severe symptoms, antiviral medications may help lessen the duration and severity of the flu and reduce complications, especially if given within a day or two of the beginning of symptoms. Generally, antiviral medications are reserved for people who are really sick. Widespread or indiscriminate use of antivirals can eventually lessen the protective effect of the medication as viruses build up a resistance to it.

About 1 in 4 children develops a secondary infection, such as an ear infection or pneumonia, after getting the flu. These secondary infections occasionally are very serious. Call your child's medical provider if your child has a fever that goes away and then comes back, or if symptoms seem to be getting worse.

What you can do The best way to prevent the flu is to receive the flu vaccine, available to everyone 6 months of age or older. If your whole family receives the vaccine, you're less likely to get the flu and pass it to one another.

You can also encourage family members to take commonsense precautions against infections:

- Wash your hands frequently.
- Keep heavily used surfaces clean.
- Cough or sneeze into a tissue or the crook of your elbow (discard used tissues promptly).
- Don't share eating or drinking utensils or toothbrushes.
- Avoid cross-contamination between sick family members by not kissing each other on the hands or mouth.
- Avoid other people who have the flu.
- Avoid crowds at peak flu season, when the chances of coming into contact with influenza viruses are greater.

If your child does develop influenza, encourage plenty of rest, fluids and hugs. If your son or daughter seems uncomfortable, acetaminophen (Tylenol, others) can help ease aches and pains, as well as

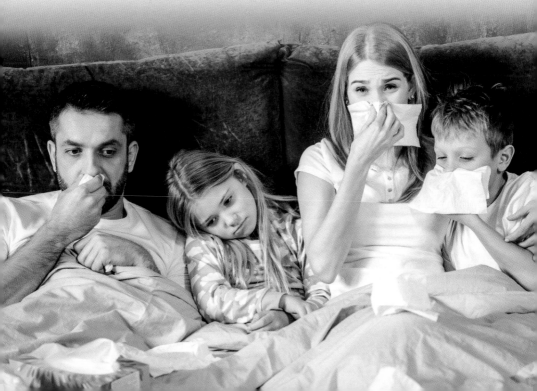

reduce fever. Don't give your child aspirin, which can cause serious side effects in kids who have a viral infection. Keep your child home from child care or school at least 24 hours after the fever has passed.

HAND-FOOT-AND-MOUTH DISEASE

Hand-foot-and-mouth disease is a mild, contagious viral infection common in young children. It's characterized by sores in the mouth and a rash on the hands and feet. It typically results from infection with coxsackievirus A16.

The illness spreads through person-to-person contact with an infected child's nasal secretions, saliva or stool. Hand-foot-and-mouth disease is often seen in child care settings because of frequent diaper changes and toilet training, and because little children often put their hands in their mouths. Exposure to fluid from ruptured blisters or from respiratory droplets sprayed into the air after a cough or sneeze also can spread the infection.

Although your child is most contagious with hand-foot-and-mouth disease during the first week of the illness, the virus can remain in his or her body for weeks after its signs and symptoms are gone. That means your child still can infect others. So it's important to have your child wash his or her hands frequently and sneeze or cough into a tissue or into his or her elbow.

Hand-foot-and-mouth disease isn't related to foot-and-mouth disease (sometimes called hoof-and-mouth disease), which is an infectious viral disease found in farm animals. You can't contract hand-foot-and-mouth disease from pets or other animals, and you can't transmit it to them.

How to recognize it Hand-foot-and-mouth disease may cause all of the following signs and symptoms or just some of them:

▶ Fever
▶ Sore throat
▶ Feeling of being unwell (malaise)
▶ Painful, red, blister-like lesions on the tongue, gums and inside of the cheeks
▶ A red rash, without itching but sometimes with blistering, on the palms, soles, and sometimes the buttocks, legs and arms
▶ Irritability in younger children
▶ Loss of appetite

The usual period from initial infection to the onset of signs and symptoms (incubation period) is three to six days. A fever is often the first sign of hand-foot-and-mouth disease, followed by a sore throat and sometimes a poor appetite and malaise. One or two days after the fever begins, painful sores may develop in the front of the mouth or throat. A rash on the hands and feet and possibly on the buttocks and genital area can follow within one or two days. Less commonly, the rash may be present on arms and legs as well.

How serious is it? Hand-foot-and-mouth disease is usually a minor illness causing only a few days of fever and relatively mild signs and symptoms. The most common complication of hand-foot-and-mouth disease is dehydration. Sores in the mouth and throat can make swallowing painful and difficult. Make sure your child frequently sips fluids during the course of the illness to prevent dehydration.

In rare cases the disease can lead to serious complications such as viral meningitis or encephalitis.

There's no specific treatment for hand-foot-and-mouth disease. Signs and symptoms usually clear up in seven to 10 days. A topical oral anesthetic, used according to instructions, may help relieve the pain of mouth sores. Over-the-counter pain medications other than aspirin, such as acetaminophen (Tylenol, others) or ibuprofen (Advil, Motrin, others) may help relieve general discomfort.

Kids can generally go back to school after they've been fever-free for 24 hours without fever-reducing medication and they're feeling well enough to eat and drink, and participate in class.

Frequent hand-washing and avoiding close contact with people who are infected with the disease may help reduce your child's risk of infection.

When to call Contact your child's medical provider if mouth sores or a sore throat keep your child from drinking fluids. Also contact your child's provider if after a few days, your child's signs and symptoms worsen.

What you can do To help make blister soreness less bothersome and eating and drinking more tolerable, have your child:
◗ Suck on ice pops or ice chips
◗ Eat ice cream or sherbet
◗ Drink cold beverages, such as milk or ice water
◗ Avoid acidic foods and beverages, such as citrus fruits, fruit drinks and soda
◗ Avoid salty or spicy foods
◗ Eat soft foods that don't require much chewing
◗ Rinse his or her mouth with warm water after meals

If your child is able to rinse without swallowing, swishing with warm salt water may be soothing. Have your child do this several times a day or as often as needed to help reduce the pain and inflammation of mouth and throat sores caused by hand-foot-and-mouth disease.

HEADACHES

Like adults, children can develop different types of headaches, including migraine or stress-related (tension) headaches. Children may also experience chronic daily headaches.

Headaches tend to become more common once a child reaches his or her teens, but they can develop in childhood and early adolescence. Among girls, headaches are often more prevalent during and after puberty.

Only rarely are childhood headaches related to a serious disorder. However, it's important to pay attention to your child's headache symptoms and consult your child's medical provider if the headaches worsen or they occur frequently.

A number of factors can cause your child to develop headaches. They include:
◗ *Unhealthy habits.* Most of the time, headaches occur due to irregular meals, dehydration, not getting enough sleep, overuse of electronic devices, lack of exercise and over-scheduling.
◗ *Illness and infection.* Common illnesses such as colds, flu, and ear and sinus infections are some of the most frequent causes of headaches in children. More-serious infections, such as meningitis or encephalitis, also can cause headaches, but these headaches are usually severe and accompanied by other signs and symptoms, such as a fever, severe sensitivity to light and neck stiffness.
◗ *Head trauma.* Bumps and bruises can cause headaches. Although most head injuries are minor, seek prompt medical attention if your child falls hard on his or her head or gets hit hard in the head. Also contact a doctor if your child's head pain steadily worsens after a head injury.

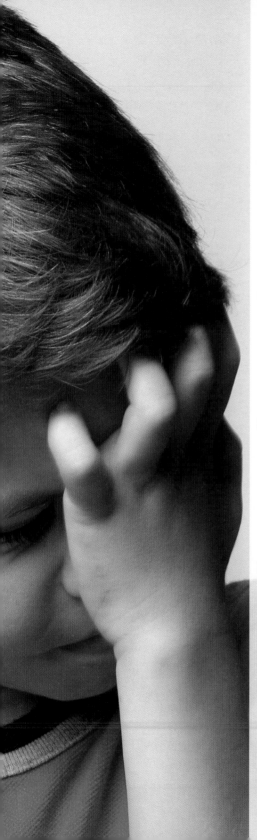

▶ *Emotional factors.* Stress and anxiety — perhaps triggered by problems with peers, teachers or parents — can play a role in children's headaches. Children with depression may complain of headaches, particularly if they have trouble recognizing feelings of sadness and loneliness.

▶ *Genetic predisposition.* Some children may be susceptible to headaches because of their genetic makeup. Headaches, particularly migraines, tend to run in families.

▶ *Vision issues.* Children with vision disorders who may be in need of glasses may complain of a headache.

▶ *Certain foods and beverages.* Nitrates — a type of food preservative found in cured meats, such as bacon, bologna and hot dogs — can trigger headaches, as can the food additive MSG. Also, too much caffeine — contained in soda, chocolate, coffee and tea — can cause headaches.

▶ *Medications.* Some medications can cause headaches as a side effect. In addition, frequent use of pain relievers such as acetaminophen or ibuprofen for headaches — more than three or four times per week — can cause what's called a medication overuse headache (previously called a rebound headache).

▶ *Problems in the brain.* Rarely, a brain tumor or abscess or bleeding in the brain can press on areas of the brain, causing a chronic, worsening headache. Typically in these cases, however, there are other symptoms in addition to persistent headaches, including persistent nausea and vomiting, lack of coordination, double vision, abnormal eye movements, seizures, behavioral changes, motor weakness, or regression in developmental milestones.

How to recognize it While children get the same types of headaches that adults do, their symptoms may differ.

Migraine Migraines in children can cause:

- Pulsating, throbbing or pounding head pain
- Pain that worsens with exertion
- Nausea
- Vomiting
- Abdominal pain
- Extreme sensitivity to light, sound and movement

Even young children can have migraines. A child who hasn't yet developed adequate communication skills may cry and hold his or her head to indicate severe pain. He or she may not eat or may be extremely restless or irritable.

Some children may not have head pain but may experience repeated attacks of abdominal pain and vomiting along with other migraine-type symptoms such as sensitivity to light and sound, followed by periods of feeling completely better. Migraines are often aggravated by physical activity and improved by sleep.

For most children, migraine pain is bilateral and may last for two to 72 hours.

Tension-type headache Tension-type headaches in children can cause:

- A pressing tightness in the muscles of the head or neck
- Mild to moderate steady pain on both sides of the head
- Pain that doesn't worsen during physical activity

Unlike a migraine, this type of headache isn't accompanied by nausea or vomiting. Tension-type headaches can last from 30 minutes to several days. Younger children may withdraw from regular play and want to sleep more.

Cluster headache Cluster headaches are uncommon in children. They usually:

- Occur in groups of five or more episodes, ranging from one headache every other day to eight a day
- Involve sharp, stabbing pain on one side of the head that lasts less than three hours
- Are accompanied by tearing from the eyes, changes in pupil size, eyelid swelling, congestion, a runny nose, forehead and facial flushing, or restlessness or agitation

Chronic daily headache Doctors use the term *chronic daily headache* for migraine and tension-type headaches that occur more than 15 days a month for more than three months in a row.

How serious is it? Headaches in children usually aren't serious, and they can often be treated at home with over-the-counter pain medications and lifestyle measures. Rest, decreased noise, plenty of fluids and balanced meals may help relieve a headache.

If your child is older and has frequent headaches, measures to help him or her relax and manage stress also may help.

Medications Acetaminophen (Tylenol, others) or ibuprofen (Advil, Motrin, others) can typically relieve headaches in children. They should be taken at the first sign of a headache. Use caution when giving aspirin to children. Although aspirin is approved for use in children older than age 2, it's been linked to Reye's syndrome, a rare but potentially life-threatening condition in children. Talk to your child's medical provider if you have concerns.

Prescription drugs called triptans are sometimes used to treat migraines. They're effective and can be used safely in children older than 6 years of age. If your child experiences nausea and vomiting with a migraine, your child's medical provider may prescribe an anti-nausea drug as well.

If your child is experiencing frequent headaches, your child's doctor may prescribe a daily preventive (prophylactic) medication to reduce the frequency and intensity of the headaches.

Medication strategies differ from child to child, however. Be sure to discuss the use of medication with your child's medical provider.

Behavioral therapies Stress can act as a trigger for headaches or make a headache worse. Depression and other mental health disorders also can play a role. In such situations, your child's medical provider may recommend behavioral therapies, such as:

▶ *Relaxation training.* Relaxation techniques might include deep breathing, yoga and meditation. Another technique is progressive muscle relaxation, which is accomplished by tensing one muscle at a time, and then completely releasing the tension, until every muscle in the body is relaxed. An older child might be able to learn relaxation techniques using books or videos, or by taking a class.

▶ *Biofeedback training.* Biofeedback teaches your child to control certain body responses that help reduce pain. During a biofeedback session, your child is connected to devices that monitor and give feedback on body functions, such as muscle tension, heart rate and blood pressure.

Your child then learns how to reduce muscle tension and slow his or her heart rate and breathing. The goal of biofeedback is to help your child enter a relaxed state to better cope with headache pain.

▶ *Cognitive behavioral therapy.* This type of therapy can help your child

---

SAFE USE OF PAIN MEDICATIONS

Over-the-counter pain relievers, such as acetaminophen (Tylenol, others) and ibuprofen (Advil, Motrin, others), are usually effective in reducing headache pain. Before giving your child pain medication, keep these points in mind:

▶ Read labels carefully and use only the dosages recommended for your child.
▶ Don't give doses more frequently than recommended.
▶ Don't give your child an over-the-counter pain medication more than two or three days a week. Daily use can trigger a medication overuse headache (see page 342).
▶ Use caution if giving aspirin to children or teenagers. Although aspirin is approved for use in children older than age 2, it's not recommended for children and teenagers recovering from chickenpox or flu-like symptoms. This is because aspirin has been linked to Reye's syndrome, a rare but potentially life-threatening condition. Talk to your child's doctor if you have concerns.

For information on dosages of acetaminophen and ibuprofen by age and weight, see the charts on pages 478 and 479.

learn to manage stress and reduce the frequency and severity of headaches. A therapist helps your child learn ways to recognize potentially stressful situations and to view and cope with life events more positively.

When to call Most headaches aren't serious, but seek prompt medical care if your child's headaches:
▶ Wake your child from sleep
▶ Worsen or become more frequent
▶ Change your child's personality
▶ Follow an injury, such as a blow to the head
▶ Feature persistent vomiting or vision changes
▶ Are accompanied by a fever and neck pain or stiffness

What you can do The following steps may help prevent headaches or reduce the severity of headaches in your child:
▶ *Rest and relaxation.* Encourage your child to rest in a dark, quiet room. Sleeping often resolves headaches in children.
▶ *Use a cool, wet compress.* While your child rests, place a cool, wet cloth on his or her forehead.
▶ *Offer a healthy snack.* If your child hasn't eaten in a while, offer a piece of fruit, whole-wheat crackers or low-fat cheese. Not eating can make headaches worse.
▶ *Practice healthy behaviors.* Behaviors that promote general good health can help prevent headaches for your child. These lifestyle measures include getting at least nine hours of sleep every night, avoiding screen time one to two hours before bedtime, staying physically active, eating healthy meals and snacks, drinking four to eight glasses of water daily, and avoiding caffeine.

▶ *Reduce stress.* Stress and busy schedules may increase the frequency of headaches. Be alert for things that may cause stress in your child's life, such as difficulty doing schoolwork or strained relationships with peers. If your child's headaches are linked to anxiety or depression, consider talking to a counselor or your child's medical provider.
▶ *Keep a headache diary.* A diary may help you determine what causes your child's headaches. Note when the headaches start, how long they last and what, if anything, provides relief.
▶ *Avoid triggers.* Avoid any food or drinks containing ingredients such as caffeine or artificial sweeteners, that seem to trigger headaches. Your headache diary can help you determine what prompts your child's headaches so you know what to avoid.
▶ *Follow the plan.* Your child's medical provider may recommend preventive medication if your child's headaches are severe, occur daily and interfere with your child's normal lifestyle. Certain medications taken at regular intervals may reduce the frequency and severity of headaches.

HIVES

Hives is the common name for a skin reaction that produces slightly raised areas of pink or red skin that are usually very itchy. The medical term for the condition is urticaria. These affected areas can range in size from small spots to large blotches.

Many things can trigger hives, including an allergic reaction to food or medication, a viral infection, insect bites and stings, airborne allergens, cold weather, changes in body temperature, sun exposure, or stress. Oftentimes, the cause is a mystery; there's no clear explanation for what causes the rash to develop.

How to recognize it Hives are characterized by splotchy, red, raised areas of skin, often with pale centers. The red areas may be irregular in shape, and they often itch or are uncomfortable. Hives can appear all over your child's body, or the rash may be concentrated in one area. And they may change locations. Some areas may enlarge and merge into each other.

Hives symptoms may last for a few hours and disappear or they may come and go for a few days or a few weeks.

How serious is it? Fortunately, hives usually are harmless and temporary. Sometimes, however, the rash may be accompanied by sudden difficulty breathing or swallowing, a swollen tongue, a sudden onset of vomiting or diarrhea, or an increased heart rate. Hives along with these symptoms may be a sign of a serious allergic reaction (anaphylaxis). Anaphylaxis requires emergency care (see page 308).

When to call If your child develops hives, contact his or her medical provider about how best to treat the condition. It's especially important to contact a provider if your child:

- Develops hives while taking medication (discontinue the medication until you've talked with your child's medical provider)
- Seems to have soreness in his or her joints
- Has hives for more than a few days
- Has hives that stay fixed in the same area of the body for 24 to 48 hours

Seek emergency medical assistance if your child develops signs of anaphylaxis, such as sudden difficulty breathing or swallowing, vomiting, diarrhea or rapid heart rate. Your child may need an injection of epinephrine to reduce the swelling.

What you can do Children with hives often look much worse than they feel. To keep your child as comfortable as possible, give your child an oral antihistamine. This will help relieve the itch and discomfort. You may need to maintain an antihistamine dosage schedule over the course of a week or so, as hives can go away and then come back.

Keep your child dressed in light, loose clothing and avoid bathing him or her in hot water. Lukewarm water is less likely to worsen the itching. Trim your child's fingernails to avoid scratching.

If your child frequently develops hives, keep a log of the outbreaks. Each time he or she develops a rash, jot down the foods he or she ate that day, what activity he or she was involved in, and where he or she was. By tracking this information, you may be able to identify a pattern to help determine a cause. Hives can happen within moments of exposure to the trigger, but they may not appear until a couple of hours later.

IMPETIGO

Impetigo is a common and highly contagious skin infection that mainly affects young children and infants. It usually appears as a red, coin-shaped rash covered in a flaking, honey-colored crust. Less commonly it can develop into blisters. It tends to occur on the face, especially around a child's nose and mouth, and on the hands and feet.

Impetigo typically develops when bacteria enter the skin through cuts or insect bites. But it can also develop in skin that's perfectly healthy. The condition is most common in children ages 2 to 5. It spreads easily in crowded places such as child care settings and schools. It also tends to be more common during the summer when the weather is warm and humid.

Keeping your child's skin clean is the best way to prevent this type of infection. Treat cuts, scrapes, insect bites and other wounds right away by washing the affected areas and applying antibiotic ointment to prevent infection.

How to recognize it Your child might have impetigo if you notice:

▶ Round, red sores that quickly rupture, ooze for a few days and then form a yellowish-brown crust

▶ Mild itching

▶ Painful fluid- or pus-filled sores that turn into deep ulcers (This is the more serious form of impetigo.)

How serious is it? Impetigo usually clears on its own within a few weeks. But because impetigo can sometimes lead to a more severe infection, your child's medical provider may choose to treat impetigo with an antibiotic ointment or oral antibiotics.

To prevent the spread of the infection, it's important to keep your child home from child care or school until he or she is no longer contagious — usually 24 hours after beginning treatment with an antibiotic.

When to call If you suspect that your child has impetigo, ask your child's medical provider for advice on treatment. If the infection is mild, the medical provider may recommend only hygienic measures. Keeping the skin clean can help mild infections heal on their own.

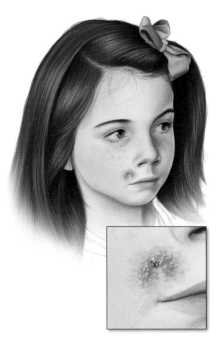

Impetigo is a bacterial infection of the skin that starts with a round, red sore that blisters briefly, oozes and forms a thick crust.

If your child is uncomfortable, or the sores are oozing or widespread, make an appointment to have the sores examined. Severe or widespread impetigo may need to be treated with oral antibiotics. Be sure your child finishes the entire course of medication, even if the sores have healed. This helps prevent the infection from recurring and makes antibiotic resistance less likely.

What you can do For minor infections that haven't spread to other areas, try the following:

▶ Soak the affected areas of skin with warm water or a vinegar solution — 1 tablespoon (½ ounce) of white vinegar to 1 pint (16 ounces) of water. This keeps the area clean, helps rid the crust of germs and helps the crust naturally detach over time.

After the crust has fallen away, apply an over-the-counter antibiotic ointment three times daily. Wash the skin before each application and pat it dry.

▶ Trim your child's nails to prevent scratching and spreading of the infection. Applying a nonstick dressing to the infected area can help, too.

▶ Encourage your child not to touch the infected area.

To help keep the infection from spreading to others, hand-washing is important. Have your child wash his or her hands frequently and you do the same. It's especially important that you do so after applying antibiotic ointment to the sores. Also, wash your child's towels and washcloths every day and don't share them or other items, such as blankets, with family members.

INSECT BITES AND STINGS

For a child, being bit or stung by an insect can be scary and painful. Fortunately, bites and stings typically produce only a minor skin reaction that's often accompanied by itching.

Sometimes, however, a child can have a more significant reaction that includes redness and swelling. This is called a local reaction. A small number of children experience a severe allergic reaction to stings from certain insects, especially bees, wasps and hornets. This severe reaction is called anaphylaxis and requires emergency treatment (see page 308).

How to recognize it Bites and stings may come from:

▶ *Bees, wasps and hornets.* In most children, stings cause initial pain and become red and swollen within the first several hours.

▶ *Mosquitoes.* Most often the site simply itches and may swell slightly.

▶ *Deerflies, horseflies, fire ants, harvester ants, beetles and centipedes.* These bites can cause painful red bumps that may blister or cause swelling.

How serious is it? Most children will have only a mild reaction to bites and stings. But some children are more sensitive than are others to insect venom, especially that of a stinging insect. In these kids, stings can cause anaphylaxis. Signs and symptoms of anaphylaxis include severe shortness of breath; swelling; itching or hives; sudden vomiting, diarrhea or dizziness; increased heart rate; and low blood pressure.

When to call Signs and symptoms of a bite or sting usually disappear in a day or two. If you're concerned, even if the reaction is minor, contact your child's medical provider. Seek immediate care if your child:

▶ Has received multiple stings from a bee, wasp or hornet and has severe swelling

▶ Has increased swelling and redness around the sting or bite after the first six to eight hours

▶ Develops hives all over the body or in an area separate from the sting itself

Also seek emergency care if your child has signs or symptoms of anaphylaxis. For a severe reaction, your child may need an injection of epinephrine to reduce the swelling.

What you can do If a stinger is noticeable, remove it from your child's skin as soon as possible. Use a credit card, firm piece of paper or other thin dull edge to scrape the stinger away. Avoid pinching or squeezing the stinger, as this may release more venom into the skin.

INSECT SPRAY AND CHILDREN

DEET is the most common chemical found in insect repellents. DEET shouldn't be used on children younger than 2 months of age. In children older than 2 months, the American Academy of Pediatrics (AAP) recommends using the lowest effective concentration for the amount of time your child spends outside.

The higher the concentration of DEET in a product, the longer the protective time it supplies. Products with 10 percent DEET provide about two hours of protection. A 24 percent DEET product provides about five hours of protection. The AAP recommends that insect repellents containing more than 30 percent DEET not be used on children.

When using a repellent on a child, apply it only once during the day and wash it off at the end of the day to avoid toxicity.

There are alternatives to DEET products. Picaridin in 5 to 10 percent concentrations is safe for young children. Oil of lemon eucalyptus is a plant-based repellent that's effective for up to 2 hours, after which you need to reapply. It's not recommended for children under 3 years of age.

Once the stinger is gone, wash the area carefully with soap and water and then apply a cool washcloth or ice pack to relieve pain and swelling. Cool compresses can also help relieve itching associated with mosquitoes, flies, ants and other insect bites.

Over-the-counter creams or ointments, such as calamine lotion or 1% hydrocortisone cream, may be applied to the site to help relieve the itching. For severe itching, your child's medical provider may recommend an oral antihistamine.

To decrease the likelihood of experiencing insect bites:

- Have your child wear lightweight clothing that covers most of his or her skin when outdoors
- Avoid areas where insects are commonly found, such as garbage cans, stagnant water (breeding ground for mosquitoes) and blooming flowers
- Use insect repellents as needed
- Don't use strong perfumes or scented soaps and lotions on yourself or your child
- Cover all picnic food, and seal picnic garbage in plastic bags
- Keep garbage cans securely covered
- Don't allow pools of stagnant water in your backyard

LICE

Lice are tiny, wingless, grayish-white insects that easily spread — especially in child care settings and among schoolchildren — through close personal contact and shared belongings. Several types of lice exist; the most common in children is head lice.

It can be difficult to prevent the spread of head lice in child care facilities and schools because there's so much close contact among children and their belongings. It's not a failure on your part as a parent or a reflection of your hygiene habits or those of your children if your child gets head lice.

Lice spread to humans through contact with the insects themselves or their eggs. Lice can't fly or walk on the ground. Transmission occurs by way of:

- *Head-to-head contact.* This may occur as children or family members play or interact closely.
- *Proximity of stored belongings.* Storing infested clothing in closets, in lockers or on side-by-side hooks at school, or storing personal items such as pillows, blankets, combs and stuffed toys close together can permit lice to spread.
- *Items shared among friends or family members.* These may include clothing, headphones, brushes, combs, hair decorations, towels, pillows and stuffed toys.
- *Contact with contaminated furniture.* Lying on a bed or sitting in overstuffed, cloth-covered furniture recently used by someone with lice can facilitate their spread. Lice can live for one to two days off the body.

Once one family member is identified as having head lice, all members of the household should be checked for lice infestation.

How to recognize it Signs and symptoms of head lice include:

- Intense itching
- A tickling feeling on the scalp
- Small red bumps on the scalp, neck, ears and shoulders
- Presence of adult lice on the scalp or in the hair. Adult lice are about the size of a sesame seed or slightly larger
- Presence of lice eggs (nits) on hair shafts. Nits attach to hair shafts using

a glue-like substance that makes them difficult to remove. They resemble dandruff but don't brush off as easily as dandruff does.

If only nits are present — with no sign of adult lice — there may not be an active infestation and treatment may not be required. This is especially true when nits are found more than a quarter of an inch away from the scalp.

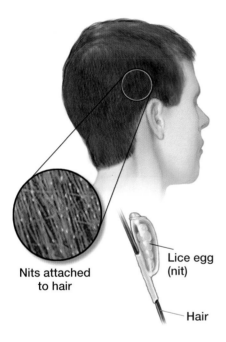

Nits attached to hair

Lice egg (nit)

Hair

How serious is it? Having head lice isn't a serious health threat, but unless it's treated properly, it can become a recurring problem.

You may be able to get rid of head lice on your child by using an over-the-counter shampoo that's specifically formulated to kill lice. Hair products containing pyrethrin (Rid) or permethrin (Nix) are usually the first option to combat lice infestations. Pyrethrin is safe for children over 2 years, and permethrin is safe for those older than 2 months. They work best if you follow the directions very

closely. Continue to check your child's hair regularly for two to three weeks to make sure all of the lice and nits are gone.

In some geographical locations, lice have grown resistant to the ingredients in over-the-counter lice products. If over-the-counter preparations don't work, your child's medical provider can prescribe shampoos or lotions that contain different ingredients.

When to call If an over-the-counter shampoo doesn't kill the lice, talk to your child's medical provider. He or she may recommend a prescription shampoo for your child. Also contact your child's medical provider if your child develops infected hives or skin abrasions from scratching.

What you can do You can get rid of head lice with a thorough treatment approach. The following steps can help you eliminate lice infestations:

Use shampoos and rinses Begin with an over-the-counter product designed to kill lice (Rid, Nix, others). Apply the product according to package instructions. You may need to repeat treatment in seven to 10 days. Rinse the medication from your child's head over a sink instead of in the shower to limit skin exposure. If an over-the-counter product doesn't work, contact your child's medical provider.

Comb wet hair Use a fine-toothed nit comb to physically remove the lice from wet hair. Repeat every three to four days for at least two weeks. Although it can be tedious, it's generally effective. This method may be used in combination with other treatments. It's usually recommended as the first line of treatment for children under 2 years.

Wash combs and brushes Use very hot, soapy water — at least 130 F — to wash combs and brushes, or soak them in rubbing alcohol for an hour.

Wash contaminated items Wash bedding, stuffed animals, clothing and hats with hot, soapy water and dry them at high heat for at least 20 minutes.

Seal nonwashable items Place them in an airtight bag for two weeks.

Vacuum Give the floor and furniture a good vacuuming. Head lice don't survive long if they can't feed. So don't spend too much time or too many resources on housecleaning.

Don't share items Don't share combs, brushes or towels; clothing such as hats, scarves, coats and headbands; or items such as headphones with other family members or friends.

School attendance Some schools have a "no-nit" policy that prohibits school attendance for any student who has even a single nit. As long as a child has been adequately treated for lice, however, this policy isn't recommended by the American Academy of Pediatrics due to the difficulty of complete nit removal.

PINK EYE

Pink eye (conjunctivitis) is an inflammation or infection of the transparent membrane (conjunctiva) that lines the eyelid and covers the white part of the eyeball. When small blood vessels in the conjunctiva become inflamed, they're more visible. This is what causes the whites of your child's eyes to appear reddish or pink.

Pink eye is commonly caused by a bacterial or viral infection. It may also occur as part of an allergic reaction. A foreign object in the eye or chemical exposure can produce inflammation of the conjunctiva as well. Chemical exposure may include chlorine in swimming pools, air pollution or a chemical splash to the eye.

Viral and bacterial conjunctivitis Most cases of pink eye are the result of a virus. Both viral and bacterial conjunctivitis can occur along with a cold or symptoms of a respiratory infection. Bacterial conjunctivitis may also result if your child wears contact lenses that haven't been properly cleaned.

Generally, viral conjunctivitis produces a watery discharge, whereas bacterial conjunctivitis produces a discharge that's thicker, pus-like, and yellow, greenish or white. One or both eyes may be affected.

Viral and bacterial conjunctivitis are very contagious. The condition often begins in one eye and then infects the other eye within a few days. It spreads through direct or indirect contact with the liquid that drains from an infected eye.

Allergic conjunctivitis Allergic conjunctivitis is a response to an allergy-causing substance such as pollen. Special cells (mast cells) located in the mucous lining of the eyes and airways release inflammatory substances, including histamines, when they sense an allergen is present. The release of histamine can produce a number of allergy-related signs, including red or pink eyes. Generally, both eyes are affected.

If your child has allergic conjunctivitis, he or she may experience itching, tearing and inflammation of the eyes — as well as sneezing and watery nasal discharge.

How to recognize it Common signs and symptoms of pink eye include:
- Redness in one or both eyes
- Tearing in the eye
- A discharge that forms a crust during the night and may prevent the eye or eyes from opening in the morning

---

PREVENTING PINK EYE SPREAD

To prevent other family members from getting the infection, practice good hygiene:
- Don't touch your eyes with your hands.
- Wash your hands often.
- Use a clean towel and washcloth daily.
- Don't share towels or washcloths.
- Change pillowcases often.

If possible, keep your child at home until the eye discharge has stopped. Viral conjunctivitis generally doesn't require treatment, so treat it as you would a common cold. Check with your doctor if you have questions about when your child can go back to school or child care. Some schools or child care centers require that your child wait at least 24 hours after starting treatment before returning. In cases of viral conjunctivitis, in which treatment typically isn't needed, a note from your doctor can explain the situation.

- A gritty feeling in one or both eyes
- Itchiness in one or both eyes

How serious is it? Although pink eye can be irritating, it rarely affects your child's vision. Treatment varies depending on the cause.

Viral and bacterial conjunctivitis Most cases of viral conjunctivitis get better on their own with basic steps that you can take at home including using artificial tears, cleaning your child's eyelids with a wet cloth, and applying cold or warm compresses several times daily. If your child wears contact lenses, he or she should stop wearing them until the infection is gone. Typically, viral conjunctivitis needs time to run its course — generally one to two weeks. Eye redness should gradually clear on its own. Antibiotics can't treat a virus and, therefore, they aren't recommended to treat viral conjunctivitis.

If your child has a bacterial infection, he or she may need antibiotic eyedrops, although not in every case. Mild bacterial conjunctivitis may get better on its own within a few days. If it doesn't, see your child's medical provider.

Allergic conjunctivitis If your child's conjunctivitis is due to allergies, his or her medical provider may prescribe one of many different types of eyedrops. These may include medications that help control allergic reactions, such as antihistamines and mast cell stabilizers, or drugs that help control inflammation, such as decongestants, steroids and anti-inflammatory drops.

Over-the-counter anti-inflammatory medications or eyedrops that contain antihistamines also may be effective. Ask your child's provider which product to use.

When to call Contact your child's medical provider if symptoms don't improve. This could indicate a bacterial infection, possibly requiring an antibiotic. Also contact your child's medical provider or seek urgent care if he or she complains of eye pain, light sensitivity, blurred or disrupted vision, or the feeling that something is stuck in his or her eye (foreign body sensation).

What you can do To help your child cope until the condition clears up:
- *Apply a compress to the eyes.* To make a compress, soak a clean, lint-free cloth in water and wring it out before applying it gently to his or her closed eyelids. Generally, a cool water compress will feel the most soothing, but you can also use a warm compress if that feels better to your child. If pink eye affects only one eye, don't touch both eyes with the same cloth. This reduces the risk of spreading pink eye from one eye to the other.
- *Try eyedrops.* Over-the-counter eyedrops called artificial tears may help relieve symptoms. Some eyedrops contain antihistamines or other medications that can be helpful for people with allergic conjunctivitis.
- *Stop wearing contact lenses.* If your child wears contact lenses, he or she should stop wearing them until the condition is cleared up. Throw away the lenses he or she was wearing when the conjunctivitis developed, as well as the cleaning solution and lens case, in case they became infected.

STOMACHACHES

Stomachaches and children seem to go hand in hand. Often, the pain is due to indigestion, constipation or the beginning of a bout with a stomach virus.

Sometimes, a child may complain of intermittent stomachaches that tend to occur in specific situations or at certain times of the day. This pain may be associated with stress or fear concerning a social situation or school issue. In many children, these types of stomachaches gradually disappear, but some children experience recurrent bouts over several years.

Occasionally, a sudden severe stomachache can be a symptom of a more-serious condition such as appendicitis or inflammatory bowel disease.

While most stomach pain typically isn't something to worry about, contact your child's medical provider if the pain gets worse, is accompanied by other symptoms such as a high fever or significant vomiting or diarrhea, or lasts longer than a week — sooner if the pain is severe.

How to recognize it Usually, your child will let you know if he or she has a stomachache. What can sometimes be difficult is determining the cause of the pain.

Specific cause Stomach pain associated with a specific physical cause may be accompanied by the following:
▶ Pain that awakens your child at night
▶ Vomiting, diarrhea, bloating or gas, rash, or fever
▶ Changes in bowel or bladder function
▶ Pain when the abdomen is pressed (abdominal tenderness)
▶ Blood in the vomit, stool or urine, which requires prompt evaluation

Common conditions that can produce stomach pain include constipation, gas, or a food intolerance. Some kids experience a stomachache after drinking milk or eating ice cream, cheese or other foods that contain milk. They may have lactose intolerance, a condition in which their bodies aren't able to digest the sugar (lactose) in milk. Children who are lactose intolerant experience cramping pain, bloating, gas or diarrhea after eating or drinking lactose-containing products.

Less common causes of stomach pain include inflammatory bowel disease, celiac disease, a urinary tract infection or other infection. Sometimes a child with strep throat will complain of a stomachache and fever rather than a sore throat.

Nonspecific cause Stomach pain that doesn't have a known cause may have these characteristics:
▶ The pain is difficult for your child to describe or locate.
▶ The pain is unrelated to meals, activity or bowel movements. The pain may occur without other symptoms or with vague symptoms such as nausea, dizziness and fatigue.
▶ The pain typically is short-lived.
▶ The pain isn't accompanied by a fever, rash, joint pain or swelling.

Stomach or abdominal pain that can't be explained by any visible or detectable abnormality after a thorough examination is referred to as functional, or non-specific, abdominal pain.

Functional abdominal pain may be triggered by stress or anxiety. It can develop during periods of change or stress within a family — such as the birth of a new sibling, a family member's illness, a parent being away from home, or a move to a new city or school. In some cases, a child can develop chronic abdominal pain.

Another theory is that some kids have a heightened sensitivity to nerve impulses that makes them more prone to feel pain during periods of emotional stress or with daily occurrences, such as movement of gas and stool through their bowels.

What's important to remember is that the pain can be real, even though there's no obvious cause. Functional abdominal pain doesn't mean that children aren't experiencing pain or that it's "all in their heads."

Pay attention to psychological or emotional concerns that might be making the pain worse. Your child's medical provider or a child therapist, psychologist or psychiatrist can suggest ways to help your child talk about his or her troubles. These providers can also offer tips on how to respond to your child's pain in a manner that doesn't support continuation of the pain. If, for example, you're constantly worried about your child's pain, your child may become more anxious and the pain may worsen.

How serious is it? In most cases, a stomachache is short-lived and gets better without treatment. A more severe stomachache sometimes can be a warning of a more serious illness, and a persistent stomachache may signal a chronic condition.

For some children, recurrent stomachaches can interfere with normal daily functioning, including attending school. In this type of situation, goals of treatment are to lessen the pain and help your child return to normal activities such as school and playing with friends. Be aware that it may take some time to figure out what's causing the pain and determine the best treatment.

Treatment for functional or nonspecific abdominal pain may include:

Relaxation techniques Older children and adolescents with functional abdominal pain can learn muscle relaxation techniques and deep-breathing exercises.

CONSTIPATION AND BELLY PAIN

Constipation is a common cause of abdominal pain in children. If your child isn't getting enough fluids or eating enough fiber, constipation is more likely to occur.

Each child's bowel patterns are different; become familiar with your child's normal bowel patterns. If your child doesn't have normal bowel movements every few days or is uncomfortable when stools are passed, he or she may need help in developing proper bowel habits.

To help prevent constipation:

▶ Encourage your child to drink plenty of water.
▶ Make sure your child eats high-fiber foods each day. Foods high in fiber include fresh fruits and vegetable, whole-grains and beans.
▶ Help your child set up a regular toileting routine.
▶ Encourage your child to be physically active. Exercise along with a balanced diet helps prevent constipation in addition to being a foundation for a healthy, active life.

How much fiber should your child get? The American Academy of Pediatrics recommends this formula for children and teens between the ages of 2 and 19: Your child's age plus 5 grams. For example, if your child is 10 years old, he or she should consume 15 grams of fiber daily (age 10 + 5 grams = 15 grams).

These techniques performed daily may help reduce stress and anxiety. They can also be used during times of pain.

Behavioral therapies These are designed to help reduce anxiety and stress and help your child better tolerate the pain. Common types of behavioral therapies include cognitive behavioral therapy, biofeedback, psychotherapy and hypnosis.

When to call Contact your child's medical provider if you have any concerns about your child's abdominal pain. Also, call if your child experiences any of the following:
- Pain that lasts one week or longer, even if it comes and goes and is mild
- Pain that doesn't improve in 24 hours or gets more severe or frequent
- Pain that's accompanied by vomiting for more than 12 hours or diarrhea for more than two days
- Pain that's accompanied by a burning sensation during urination

See your child's medical provider immediately or seek urgent care if your child has:
- Severe pain lasting more than an hour
- Pain along with blood in the urine or a change in the color of urine
- Pain in the scrotum or testicle
- Pain located or moving to the right lower part of your child's abdomen that makes it hard for your child to stand up straight, walk or hop
- Pain that comes and goes for more than a day
- Pain that's becoming more severe and constant
- Bloody stools, severe diarrhea, or recurrent or bloody vomiting
- Severe pain accompanied by fever
- Refused to eat or drink anything for a prolonged period

- Changes in behavior, including lethargy or decreased responsiveness

What you can do If your child complains of a stomachache, try these tips to see if the pain improves:
- Have your child lie quietly and rest.
- Offer sips of water or other clear fluids.
- Suggest that your child go to the bathroom and try to poop.
- Avoid solid foods for a few hours. Then try small amounts of mild foods such as rice, applesauce or crackers. Avoid foods and beverages that can be irritating to the stomach, such as fried or greasy foods, tomato products, dairy products, or carbonated or caffeinated beverages.

Stress-related pain If you think that your child's stomachaches may be related to stress and anxiety, make sure to provide your child with positive attention, especially during periods of change. One way that you can do this is to schedule regular time devoted solely to your child — the two of you alone together talking or doing a fun activity. Scheduled time together is preferable to random times spent together in the car or with other siblings. Being together only when your child complains of a stomachache teaches your child that this is the way to get your attention and spend time with you.

STOMACH VIRUS (GASTROENTERITIS)

Diarrhea and vomiting — not fun. No one wants a stomach bug in the house, but when it happens, it can make for an unpleasant few days. Luckily, it doesn't usually last long and most of the time requires only rest and plenty of fluids.

Although a bout of diarrhea and vomiting is often referred to as the stomach flu, this isn't the same as the flu (influenza). Influenza affects the respiratory system — the nose, throat and lungs. Stomach flu is more accurately called gastroenteritis, which means inflammation of the lining of the stomach and intestinal system. It's often due to infection by a virus, but bacteria and, rarely, parasites also can cause gastroenteritis.

These infectious causes of gastroenteritis are all contagious. As long as your child has diarrhea, he or she is considered contagious. It's best to keep your child at home and away from others until diarrhea and vomiting improve. Diarrhea-causing germs are passed from hand to mouth, which means that proper hand-washing is key to keeping germs in check.

How to recognize it Diarrhea — frequent, runny bowel movements — is the primary sign of gastroenteritis. An occasional instance of runny poop is within the range of normal.

But if your child has a stomach bug, he or she may be making multiple trips to the toilet for a day or two. Other signs and symptoms of gastroenteritis include a fever, loss of appetite, nausea, vomiting, painful stomach cramps and muscle aches.

A sudden onset of watery diarrhea is probably due to a viral infection. A sudden onset of watery diarrhea with signs of blood in it, along with a fever, is likely a result of a bacterial infection. Chronic watery diarrhea may be due to parasites or an underlying illness, such as irritable bowel syndrome or celiac disease.

How serious is it? For most kids, the biggest complication of diarrhea and vomiting is loss of fluids leading to dehydration. Helping your child stay hydrated while he or she is sick can prevent this.

Most cases of gastroenteritis can be treated at home with rest and plenty of fluids. Antibiotics won't help viral infections. Even with bacterial causes, antibiotics are effective in only certain infections, such as those acquired while traveling. In some cases, antibiotics may increase the risk of complications such as hemolytic uremic syndrome, a condition that damages red blood cells. Furthermore, indiscriminate use of antibiotics can contribute to the rise of drug-resistant bacteria. Parasitic infections are generally treated with anti-parasitic medications.

When to call See your child's medical provider right away if your child:
▶ Has a fever of 102 F or higher
▶ Seems lethargic or very irritable
▶ Is in a lot of discomfort or pain
▶ Has bloody diarrhea
▶ Develops a rash or bruising
▶ Has changes in urine color or blood in his or her urine
▶ Seems dehydrated — watch for signs of dehydration in sick children by noting how much they drink and urinate compared with when they're not sick (urinating less than three times in 24 hours often indicates dehydration)
▶ Refuses to eat or drink anything for more than eight hours
▶ Has symptoms that last more than three days

What you can do When your child has diarrhea or is throwing up, or especially when both are present, the most important goal is to replace lost fluids and salts (see page 321). These suggestions may help.
▶ *Help your child rehydrate.* Give your child an oral rehydration solution (Pedialyte) available at pharmacies

PROPER HAND-WASHING

One of the best ways to keep from getting sick is to have good hand hygiene — which is another way of saying wash your hands often and well. Washing your hands gets rid of germs that your hands pick up throughout the day — whether from preparing food, taking out the garbage or using the toilet — and prevents them from being transmitted to your mouth, eyes or nose, or to other people. To get the most protection out of hand-washing, follow these tips from the Centers for Disease Control and Prevention. Show your children how to do it, too.

- Wet your hands with clean, running water. It can be warm or cold — evidence shows that the temperature doesn't really matter.
- Lather well with liquid, foam or bar soap. Soap is better than water alone because elements in the soap help lift the dirt and germs away from the skin. No need for antibacterial soaps, as they are no more effective than plain soap at getting rid of germs.
- Rub your hands vigorously for at least 20 seconds — or hum the "Happy Birthday" song through twice. Remember to scrub all surfaces, including the backs of your hands, your wrists, between your fingers and under your fingernails.
- Rinse well with clean, running water to wash away the soap and germs.
- Wet hands are more germ-friendly than dry ones. Dry your hands thoroughly with a clean or disposable towel or air dryer. Some evidence suggests that disposable towels are more hygienic than air dryers.

If soap and water aren't available, an alcohol-based sanitizer that contains at least 60 percent alcohol is an acceptable substitute for disinfecting your hands.

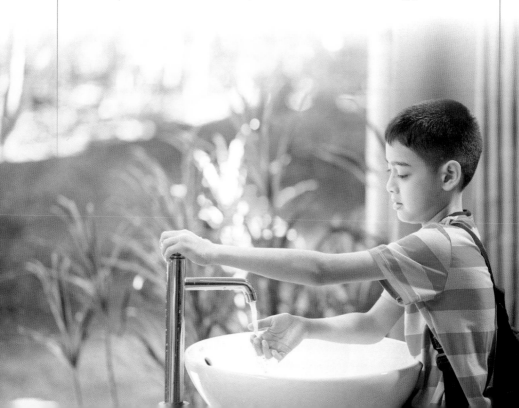

without a prescription. Call your child's medical provider if you have questions about how to use it. Giving your child apple juice or a sports drink diluted with water (half and half) may help with mild dehydration. Avoid carbonated beverages and sodas.

▶ *Try ice chips or small sips of water.* If your child is feeling nauseated or vomiting, avoid giving too much fluid at once. Take a 30- to 60-minute break from oral rehydration. After his or her stomach is rested, encourage him or her to suck on ice chips or an ice pop, or to take small sips of water or clear fluid every five minutes. If vomiting returns, rest the stomach again for an hour and start over with smaller amounts. After four hours with no vomiting, you can double the amount of fluids.

▶ *Make sure your child gets plenty of rest.* Stomach bugs can make your child feel weak and tired. Find him or her a comfortable place to rest — preferably one that has convenient access to the bathroom.

▶ *Get your child back to a normal diet slowly.* As your child's appetite returns, you can gradually return him or her to a normal diet. Generally, wait eight hours — with no vomiting — before giving food. Bland, easy-to-digest foods — such as toast, rice, bananas and potatoes — are often recommended, although there's no solid evidence that these kinds of restrictions are helpful. More importantly, make sure your child is getting enough nutrients, focusing on complex carbohydrates, lean meats, yogurt, and fruits and vegetables. Foods that are high in fat are harder to digest, so avoid those.

▶ *Avoid giving medications.* There's generally no need to give your child over-the-counter anti-diarrheal medications, unless advised by your doctor. Anti-diarrheal medications can slow down the gastrointestinal system and make it harder for your child's body to eliminate the virus or bacteria.

▶ *Avoid spreading the bug.* Keep your sick child's personal items and eating utensils separate from everyone else's in the house. Wash your hands thoroughly after using the bathroom or helping your child use the toilet. Make sure everyone in the family washes their hands, too. Disinfect hard surfaces — such as counters, faucets and doorknobs — with a bleach-containing cleaning agent or a mixture of 2 cups of bleach to 1 gallon of water.

SUNBURN

A child's skin is especially susceptible to sunburn. A sunburn can occur with only 10 to 15 minutes of sun exposure. Sunburn can also happen on a cloudy or a cool day. It's not the visible light or the heat from the sun that burns the skin but invisible ultraviolet (UV) light. In addition, the lighter the color of your child's skin, the more sensitive the skin is to UV rays. That doesn't mean, however, that children with darker skin can't experience a sunburn.

Most sun damage occurs in the childhood years. You certainly don't want to keep your child from playing outdoors because exercise and play are good for your child. But at the same time, it's important to be sun smart. You can help prevent sun damage by spending time in shady areas outside (or using an umbrella), using sunscreen appropriately, and dressing your child in hats and sun-protective clothing.

How to recognize it You may not realize that your child has sunburn because the pain and redness may not appear for several hours. Sunburn typically causes red, tender or swollen skin that's usually warm to the touch. If the sunburn is more severe, the skin can blister.

How serious is it? Sunburn — even a mild burn — isn't healthy for the skin. Children can develop blisters, a fever, chills and nausea with sun exposure that may not affect an older person.

When to call If your child's burn is just red, warm and a bit painful, you can probably treat it yourself. Contact your child's medical provider if the sunburn blisters or if your child develops a fever or chills, begins vomiting, or acts ill.

What you can do Treat the sunburn by gently applying cool compresses every few hours, taking care not to allow your child to become chilled. Apply moisturizer to the sunburn to aid in healing. A lotion or gel that contains aloe vera may be soothing. In addition, encourage your child to drink plenty of fluids.

Give your child acetaminophen (Tylenol, others) to relieve the pain if needed. Don't use anesthetic lotions or sprays that you apply to the skin without the approval of your child's medical provider. Some products sting, and your child's skin may react to the spray. Benzocaine in particular can have rare but serious side effects in young children.

It's also important that you take steps to prevent sunburn:

▶ Before going outside, apply sunscreen generously to all exposed skin. Use a broad-spectrum sunscreen, which protects against UVA and UVB rays, with a sun protection factor (SPF) of at least 30.

- Reapply every two hours — or more often if your child is swimming or perspiring. Don't forget the back of the neck, ears, nose, lips and tops of the feet.
- Use sunscreen even on cloudy days. Clouds block only a small portion of UV rays.
- Use extra caution at the pool or beach (and even snow). UV rays reflect off of snow, water and concrete, increasing exposure. If possible, keep your child out of the sun when UV rays are strongest. This is generally between 10 a.m. and 4 p.m.
- Find shade under a tree or umbrella.
- When possible, dress your child in comfortable lightweight clothing that covers the body. Select clothes made with a tight weave, which provides more protection than clothes made of a looser weave. Or you can look for protective clothing labeled with an ultraviolet protection factor (UPF). The higher the number the better.
- Have your child wear a hat with a 3-inch brim or a bill facing forward.

URINARY TRACT INFECTION

Urinary tract infections (UTIs) are a fairly common childhood problem. The urinary tract includes the kidneys and ureters, the bladder, and the urethra, the small tube that drains urine from the bladder and out of the body.

Most infections involve the lower urinary tract — the bladder and the urethra — and are called bladder infections. When bacteria enter the tract, an infection can result. *Escherichia coli* (*E. coli*)

bacteria normally found in stool account for approximately 80 percent of UTIs in children. Less common causes of a UTI include other types of bacteria, a fungus or a virus.

Urine is naturally sterile — it doesn't have any bacteria in it. However, bacteria are plentiful elsewhere in the body — on the skin, in the bowels and in stool. It's not uncommon for bacteria from these locations to migrate to and travel up the urethra and into the bladder. Inside the warm environment of the bladder, the bacteria can multiply quickly if the body doesn't get rid of the organisms through urination. The one-way flow of urine out of the kidneys and bladder keeps bacteria from accumulating in the urinary tract and producing an infection.

Sometimes, however, this natural defense fails. Factors that can make a child more prone to a urinary tract infection include:

- Waiting too long to go to the bathroom
- Not fully emptying the bladder
- In girls, not wiping front to back to avoid introduction of stool bacteria into the urethral opening
- Constipation that interferes with urine flow
- Having a bladder catheter for a prolonged period
- A weakened immune system
- A family history of UTIs
- In boys, being uncircumcised
- An anatomic abnormality from birth that interferes with the normal flow of urine

How to recognize it Signs and symptoms of a UTI may include:

- An inability to urinate or ability to pass only a few drops
- A sensation of pain or burning when urinating

- Cloudy, dark, bloody or foul-smelling urine
- A need to urinate more often than usual
- A fever
- Pain in the low stomach area or back
- Difficulty controlling the flow of urine, resulting in "accidents" or wetting the bed

How serious is it? Most children who experience a UTI have no long-term damage, but it's important to seek treatment right away to prevent a kidney infection. A kidney infection can develop when a bladder infection moves upstream from the bladder to one or both kidneys. Kidney infections are often very painful and can cause serious health problems, including kidney damage.

A UTI is typically treated with antibiotics to kill the bacteria causing the infection. Your child's symptoms should begin to improve within one to two days after starting the medication.

Make sure your child takes the medication exactly as directed to fully clear the infection and prevent it from coming back. In some cases, tests may be needed once the infection is gone, particularly if your child had a kidney infection. The tests are performed to make sure there are no abnormalities in the urinary tract that are making your child more prone to UTIs. They're also done to ensure there hasn't been any kidney damage.

If your child has recurrent UTIs, his or her medical provider might recommend that your child take an antibiotic daily to prevent future infections.

When to call If you're concerned that your child has a UTI, see your child's medical provider within 24 hours. Waiting to start treatment can increase the risk of a kidney infection.

What you can do It's important to teach your child habits that protect the urinary tract from irritation and infection.

Hygiene After each bowel movement, girls should wipe from front to rear — not rear to front. This keeps germs from spreading from the anus to the urethra. Uncircumcised boys should know how to gently retract the foreskin covering the penis and cleanse the area.

Bladder emptying Teach your child not to "hold it in" if he or she needs to pee. Some children ignore the sensation of a full bladder because they don't want to stop what they're doing to take the time to go to the bathroom. Urine that sits in the bladder too long gives bacteria a good place to grow.

Liquids Make sure your child drinks plenty of liquids, preferably water, each day. Having to pee helps to flush bacteria from the urinary tract. Some children simply don't urinate enough.

Constipation It's also important that your child has regular bowel movements to prevent constipation. Hard stools can press against the urinary tract and block the flow of urine (see page 325). A diet that includes adequate fiber and plenty of liquids can help prevent constipation.

Clothing Have your child wear cotton underwear and avoid tightfitting pants, shorts or leggings. This helps prevent a buildup of moisture around the urethra. After swimming, have your child change into dry clothes instead of sitting around in a wet suit.

Baths and soaps Avoid bubble baths, perfumed soaps, and other substances that may irritate the genitals and urethra.

VIRAL RASHES

Rashes can result from a variety of viral illnesses. Some of the most common viral rashes in children include:

Chickenpox Chickenpox (varicella) causes itchy red spots that quickly fill with a clear fluid to form blisters. The blisters eventually rupture and crust over. The initial rash tends to break out on the face, scalp, chest and back and may spread to the arms and legs. Spots continue to appear for several days and your child may also experience a fever, loss of appetite, tiredness and headaches.

The chickenpox rash appears 10 to 21 days after your child has been exposed to the virus, and the infection usually lasts about five to seven days. Your child is contagious until the rash crusts.

The crusted sores may itch as they heal. Try to keep your child from scratching them. Scratching can cause scarring and increase the risk that the sores will become infected. Keep your child's nails trimmed.

Chickenpox occurs primarily in children, but adults who aren't immune can get it, too. The incidence of chickenpox has declined drastically since the development of a chickenpox vaccine. The vaccine is given in two doses to children age 1 or older (see Chapter 6).

If you think your child has chickenpox, contact your child's medical provider. In otherwise healthy children, chickenpox typically requires no medical treatment and the disease is allowed to run its course. However, a medical provider can prescribe medications, if necessary, to lessen the severity of chickenpox and treat complications.

Contact your child's medical provider immediately if the rash spreads to one or both eyes, or the rash becomes warm or tender, which indicates a possible bacterial skin infection. Also call right away if your child's fever is higher than 102 F and is accompanied by other signs and symptoms such as dizziness, vomiting, tremors or coughing with difficulty breathing. Rarely, chickenpox can lead to serious complications such as pneumonia and encephalitis, an infection of the brain — which is why vaccination is so important.

Roseola Roseola is a viral infection that typically affects young children. It usually begins with a sudden, high fever that lasts several days. When the fever goes down, a rash appears on the trunk and neck and may last from a few hours to a few days. The rash consists of many small pink spots or patches. The spots are generally flat and there may be a white ring around some of them.

Some children develop a very mild case of the illness and hardly seem to be ill, while others experience a full range of signs and symptoms, including a sore throat and runny nose or cough.

The rash generally causes little discomfort and in most cases the illness isn't serious. It usually disappears on its own without treatment, but acetaminophen (Tylenol, others) or ibuprofen (Advil, Motrin, others) can help relieve the fever and discomfort. Keep your child home and away from other children until he or she has been without a fever for 24 hours. Occasionally, young children experience convulsions caused by the high fever (febrile seizure). Contact your child's medical provider or seek urgent care immediately if this happens.

Fifth disease Fifth disease is a common, mild infection in children. It's caused by a virus called human parvovirus B19. Doctors often refer to the illness as parvovirus infection.

The primary sign of fifth disease is the appearance of bright red, raised patches on both cheeks, resembling slap marks. A pink, lacy, slightly raised rash may also develop on the arms, trunk, thighs and buttocks. The rash may come and go for up to three weeks. Some children develop a slight fever and other mild, cold-like symptoms. Once the rash appears, your child is no longer contagious.

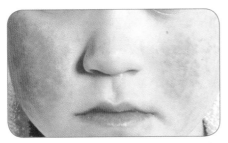

Fifth disease (parvovirus) is a mild viral infection that causes bright red, raised patches on both cheeks.

In most children, the infection is mild and requires little treatment. Acetaminophen (Tylenol, others) or ibuprofen (Advil, Motrin, others) may relieve the fever and discomfort. Pregnant women who suspect they've been exposed to the virus should contact their doctor because there's a chance a fetus could develop serious complications.

Measles (rubeola) Measles (rubeola) typically begins with a high fever — often as high as 104 to 105 F. Other signs and symptoms may include a cough, sneezing, runny nose, sore throat and red, watery eyes. Three to five days later, a red, blotchy rash appears on the face and hairline and behind the ears. The rash often spreads down the neck to the trunk, arms and legs. The rash may begin as fine, red spots that increase in size. Sometimes,

small, white spots may appear on the inside lining of the cheeks. The rash usually lasts about a week.

Measles occurs primarily in children, but adults are susceptible, too. A vaccine to prevent measles has significantly reduced the incidence of this disease. A key way to prevent measles is to make sure your child is current with his or her vaccinations.

Contact your child's medical provider if you think your child may have the disease or your child has been exposed to measles and is unvaccinated or has a weakened immune system. Measles is highly contagious, and you want to keep your child isolated from about four days before to four days after the rash breaks out. Over-the-counter medications such as acetaminophen (Tylenol, others) and ibuprofen (Advil, Motrin, others) can help control the fever. Have your child drink plenty of water or an oral rehydration solution to replace fluids lost to sweating and avoid dehydration (see page 321).

Complications that can develop from measles include ear infection, bronchitis or pneumonia. In rare cases, inflammation of the brain (encephalitis) can follow the measles.

WARTS

Warts are raised round or oval growths that may be lighter or darker than the skin around them. Some have tiny black dots in them, often called "seeds," which are small, clotted blood vessels.

Warts can appear anywhere on your child's body, but most often they develop on the hands or near the fingernails, as well as on the face, toes, and around the knees and elbows. Warts can also develop on the soles of your child's feet. This type of wart is known as a plantar wart.

Warts are caused by an infection with the human papillomavirus (HPV). This virus is typically transmitted by touch and often enters the body through breaks in the skin. There are hundreds of HPV types. Most cause relatively harmless conditions such as common warts. Some HPV types can cause serious disease, such as cancer of the cervix, but these are different from the types that cause warts.

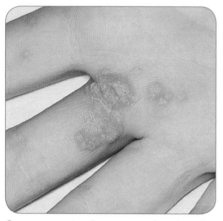

Common warts often grow on hands or fingers. They're small, grainy bumps that are rough to the touch. They're usually flesh-colored, white, pink or tan.

Anyone can get warts, but some people are more prone to them than others. Warts are most commonly found in children and teens, especially those who bite their nails or pick at hangnails. Warts are also more common in people with weakened immune systems.

Your child can get warts from skin-to-skin contact with someone who has warts. If your child has warts, he or she can spread the virus to other places on his or her body. Your child may also develop warts by touching something that another person's wart has touched, such as a towel or sports equipment. Walking barefoot around public swimming pools may increase your child's risk of developing plantar warts.

How to recognize it In children, warts usually occur on the fingers or hands. They may appear as small fleshy or grainy bumps that are rough to the touch. They can be flesh-colored, white, pink or tan. They may be sprinkled with black pinpoints.

How serious is it? Warts generally aren't serious. In children, about two-thirds of warts go away on their own without treatment. But it can take months to years for a wart to disappear, and during this time it may enlarge or new warts may develop. A wart also can be painful, and some children are embarrassed by them.

The earlier treatment begins, the greater the chances are of completely getting rid of warts. Treatment depends on where the wart is located, how much it bothers your child and how quickly you want to get rid of it. You can try to remove the wart yourself with an over-the-counter product or you can seek treatment from your child's medical provider.

Over-the-counter products You can purchase nonprescription wart removal products, such as salicylic acid, as a patch or a liquid. Look for a 17 percent salicylic acid solution. These products require daily use for several weeks, oftentimes two to four months.

For best results, first soak your child's wart in warm water for 10 to 20 minutes. Use a new nail file or emery board (you can cut them in half) to gently slough off dead skin from the surface of the wart. Throw the contaminated file or emery

DOES DUCT TAPE WORK?

Duct tape, the popular repair tape available at most home improvement stores, has been used to treat skin warts. It's not clear how duct tape works — or even if it's an effective treatment for that matter. Some studies have found duct tape effective while others have not.

If you choose to try duct tape on your child's wart, silver duct tape is preferred over clear tape because it sticks to the skin better. Cover the wart with a strip of tape and leave it in place for six days. After removing the tape, soak the wart in warm water for 10 to 20 minutes and then use a fresh nail file or emery board to gently slough off the dead skin. Leave the wart uncovered for one night, then reapply the tape for another six nights.

It can take some time for duct tape to work — several months in some cases. If you don't see any improvement in your child's wart within six to eight weeks, it's unlikely that duct tape will help.

board away when finished; don't reuse it. Apply the medication and let it dry. Cover with tape or duct tape. Repeat nightly or as directed. If the skin becomes irritated, discontinue treatment until soreness or redness goes away.

Medical care Many parents prefer to have a medical provider treat the condition, especially if the wart is spreading or the parent or the child is bothered by the wart. Your child's medical provider may suggest a prescription-strength chemical to apply to the wart. Other options include scraping or cutting away (cauterizing) the wart or freezing it with liquid nitrogen. These approaches are usually recommended if your child has multiple warts or warts that keep coming back. Sometimes a combination of methods is used to try to prevent warts from recurring. In rare cases, a doctor may recommend surgery to remove a wart.

Generally, the approach that's least painful is the preferred method, especially when treating young children. The goal of treatment is to destroy the warts. However, even with treatment, warts can recur or spread.

When to call See your child's health medical provider if:
▶ You aren't sure whether the growths are warts.
▶ The warts are painful, change in appearance or color, or are bothersome.
▶ The warts don't respond to over-the-counter treatments.
▶ Your child has a weakened immune system.

What you can do To reduce your child's risk of developing a wart or having an existing wart spread:
▶ *Don't let your child pick at the wart.* Picking may spread the virus.

- *Try to keep your child from biting his or her fingernails.* Warts occur more often in skin that's been broken. Nibbling the skin around the fingernails opens the door for the virus.
- *Encourage hand-washing.* It's especially important that your child washes his or her hands after touching a wart. Hand-washing after touching common surfaces such as shared sports equipment or towels may also help prevent the spread of the virus.
- *Promote footwear.* Don't let your child walk barefoot around swimming pools and locker rooms.

PART 6

Complex needs

CHAPTER 21

Attention-deficit/ hyperactivity disorder

Active … or hyperactive? A little flighty … or chronically forgetful? Most of the signs and symptoms of attention-deficit/hyperactivity disorder (ADHD) — interrupting conversations, difficulty taking turns, forgetting items at home or school, fidgeting, or getting bored quickly — are part of every child's playbook. But for a child with ADHD, these signs and symptoms are chronic disrupters, causing problems at home, at school and with others.

Talking to a doctor or other medical provider and getting a proper diagnosis can help relieve the frustration and helplessness many parents feel not knowing how to cope with their child's behavior. It's also important to know that most kids can go on to lead successful lives with proper treatment, especially if treatment is started as early as possible. ADHD can't be cured, but it can be effectively managed.

As a parent, the key things you can do for your child with ADHD is partner with your medical team in a treatment plan, show your child unconditional love, help build your child's sense of self-worth, and learn how to speak up for your child's needs.

WHAT IS ADHD?

ADHD is a medical condition that develops in childhood. It affects how the brain develops and how it directs neurobehavioral functions such as attention, energy levels, behaviors and emotions. Studies of brain images show key differences between children with ADHD and those without ADHD, both in how the brain is structured and how different parts of the brain are activated. Researchers aren't sure what causes these differences, though there's strong evidence that it runs in families. For instance, a child with a parent or sibling with ADHD is five times more likely to have the condition than a child with no family history of it.

ADHD isn't caused by poor parenting or eating too much sugar. Environmental factors such as diet, activity and parenting techniques may affect behavior, but they don't cause a child to have ADHD.

Before 1994, the term *attention deficit disorder (ADD)* was used to describe someone with mostly attention difficulties. Now, the umbrella term *attention-deficit/hyperactivity disorder (ADHD)* is used for someone with any symptoms of ADHD, whether the person is inattentive, hyperactive or both.

Children with symptoms of ADHD may have a hard time paying attention and concentrating. They may also have difficulty sitting still and controlling sudden impulses. These behaviors can affect nearly every aspect of life.

Based on feedback from parents and medical records, ADHD appears to occur in as many as 1 in 10 school-age children. About half the kids with ADHD will continue to experience these symptoms as adults.

ADHD — especially when untreated — can have a profound impact on a child's life, as well as on the child's family. ADHD has been linked to troubled relationships, poor school performance, accidental injuries and low self-esteem.

It's not uncommon for ADHD to be accompanied by other disorders, including learning disabilities, oppositional defiant disorder, anxiety and depression. ADHD has also been associated with a greater risk of substance and alcohol use, mental health concerns, and legal problems later in life.

Is it normal or ADHD? Most healthy children are inattentive, hyperactive or impulsive at one time or another. It's part of being a kid.

Preschoolers in general have short attention spans and are unable to stick with one activity for long. Even in older children and teenagers, attention span can vary. A child's concentration depends on a number of factors, including his or her level of interest in what's going on and the amount and quality of sleep the child is getting.

The same is true of hyperactivity. Young children are naturally energetic and may become even more active when they're tired, hungry, anxious or in a new environment. Some children simply have a higher activity level than others do.

Observe your child closely at home and in other environments, including school or social settings. In addition, try to gather information from a variety of sources, such as babysitters, child care staff, teachers and your child's medical provider.

A child who occasionally acts up or gets called out for being a chatterbox probably doesn't have ADHD. If your child has problems in school but gets along well at home or with friends, he or she may be struggling with something other than ADHD. The same also holds true if your child is hyperactive or inattentive at home, but his or her schoolwork and friendships remain unaffected.

When a child has ADHD, his or her behaviors are out of step with those of his or her peers and don't result from a separate medical problem. Furthermore, these behaviors are excessive and persistent enough to interfere with your child's daily life at home, at school and with other people.

What to watch for Signs and symptoms of ADHD generally start before age 12. They typically become noticeable around age 4. Signs and symptoms can be mild, moderate or severe. ADHD occurs more often in boys than in girls, and behaviors between the two may vary. For example, boys may be more hyperactive and girls may be more inattentive.

SIGNS AND SYMPTOMS OF ADHD

A child may have signs and symptoms of inattentiveness or hyperactivity and impulsiveness. Many children have a mix of both.

Inattentiveness

A child who shows a pattern of inattentiveness often:

- Fails to pay attention to details or makes careless mistakes in schoolwork
- Has trouble staying focused during tasks or at play
- Doesn't seem to listen, even when spoken to directly
- Has difficulty following through on instructions and fails to finish schoolwork or chores
- Has trouble organizing and following through on tasks and activities
- Avoids or dislikes tasks that require focused mental effort, such as homework
- Frequently loses items needed for tasks or activities
- Is easily distracted
- Forgets to do routine daily activities and needs many reminders

Hyperactivity and impulsiveness

A child who shows a pattern of hyperactive and impulsive signs and symptoms often:

- Fidgets or taps his or her hands or feet, or squirms in the seat
- Has difficulty staying seated in the classroom or in other situations
- Appears to be in constant motion
- Runs around or climbs in situations where it's not appropriate
- Has trouble playing or doing an activity quietly
- Talks too much
- Blurts out answers, interrupting the questioner
- Has difficulty waiting for his or her turn
- Interrupts or intrudes on others' conversations, games or activities

WHAT OTHER ISSUES ARE ASSOCIATED WITH ADHD?

Children with ADHD often have other health conditions, such as:

Learning disorders Up to half the children with ADHD have some type of learning disorder (see Chapter 22). Children with ADHD and learning disorders are more likely to repeat a grade in school. Having a learning disorder doesn't mean a child is less intelligent than other children, however.

Oppositional defiant disorder (ODD) ODD is a pattern of negative, defiant and hostile behavior toward parents, teachers or others in authority (see Chapter 20). ODD tends to occur more often in children who are impulsive and hyperactive.

Mood disorders Children and adults with ADHD have an increased risk of developing depression or bipolar disorder, particularly when there is a family history of such disorders. See Chapter 20 for more on mood disorders.

Anxiety disorders Anxiety disorders tend to occur fairly often in children with ADHD. These disorders may cause overwhelming worry and nervousness, as well as physical symptoms, such as a rapid heartbeat, sweating and dizziness (see Chapter 20).

Sleep disorders Up to half the children with ADHD have sleep problems, especially difficulties with falling asleep and staying asleep. Sleep problems can be a symptom of ADHD. An existing sleep problem may be made worse by ADHD or may make the symptoms of ADHD worse.

Tic disorders Children with ADHD are more likely than other children to have disorders that can cause involuntary twitches (tics).

Autism ADHD may occur alongside autism. Autism is a brain-related disorder that causes problems with social interaction and communication (see Chapter 23).

It's important that each condition be diagnosed and treated separately from ADHD, since treatment will vary from condition to condition. Treating these other conditions may help improve symptoms of ADHD, although it won't replace the need to treat ADHD.

Symptoms of ADHD generally fall into three categories. In some kids, the majority of symptoms relate to inattentiveness. Other kids have mostly hyperactive or impulsive symptoms. But most children with ADHD have a combination of inattentiveness, hyperactivity and impulsiveness.

Signs and symptoms such as hyperactivity and impulsiveness are often readily noticeable, even in young children. However, signs and symptoms such as inattentiveness and poor organizational skills may go unnoticed until the elementary and middle school years, as school performance drops and a child is unable to keep up with his or her peers.

As a result, children with inattentive ADHD are often diagnosed later in childhood compared with those with hyperactive-impulsive or combined ADHD. Into the teen years, symptoms trend toward restlessness, fidgeting, inattentiveness and impulsiveness.

HOW IS ADHD DIAGNOSED?

Several types of medical providers can diagnose ADHD, including medical doctors, psychologists, psychiatrists and nurse practitioners. There's no single test for ADHD. Instead, diagnosis involves a comprehensive evaluation that includes:

▶ A complete personal and family history of medical conditions

▶ Information from you and other caregivers, and your child's teacher (this may include filling out questionnaires)

▶ A physical exam to rule out other conditions that may be causing or contributing to symptoms, such as vision or hearing problems

▶ Tests for learning or emotional problems, if needed

Your medical provider may ask you a number of questions: Has your child had symptoms for at least six months? How long have symptoms been present? Have you noticed that his symptoms occur in two or more settings, such as home, school and social situations? How does her behavior compare to behaviors of her peers? For example, is your child able to quietly focus on a task alongside classmates, or does she tend to hop up and move to another activity before others have finished?

Because ADHD is diagnosed mainly by reviewing your child's history and observing symptoms, the more details you can give your child's medical provider, the better. To provide the fullest picture of your child, write down your concerns and observations and bring them to your child's appointment.

Preschoolers and ADHD At the preschool age, behaviors related to ADHD — high energy, impulsiveness, short attention span — are common. It can be difficult to sort out what's typical for this

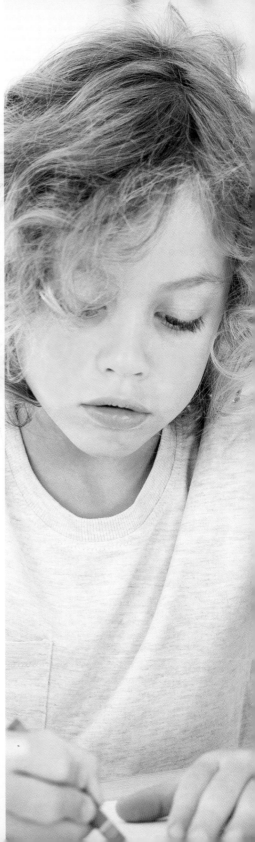

age from what might be related to ADHD. It can also be a challenge to separate ADHD symptoms from developmental delays and other conditions that may become evident around this time. To evaluate preschoolers and younger children for ADHD, medical providers may ask for help from other specialists, such as a psychologist or psychiatrist, speech pathologist, or developmental pediatrician.

Preschoolers with ADHD often have difficulties at school or child care because of their disruptive behavior. If your child's behavior is concerning to you, talk with his or her teacher or child care provider. Someone who spends time with children on a regular basis can offer insight about what's typical behavior. Bring it up with your child's medical provider, as well.

UNDERSTANDING TREATMENT

Although there's no cure for ADHD, symptoms can be managed effectively with proper treatment. A treatment plan tailored to your child's age and symptoms can help your child overcome the social, emotional and academic gaps that can occur because of ADHD.

For school-age children, the mainstay of treatment for ADHD is medication

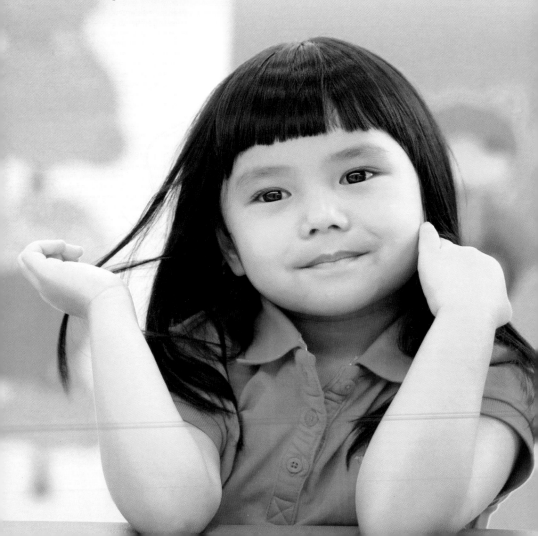

along with behavioral management and counseling. Research suggests that children who receive medication combined with behavioral treatment experience significant improvement in behavior and relationships at home and in school.

For children under age 6, the American Academy of Pediatrics recommends beginning with parent-child behavior therapy sessions rather than medication, although medication may be considered if behavioral therapy isn't helping.

Finding what works for your child requires working closely with your child's medical team and school teachers, being open to treatment possibilities, and monitoring your child's response to treatment. It's also important to take into consideration factors such as your child's developmental stage, temperament and specific signs and symptoms.

Successful treatment is a team effort. A solid support network can increase your child's chances of effectively managing ADHD. The best treatment strategies for ADHD are the result of a partnership involving you, your child, medical providers, teachers, child care providers, counselors and other key players in your child's life.

You might wonder whether a child with ADHD needs to be treated. Most medical experts in the field recommend that a child diagnosed with ADHD receive appropriate treatment as early as possible. Treatment can help prevent or limit complications of ADHD, such as getting in trouble for behavior the child can't always control, having difficulty making friends, doing poorly at school, dropping out of school, having emotional difficulties, and becoming dependent on alcohol or other drugs.

Parents who opt for treatment that includes medications and behavioral therapy often find that the treatment eases their child's symptoms and allows him or her to enjoy home life and improved family relationships, perform better at school, make and keep new friends, and increase his or her self-esteem.

MEDICATIONS

Medications are an important and effective part of treatment for ADHD. They can help turn on parts of the brain that are less active in people with ADHD than in people who don't have ADHD.

It may take some time to find the best medication at the right dose for your child. Most medical providers start children at a low dose and increase the amount at regular intervals until the ADHD symptoms are under control. Your child's dosage may also need to be adjusted as your child matures or if bothersome side effects occur.

The two main kinds of ADHD medications are stimulants and nonstimulants.

Stimulants These are considered the most effective medications for ADHD. Stimulants work to modulate levels of neurotransmitters associated with motivation, attention and movement. Methylphenidate (Ritalin, Metadate, others) is a commonly prescribed stimulant. Medications containing forms of amphetamine (Adderall, Dexedrine, others) also are examples of stimulants. Studies show that stimulants help improve the signs and symptoms of inattentiveness and hyperactivity in about 80 percent of children with ADHD.

The advantages of stimulant medications include a proven track record and the fact that they work quickly. In fact, their effects may be noticeable as early as 30 minutes after your child takes a dose.

ARE MEDICATIONS SAFE?

Deciding to use medication to treat your child's ADHD can be a difficult decision for a parent to make. You may wonder if medication will turn your child into a zombie, if your child may become addicted to the medication, or if taking medication may open a gateway to more-dangerous substance use down the road.

The goal of stimulant treatment is to improve your child's concentration skills with just the right dose of ADHD medication. When taken as prescribed, stimulants make most children with ADHD feel more calm and better able to focus, and don't lead to problems.

It's true that some people misuse or abuse stimulant medications. As a result, the medication is a controlled substance and must be used and stored appropriately. Make sure you supervise your child's daily dosing, that medication is kept locked in a childproof container, and that you personally deliver any medication to your child's school nurse or health office.

If your child complains about a medication's side effects or you notice a personality change, such as irritability or flat emotions, your child's dose may be too high. Talk with your child's medical provider about changing the dose.

Though many children with ADHD ultimately have ADHD as adults, some do eventually outgrow ADHD symptoms and stop taking medication. Others learn ways to control symptoms without medication. Most children need to keep taking ADHD medication throughout their school years, though. Some people continue taking ADHD medication when they're adults.

Your child's medical provider may have your child start out with a low dose on a weekend so that you have time to observe your child's response to the medication. You may need to try a different dosage or another medication before you find the regimen that most improves symptoms with the fewest side effects.

There have been some concerns about growth delays with long-term use of stimulant medications, but this is rarely a problem. Stimulants may decrease appetite during the day, so it's important to make sure your child is eating an adequate amount of total calories. For example, this might mean eating a bigger breakfast, before the medication takes effect.

Nonstimulant medications Research shows that taking stimulant medications most effectively controls symptoms of ADHD. However, nonstimulants may be an option if your child can't take stimulants because of health problems or if stimulants cause severe side effects. Nonstimulant medications work more slowly than stimulants do and may take several weeks before they take full effect.

Nonstimulants include medications such as atomoxetine (Strattera), a type of selective norepinephrine reuptake inhibitor. It works by increasing the levels of norepinephrine, a chemical in the brain that helps control behavior. High blood pressure drugs such as guanfacine (Intuniv) and clonidine (Kapvay) and the antidepressant bupropion (Wellbutrin) are sometimes helpful, as well.

Medication side effects Many children who take medication for ADHD experience some side effects, but these are usually mild. Side effects may go away if the medication is swapped for another or the dosage is adjusted. If you notice side effects that you think may be from ADHD medication, tell your child's medical provider promptly.

Stimulant side effects The most common side effects from stimulants include loss of appetite, sleep problems, and irritability or social withdrawal.

A small number of children have an increase in tics when they start taking stimulant medication. Tics are sudden, brief, intermittent movements, such as facial grimaces or twitches. Stimulant medication doesn't cause tics, but it can make an existing tic disorder more obvious.

Stimulants carry a small risk of damage to the liver. Also, they generally aren't recommended for children who have heart defects, heart disease or other serious heart problems because stimulants may increase the risk of a heart attack, stroke or death.

Concerns have been raised that there may be a slightly increased risk of suicidal thinking, hallucinations or aggressive behavior in children taking stimulants. If you notice worrisome signs or symptoms, such as depression, panic or hostility, let your child's medical provider know. If your child mentions suicide, contact your child's medical provider right away.

Some parents worry that taking medication for ADHD will change their child's personality. Even though it's called a stimulant, the medication typically has a calming effect. It shouldn't cause significant changes in personality or take away

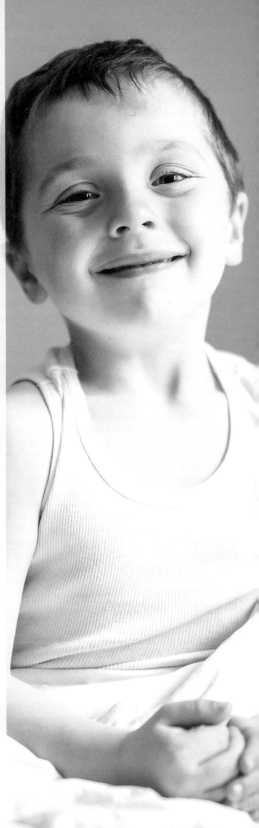

DO ALTERNATIVE THERAPIES WORK FOR ADHD?

Some parents look to complementary and alternative therapies to treat their child's ADHD, perhaps hoping to avoid the side effects of medication or maybe because they believe natural is better. Some of the more popular treatments include special diets, omega-3 fatty acids, herbal supplements, vision therapy, exercise and neurobiofeedback.

So far, most of these treatments have not been shown to be effective for ADHD, and some may even be harmful — especially for children. There is some evidence that omega-3 polyunsaturated fatty acids may improve ADHD symptoms, but further research is necessary to confirm their usefulness.

There's little evidence that elimination diets, where individual foods are removed and reintroduced later, are helpful. Though it's beneficial to minimize sugar consumption in general, sugar hasn't been proved to worsen ADHD symptoms.

In the end, natural approaches recommended to complement ADHD treatment are the same as for any child: plenty of exercise, enough sleep, and a nutritious diet that includes whole grains, fruits, vegetables, low-fat dairy products and lean proteins. These healthy habits set the stage for all children to be ready to learn with confidence and enjoy healthy relationships.

your child's individuality. If you feel your child's personality changes in negative ways when he or she takes ADHD medication, talk to your child's medical provider. Switching medications or adjusting dosages may help.

Nonstimulant medication side effects Atomoxetine has been associated with nausea, vomiting, tiredness, abdominal pain, headaches and weight loss in younger children. Atomoxetine also carries a small risk of suicidal thinking, similar to the risk of taking a stimulant.

Common side effects of alpha agonists guanfacine and clonidine include a drop in heart rate and blood pressure, fainting, dizziness, drowsiness, fatigue, irritability, constipation, and dry mouth. Talk to your child's medical provider if side effects cause discomfort or are concerning, so the regimen can be adjusted.

Managing side effects A few tweaks to your child's routine may help prevent or minimize some of the most common side effects of ADHD medications.

Loss of appetite If your child is having a hard time eating:

▶ Make sure your child takes the medication exactly as directed by your child's medical provider. Taking it consistently over time makes loss of appetite less likely.

▶ Ask the medical provider if your child can wait until after breakfast to take the medication. That may make your child hungrier at the morning meal.

▶ Serve a larger meal in the evening when the medication is wearing off.

▶ Have healthy high-calorie foods on hand for your child to eat when he or she is hungry. Examples include nuts, granola, peanut butter and cheese.

GIVE YOURSELF A BREAK

Caring for a child with ADHD can challenge the whole family. Family members may have a hard time living with someone who may be demanding or aggressive. Siblings often get less attention than the child with ADHD. Stress can take its toll on everyone and make each family member feel mentally and physically worn out.

If you're the parent or caregiver of a child with ADHD, give yourself a break if possible. Take time to care for your relationships, including your spouse or partner and your other children. Ask friends or relatives to help with the kids when you need time alone with someone, or just time to yourself. Some parents find it helpful to join a support group for families with ADHD. Group members, all in similar situations, confidentially share information about coping with ADHD.

Don't feel guilty for spending time away from your child. You'll be in a better position to care for your child if you're rested and relaxed!

Trouble falling asleep If your child is having difficulty sleeping:

- Stick to a regular wake-up time, even during weekends.
- Follow a bedtime routine every evening. Include calming activities, such as bathing or reading.
- Shut off all electronics about one hour before bedtime. That includes TV, video games, computers and cellphones. Remove electronics from your child's bedroom.
- If these changes don't help, talk to your child's medical provider. You may need to change the time when your child takes ADHD medication or the kind of medication he or she takes. Tell the provider if you notice other sleep problems, too, such as daytime drowsiness or snoring.

Irritability If your child feels irritable, moody or agitated when taking ADHD medication:

- It may be that the medication is wearing off too soon, especially if it happens in the late afternoon or evening. If you notice this side effect, talk to your child's medical provider. The timing or the type of your child's medication may need to change.

BEHAVIORAL THERAPY

Medication can help ease the symptoms of ADHD, but it doesn't address other problems, such as poor social skills or conflict at home. Children with ADHD, as well as their family members and teachers, may benefit from behavioral therapy. Studies show that children with ADHD who are treated with intensive behavioral therapy are sometimes able to take lower doses of medication. For preschoolers with ADHD symptoms, behavioral therapy is considered the initial treatment of choice.

Behavioral therapy sessions focus on establishing positive parent-child interactions. Sessions may include strategies for developing ways to understand and

WORKING WITH TEACHERS

Bringing out the best in a child with ADHD means assembling a team of players dedicated to your mission. As head coach of this team, you play a critical role in getting everyone on board with your child's game plan. Building strong, productive relationships with teachers will help you feel confident about providing a secure, thriving environment for your child — even when you're not there.

Get to know each other Getting someone to invest in your child will be much easier if you have a sturdy foundation. Schedule a sit-down with your child's teacher and give him or her a personal glimpse of your child that will help forge a personal connection and make it easier to root for your child.

Advocate and cooperate When meeting with teachers, arrive with a spirit of cooperation and openness to the teacher's style and suggestions. Let the teacher know that you want to work together with the school to help your child meet expectations. When your child needs help or runs into obstacles, a strong parent-teacher alliance built on mutual respect will work in your child's favor.

Listen and empathize A classroom full of children puts any teacher through daily, exhausting paces. On some days, a child that occasionally requires more time or attention may be tugging at the end of a taut rope. If your child has been particularly challenging or disruptive, allow the teacher a chance to blow off steam and vent. Let the teacher know that you understand and direct the conversation toward finding a solution.

Get involved Volunteering at school — in the classroom, the playground or the cafeteria — shows that you're willing to cooperate with others to give your child the best educational experience possible. A glimpse into your child's daily school routine also can provide insight into his or her daily struggles.

guide the child's behavior. These strategies may include spending special time together, reinforcing positive behavior, setting clear expectations, ignoring mildly inappropriate behavior and maintaining consistent consequences. They may also involve learning how to minimize distractions and helping the child gradually widen his or her attention span. For some children, training in social skills can be helpful.

What you can do Your child's therapist will help you target specific behaviors in your child that may need to be modified.

In addition, these general behavioral therapy techniques can help make day-to-day life easier for you and your child.

Encourage your child Show your child lots of affection; make him or her feel appreciated. Every day, try to give your child more positive than negative attention. If your child doesn't like spoken signs of affection, a smile, a pat on the shoulder or a hug can show you care. Focusing only on the negative aspects of your child's behavior can harm your relationship and affect your child's self-confidence and self-esteem.

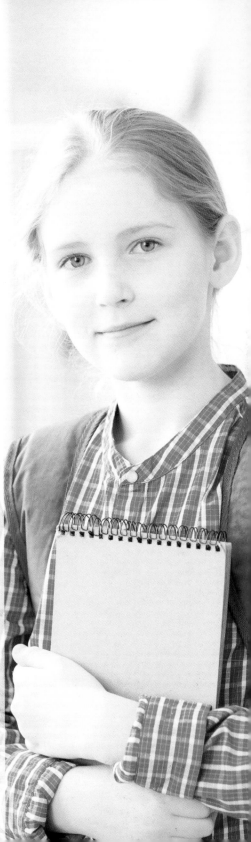

Be patient Try to remain patient and calm, even when your child is out of control. If you are calm, your child is more likely to calm down, too.

Set realistic expectations Set small goals for improvement for you and your child. Don't try to make a lot of changes at the same time.

Spend time with your child Make an effort to spend time alone together. Focus on and appreciate the pleasing aspects of your child's personality.

Keep a schedule Maintain regular times for meals, naps and bedtime. Use a big calendar to note upcoming activities. Give your child plenty of time to get ready to leave the house or change activities. Use an alarm clock or a timer as needed. When you go out, schedule your trips when the destination isn't crowded.

Offer organizational suggestions Create a daily assignment chart or notebook for your child. Find a quiet place for homework or time to calm down. Set up specific places for your child to store toys, clothes and school supplies. Encourage your child to set out tomorrow's clothes and pack a backpack the night before school. Small, achievable tasks can help a child feel successful.

Be sensitive to your child's limits Avoid situations that overwhelm your child, such as sitting through long presentations or shopping in large malls. Try to keep your child from becoming overly tired. And give him or her time and a place to "just be," with few rules or expectations.

Communicate clearly with your child Use simple words and demonstrations

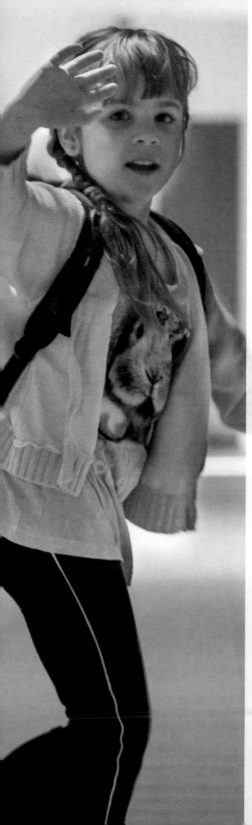

when giving directions. Speak slowly and quietly and be very specific. Give one direction at a time.

Reward and discipline effectively Have clear, firm expectations for behavior. Reward good behavior and use consistent consequences to discourage harmful actions. Awarding special privileges — an extra 15 minutes of playing a favorite game, for example — for positive behavior usually works well.

A timeout or the loss of a privilege can be an effective consequence for negative behavior. A timeout should be fairly brief, but long enough for your child to regain control of his or her behavior. The idea is to interrupt and defuse out-of-control behavior. Children with ADHD can be expected to accept the results of the choices they make.

Help with peer interactions Invite another child to your house. Supervise play and suggest activities for young children. Help older children choose activities before the friend arrives.

HELP AT SCHOOL

Your child's teacher may have been part of the evaluation process for ADHD. Once a diagnosis has been made, work closely with your child's teacher and the school to make sure your child has the resources, support and feedback he or she needs to succeed, both academically and socially.

Start by identifying special care needs your child may have based on his or her symptoms. Ask about and take advantage of any special programs your school has for children with ADHD. For example, your child may be able to take tests in the library or a less distracting environment than the classroom. Work with the school to see whether your child qualifies for special school services, such as an individualized education program (IEP) or a Section 504 plan (see page 463).

Together with your child's teacher, establish specific goals your child can strive toward. These can be based on principles learned from behavior therapy sessions — concepts that your child's teacher can help reinforce. Perhaps your child and his or her teacher will want to share a daily planner that tracks these goals, along with homework and other assignments. Also share with the teacher and relevant staff any triggers that might prompt poor behavior in your child, and work with the school to minimize these triggers.

Communicate often with your child's teachers and support their efforts to help your child in the classroom. Ask teachers to closely monitor your child's work, provide constructive feedback and be very clear when giving your child instructions. Be sure other staff members know how they can help make school a positive experience for your child.

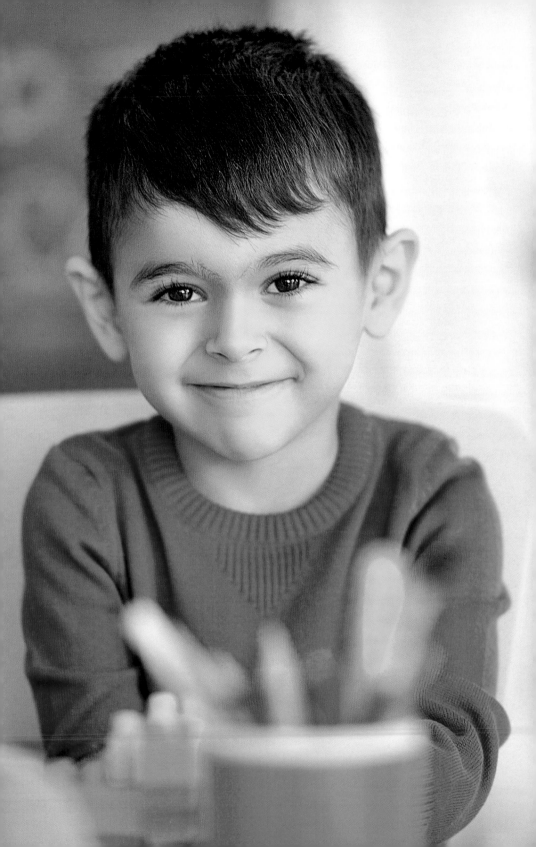

CHAPTER 22

Learning disorders

It's normal for a child to struggle with reading, writing and math skills now and then, especially when tackling new concepts. But repeated difficulties over time may indicate a learning disorder.

A learning disorder is diagnosed when a child has difficulty processing, remembering and using information, primarily with reading, math and spelling. As a result, learning disorders are marked by a level of academic achievement that is lower than expected for a child's age and developmental level.

Because they have close contact with children during school hours, teachers are often the first to recommend that a child be evaluated for a learning disorder. Parents may not realize a child has a problem until schoolwork becomes so overwhelming that their child can't keep up.

Many children who have learning disorders, also known as learning disabilities, struggle for a long time before being diagnosed, which causes them to feel inadequate, frustrated and misunderstood. This can affect a child's self-esteem and motivation at school and in other areas of life, including relationships with family and friends.

Learning disorders are likely caused by multiple factors, including differences in the brain that may be present from birth or shortly after. These differences affect how the brain handles information and can create issues with reading, writing and math. Genetics may play a role, as learning disorders have been known to run in families. Environmental factors, such as an illness or injury to the brain, also may contribute.

Children with learning disorders may have problems with other skills, including organization, time management, abstract reasoning, long- or short-term memory, attention, and motor skills. Learning disorders aren't related to how smart a child is, however.

Having a learning disorder is often a lifelong challenge — but early detection, proper support and targeted interventions can help your child navigate through school and beyond.

TYPES OF LEARNING DISORDERS

Learning disorders encompass a wide range of difficulties that can vary considerably from child to child. Some children show only subtle signs of disability, whereas in others, signs are more pronounced. Problems are frequently clustered together in terms of reading, writing and math.

Problems with reading Reading disability, also known as dyslexia, is a learning disorder characterized by difficulty in decoding the sounds of words (phonics), spelling, and recalling known words.

Some cases are mild, some more severe, but the condition often becomes apparent as a child starts learning to read. By far the most common learning disorder, dyslexia accounts for 80 percent of learning problem diagnoses.

Schools use slightly different terms than the medical community uses to describe learning disorders. These terms are based on guidelines set up by the federal government under the Individuals with Disabilities Education Act (IDEA).

When working with your child's school, it helps to know the terminology the school staff is likely to use. The IDEA term for dyslexia is specific learning disability in basic reading skills, reading fluency (speed) or reading comprehension.

Signs of dyslexia sometimes can be difficult to recognize before your child enters school, but there are some early clues you can look for. Signs that a young child may be at risk of dyslexia include problems forming words correctly, such as reversing sounds in words or confusing words that sound alike; problems remembering or naming letters, numbers and colors; and difficulty learning nursery rhymes or playing rhyming games.

THE EMOTIONAL IMPACT OF A LEARNING DISORDER

The mismatch between a child's intelligence and his or her ability to learn, in addition to the unmet expectations of parents and teachers, can make a child with a learning disorder feel frustrated, anxious and discouraged.

Adults with learning disorders often recall extraordinary efforts to do well at school that went unrecognized. Instead, they were more often pegged as lazy or unmotivated students.

When a learning disorder remains undiagnosed, it can lead to a harmful cycle for the child, as well as for parents and teachers. When a child experiences learning problems, parents and teachers may think the child simply isn't trying hard enough. They may recommend more time spent on homework, which can lead to increased stress and conflict. Unable to meet expectations, the child typically feels frustrated and anxious. He or she may become defensive about academics and act in disruptive ways to avoid looking "stupid." This tends to lead to even more stress and possibly disciplinary action on the part of caregivers and school staff. These responses further disrupt the child's ability to learn, leading to more failure and another downward turn in the cycle.

On the other hand, when a learning disorder is properly diagnosed and efforts are made to help the child overcome the difficulties presented, results are generally much more positive. Advocating for your child early on at school is a big help.

As a parent, another important thing you can do for a child with a learning disorder — as with any child — is to accept him or her wholeheartedly, without reservations. A home environment of warmth and acceptance can free a child to creatively overcome weaknesses and display unexpected strengths.

Once your child is in school, signs of dyslexia may become more apparent. These may include reading well below the expected level for his or her age, difficulty spelling, inability to pronounce unfamiliar words, and problems processing what he or she hears.

In the fourth and fifth grades, when students start reading to learn rather than learning to read, difficulty with reading comprehension may become more prominent. Kids with a reading disability may have problems paying attention during a reading task and may dislike reading in general because of the frustration it brings.

Problems with written expression
Some children have a learning disorder that's characterized by trouble putting thoughts into words or putting words onto paper (dysgraphia).

Signs of dysgraphia might include poor spelling and grammar, writing samples that don't match a child's grade or developmental level, and difficulty thinking and writing at the same time.

Some kids with dysgraphia have more difficulty with fine motor skills and the mechanics of handwriting. Difficulties might include illegible or inconsistently spaced handwriting and a cramped or improper grip on a writing tool. The

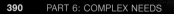

EXPLAINING A LEARNING DISORDER TO YOUR CHILD

Once you have confirmation of a learning disorder, you may be wondering how your child will react to the diagnosis. For some children, finally knowing the cause for schoolwork frustrations can be a relief.

Ask your child what he or she thinks having a learning disorder is about, and clear up any misconceptions. Until now, your child might have thought of himself or herself as "slow," "lazy" or "bad" — or heard it from someone who didn't understand him or her. Even labels such as "learning disabled" or "inattentive" describe only a small part of your child's personality.

Refrain from focusing primarily on your child's learning disorder. Instead, approach your child as a whole person. Address weaknesses but also focus on your child's strengths and assets. Allow time to find and develop your child's natural talents and gifts. To get a glimpse of possibilities, do a quick internet search with your child on famous individuals who have overcome a learning disorder.

Reassure your child that while having a learning disorder may require that more time and effort be spent for some things, every completed task is a success. Create a supportive environment that encourages your child to strive for his or her personal best, no matter how small the task or large the obstacle.

IDEA term for dysgraphia is specific learning disability in written expression.

Problems with math Dyscalculia is a learning disorder related to math concepts. Signs that a young child may be at risk of dyscalculia include trouble counting and sequencing. Once in school, signs may include difficulty solving simple math problems or organizing math problems when writing them on the page. Another sign of dyscalculia is difficulty handling money or making change.

Children with dyscalculia also have trouble understanding time-related concepts such as measuring time or telling time, or grasping calendar concepts such as days, weeks, months and seasons.

IDEA refers to mathematics learning disorders as specific learning disability in mathematics calculation or mathematics problem-solving.

SEEKING HELP FOR A LEARNING DISORDER

Early intervention is essential to remedying a learning disorder and helping your child function well at school and elsewhere. For example, early help with basic math skills in elementary school may allow a teen to tackle algebra in high school. If you or your child's teacher observes your child struggling to learn, consider having him or her evaluated for a learning disorder.

Under IDEA, federal law gives you the legal right to request a full evaluation from your child's school district. Talk to your child's principal to find out how to proceed. You can also call your local school district or visit its website to find out next steps in obtaining an evaluation.

Sometimes, a school may suggest one or more pre-referral interventions to help your child, such as a tutor or extra help in the classroom. If these services are successful in getting your child up to speed and adequately address your concerns, a special education evaluation may not be necessary.

Evaluation The special education evaluation process is usually a team effort. One or more of the following people may be involved in assessing your child along the way: your child's medical provider, your child's teacher, a school psychologist, occupational and physical therapists, a speech language pathologist, an educational specialist, a social worker, and the school nurse.

An evaluation typically includes a full account of your child's school history, classroom observations and a review of your child's academic performance. Sometimes, it involves standardized testing to measure your child's IQ or reading, writing, math and other skills. A comprehensive evaluation also considers other factors that may contribute to poor academic performance such as inattention, hyperactivity, depression or anxiety.

In some circumstances, a medical examination, including a neurological exam, may be recommended to rule out other possible causes of your child's difficulties — including intellectual or developmental disabilities — and certain brain disorders.

Moving forward If your child is eligible for special education services, the next step is to develop an individual education program (IEP) to meet your child's needs. If your child doesn't qualify for an IEP, the school may offer assistance through a Section 504 plan. This plan provides for classroom accommodations but not direct teaching services. See "Understanding special education services" on page 463.

It's important for you to understand the results of the evaluation before developing an education plan for your child. If you have questions, ask to have the evaluation results explained to you. If a more relaxed environment helps you to concentrate, consider reviewing the results at home before making any decisions.

To develop your child's education plan, you and your child's teachers or therapists will set goals specifically for your child, as well as devise strategies to reach those goals. If your child has an IEP, he or she will be assigned a case manager who will monitor your child's plan and make sure it's meeting your child's needs. Federal law doesn't require a case manager for Section 504 plans, but some school districts will provide one.

Keeping tabs on your child's progress and checking in with teachers and other professionals periodically will ensure that your child receives the necessary help to succeed.

INTERVENTION OPTIONS

Timely identification of a learning disorder can make it possible for your child to get help before he or she falls too far behind. With special education and tutoring, many children adapt their skills and perform much closer to their potential. They can achieve most academic and occupational goals if the appropriate teaching methods and motivation are found.

Types of interventions If your child has a learning disorder, school staff might recommend:

Extra help Both within and outside of the school setting, a reading specialist, math tutor or other trained professional can teach your child techniques to improve his or her academic skills. Tutors can also teach children organizational and study skills.

Therapy Depending on the learning disorder, some children might benefit from therapy. For example, speech therapy can help children who have reading issues. Occupational therapy might help improve the motor skills of a child who has writing problems. Psychotherapy or counseling can address mood or behavioral issues.

School and community programs Using evaluation results, your child's school may develop an IEP or a Section 504 plan for your child to formulate how he or she can best learn in school.

You can also find out about other programs your school or community may have to help children with learning disabilities. The federally funded Center for Parent Information and Resources maintains a website that offers a search function for finding a parent center in your state or territory. These centers provide support and services to families of children with disabilities and can give you specific state information and guidance on how to negotiate the special education system.

What to look for When assessing intervention options for your child, look for components that will maximize your child's chances for success:

- Small group or, preferably, individual instruction
- Several sessions a week
- Treatment that's aligned or overlaps with your child's school curriculum and breaks the curriculum down into smaller steps
- Time to practice learned concepts before introducing new material

- Periodic evaluation of treatment strategies during the intervention to make sure they're still effective

Many programs are marketed to families of children with learning disorders, promising new ways of improving brain function or helping a child achieve academic success. Not all of these programs, which might include online-based learning or mobile apps, are based on scientific evidence or proven effectiveness. In addition, they usually aren't covered by insurance, and some can be quite expensive.

When considering a program you think might help your child, ask yourself these questions:

- Is the program based on scientific research? Ideally, the program will be backed by scientists who specialize in understanding and measuring how the brain works (neuropsychologists).
- What are the specific benefits of the program? Are they measurable?
- Does the program teach my child something new? Does it gradually increase the level of challenge it presents?
- Does it fit our family's goals and lifestyle? Is it a good match for my child?

If you have questions or concerns about a program, talk about them with your child's case manager, teacher or medical provider, who may be able to provide additional guidance.

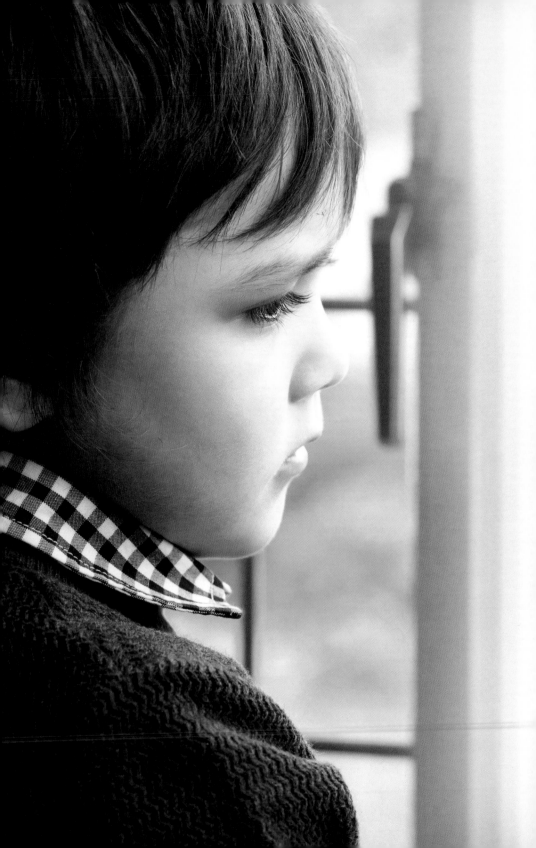

CHAPTER 23

Autism spectrum disorder

Over the past several decades, the diagnosis of autism in children has increased, likely due to a rise in the overall awareness of the disorder and a broadening of the diagnostic criteria for autism. Asperger's syndrome and pervasive developmental disorder-not otherwise specified (PDD-NOS) — two conditions that share common symptoms with autism and are treated using the same approach — now fall under the umbrella term *autism spectrum disorder*.

If your child's been diagnosed with autism, you likely understand the challenges the disorder can add to the already difficult and sometimes chaotic world of parenting. Your child's insistence on sticking with the same routine, difficulty with transitions or tendency to have severe temper tantrums, for example, can test your patience or make you feel overwhelmed. But you may also have come to realize the ways in which raising a child with autism can enrich your life, grounding you firmly in what's most important at any given moment.

This chapter will walk you through the basics of autism diagnosis and treatment, how to help your child at home, and how to care for yourself and your family.

UNDERSTANDING AUTISM

Autism is a disability that affects the brain and nervous system, interfering with a child's ability to interact socially with other people, both kids and adults. The disorder also leads to fixed and repetitive patterns of behavior, interests or activities. These signs and symptoms can severely limit or impair everyday functioning.

Still, not every child diagnosed with autism has the exact same symptoms or shows every sign. This is why *spectrum* is included in the name of the disorder. Some children with autism may experience mild symptoms, while others face more-difficult challenges in their day-to-day lives. No two children show signs or experience symptoms in the same way.

AUTISM SIGNS AND SYMPTOMS

Children with autism typically have difficulties in two key areas: (1) social interaction, and (2) patterns of behavior. To be diagnosed with autism, a child must meet all of the criteria for social interaction and at least two of the criteria for patterns of behavior.

Social interaction

Lack of mutual give-and-take

▶ Difficulty interacting with family members and friends, showing little interest in socializing.

▶ Difficulty starting a conversation or participating in one. Older children may engage in one-way conversations — talking about a topic of their own interest while showing little to no regard for the listener's interests.

▶ Trouble sharing interests and emotions with others.

Not understanding social cues

▶ Difficulty reading and comprehending gestures, facial expressions or eye contact.

▶ Poor eye contact and a lack of facial expressions.

▶ Expressing emotions or feelings in a way that is different from most peers.

Difficulty with relationships

▶ Lack of interest in friendships.

▶ Problems playing with others, adjusting behavior to others', understanding relationships.

▶ Difficulty making and keeping friends within peer groups.

Patterns of behavior

Repetitive behaviors

▶ Performs repetitive movements, such as flapping hands or flicking fingers, spinning objects such as coins, or rocking while standing.

Routines and rituals

▶ Strong adherence to regular routine. Children with autism often follow a particular routine every day or eat foods in a specific sequence. They may become extremely upset or irritable when the routine is altered in any way.

▶ Problems with transitions. Changing from one activity to another can be a particular source of frustration.

Narrow focus

▶ Intense preoccupation with a particular sensory experience, such as shiny surfaces, lights or smells.

▶ Strong focus on a narrow subject of interest. Older children may become preoccupied with schedules, the weather or phone numbers.

Reactivity level

▶ Unusual sensitivity — or lack of sensitivity — to light, sounds, tastes or touch.

In nearly all cases, children diagnosed with autism have another disorder that may have connections to their autism diagnosis. Common co-occurring conditions include congenital or genetic disorders, attention-deficit/hyperactivity disorder (ADHD), language disorders, anxiety, depression and sleep concerns.

About a third of children with autism have intellectual disability. Most have average intelligence, and a few have high intelligence. As they mature, some children with autism become more engaged with others and show fewer disturbances in behavior.

HOW AND WHEN THE DIAGNOSIS IS MADE

Most medical providers screen for autism in early childhood, looking for indicative developmental problems between 18 and 24 months of age. Usually, symptoms of autism are recognized between ages 2 and 3 years. But that doesn't mean autism isn't diagnosed at later ages.

Diagnosing a child with autism typically involves a series of screenings, information gathering and clinical evaluations. If you notice a consistent pattern of behavior and symptoms suggestive of autism in your child (see left), bring these concerns to your child's medical provider. As a parent, you play a key role in providing a description of your child's day-to-day life, particularly details related to social and communication skills, and behavior. This information will help the provider evaluate your child's condition and plan next steps.

Since genetics can play a role in autism, it helps to make note of any instances of developmental disorders such

MYTHS ABOUT THE CAUSES OF AUTISM

Autism spectrum disorder has no single known cause. In most cases, autism likely occurs due to a complex interaction between a child's genes and the environment. It's probable that this interaction affects early brain development and how nerve cells in the brain connect. Research continues in this field, and there may be other causes that have yet to be discovered.

Still, many people speculate about possible causes. For example, controversy has persisted around a suggested (then debunked) link between vaccines and autism. Scientists have investigated the question extensively. Despite numerous studies, there's no evidence that vaccines cause autism. Not vaccinating your child, however, increases your child's risk of catching and spreading serious diseases such as whooping cough (pertussis), measles and mumps.

Other claims have surfaced that what a child eats may play a role in autism. Some have proposed that specialized diets, such as a gluten-free diet, may help curb symptoms. Again, after many studies, no evidence has been found that draws any connection between diet and autism.

And, perhaps most importantly, there is absolutely no evidence to suggest that autism is caused by bad parenting.

---

as autism or intellectual disability in your family history.

Because behavior can vary considerably depending on time of day, location, familiarity with medical staff, and many other factors, it's important that your child undergo several different observations before a final diagnosis is made.

Typically, these observations are made by different clinicians. You and your child might talk with a developmental pediatrician, pediatric neurologist, medical geneticist, child and adolescent psychiatrist, speech and language pathologist, occupational or physical therapist, and a medical social worker. However, your child may not need to see all of these specialists.

To be diagnosed with autism, a child must show signs and symptoms in two key areas: difficulties with social interaction and repetitive or restrictive behaviors. These signs and symptoms must start in early childhood and negatively affect everyday function. To make the diagnosis, medical providers use a comprehensive list of criteria from the Diagnostic and Statistical Manual of Mental Disorders (DSM-5), published by the American Psychiatric Association. Your child's provider can help you understand the criteria as it applies to your child.

TALKING TO YOUR CHILD ABOUT AUTISM

Don't be afraid to talk with your child about his or her condition when the subject comes up or when your child has questions. For example, when your child doesn't understand a social situation, take advantage of it. Something as simple as not understanding a joke is an opportunity to say, "You probably didn't understand that because you have autism, and that's OK. Your speech therapist can sometimes help with stuff like that. I'll help you understand the joke." In this way, you can help your child understand his or her condition and learn how to manage it.

It's likely that some children, especially those who are 8 or older, have a sense that they're different from their peers. Focus on emphasizing your child's strengths, but also talk with your child about the challenges brought on by autism. How might your child's strengths be used to overcome or cope with the challenges? Mention that everyone is unique and all have strengths and weaknesses of their own. Also explain that autism is a common disorder, and many other children have it, too. Provide an accurate, age-appropriate and realistic definition of autism.

Importantly, don't let the disorder take over your child's life or your own. Take time to point out your child's strengths or interests that have nothing to do with your child's diagnosis. This helps your child realize that he or she isn't defined by the disorder. Let your child know that you will be there, loving and supporting him or her, no matter what challenges might come up.

TREATMENT OPTIONS

Although there's no known cure for autism, early intervention and therapy are crucial to maximizing your child's ability to function in everyday life.

COMPLEMENTARY AND ALTERNATIVE THERAPIES

Since a cure has yet to be found for autism, many parents seek complementary or alternative therapies for their children. It's possible that some of these therapies are helpful, but many have little or no research to show that they're effective. Some treatments may carry significant financial cost and be difficult to implement. And some are potentially dangerous. If you're considering a particular therapy for your child, don't hesitate to talk with your child's medical provider about the scientific evidence behind it, as well as the potential risks and benefits.

Here's a sampling of complementary and alternative therapies for autism.

Possibly helpful Some complementary therapies may offer some benefit when used in combination with evidence-based treatments. These are referred to as integrative therapies. For example:

▶ Creative therapies, such as art therapy or music therapy, focus on reducing a child's sensitivity to touch or sound. These therapies may offer some benefit when used along with other treatments.

▶ Sensory-based therapies are based on the unproven theory that children with autism have a sensory processing disorder. This causes problems tolerating or processing sensory information, such as touch, balance and hearing. Therapists use brushes, squeeze toys, trampolines and other materials to stimulate these senses.

▶ Massage may help kids relax, but there isn't enough evidence to show that it improves symptoms of autism.

▶ Pet therapy can provide pet companionship and recreation, but it's uncertain whether interaction with animals helps symptoms of autism.

Neither here nor there Some complementary and alternative therapies may not be harmful, but there's no evidence that they're helpful, either. For example:

▶ Special diets haven't proved effective for autism. And for growing children, restrictive diets can lead to nutritional deficiencies. If you decide to pursue a restrictive diet, be sure to work with a registered dietitian to create an appropriate meal plan for your child.

▶ Vitamin supplements and probiotics aren't harmful when used in normal amounts. But there's no evidence that they're beneficial for autism symptoms, and supplements can be expensive. Talk to your child's medical provider about vitamins and other supplements and the appropriate dosage for your child.

▶ Acupuncture has been used with the goal of improving autism symptoms, but it's effectiveness isn't supported by current research.

Possibly dangerous Some treatments haven't proved beneficial for autism, and they're potentially dangerous. For example:

▶ Chelation therapy is said to remove mercury and other heavy metals from the body, but there's no known link between heavy metals and autism spectrum disorder. Chelation therapy isn't supported by research and can be very dangerous. In some cases, children treated with chelation therapy have died.

- Hyperbaric oxygen treatments involve breathing oxygen inside a pressurized chamber. This treatment hasn't been shown to be effective for autism and isn't approved for this use.
- Intravenous immunoglobulin infusions haven't proved effective for autism and aren't approved for this use.

In the United States, children with autism who are younger than 3 typically are referred to early intervention services, which may include speech, occupational or physical therapy services. The goal of these services is to help your child gain developmental skills and help your family learn ways to meet your child's needs. Early intervention visits can occur at home, in a center, at preschool or through other outpatient programs. These services are administered by individual state agencies.

After age 3, services are available through the public school system, specifically through special education. Work with your school to obtain an individualized education program (IEP) or Section 504 plan for your child (see page 463). In addition to academic instruction, special education services aim to improve your child's communication and social, behavioral and daily living skills. These services may take place at a dedicated school or center, but they can also be integrated into mainstream schools.

Services available to your child will vary depending on the state in which you live. Navigating support options can seem overwhelming at times. A social worker can be a valuable resource as you begin to explore the assistance available to your child through local and state government agencies. A social worker can guide families who might be in need of financial assistance through the process of applying for social security aid.

Also visit the Center for Parent Information and Resources website. It offers a search function for finding a parent center in your state or territory. These agencies provide support and services to families of children with disabilities and can give you specific state information and guidance on how to negotiate the special education system.

In addition to the training your child receives in school, consider arranging private speech and occupational lessons at home or during the summer. This extra therapy time can help expand and reinforce intervention efforts at school while allowing you and your child's therapists to work together on a plan for how therapy can be applied at home.

As treatment progresses, take time periodically to re-evaluate therapy goals with your child's medical providers and teachers, and adjust the plan as needed.

Treatment for autism may include the following components:

Behavioral therapies Many programs address the range of social, language and behavioral difficulties associated with autism spectrum disorder. Some programs focus on reducing problem behaviors and teaching new skills. Other programs focus on teaching children how to act in social situations or communicate better with others.

Applied behavior analysis (ABA) is a commonly used method for helping children with autism and their families. It can help children learn new skills and generalize these skills to multiple situations through a reward-based motivation system. Parent training may be part of the intervention. Sessions are typically conducted in the family's home when the child is young, but then moved to a school or community setting as the child grows older.

Other therapies Depending on your child's needs, speech therapy to improve communication skills, occupational therapy to teach activities of daily living, and physical therapy to improve movement and balance may be beneficial.

A psychologist can recommend ways to address problem behavior. You might also look into social skills therapy groups, which can help your child learn the finer points of communication, including maintaining eye contact, reading facial expressions, understanding humor and learning other language subtleties.

Medications No medication can improve the core signs of autism spectrum disorder, but specific medications may help control some of the symptoms. For example, certain medications may be prescribed if your child is hyperactive; antipsychotic drugs may be used to treat severe behavioral problems; and antidepressants may be prescribed for anxiety.

When considering prescription medications for your child, ask about possible side effects and weigh those against the benefits of taking the drug. Also give some thought to the goal of taking the medication. Does treatment with medications fit in with your child's overall treatment plan? Will the benefits of taking the drug allow your child to make progress?

In the end, you are the best advocate for your child. If you do choose medications, keep a close eye on your child for possible side effects and tell your child's medical provider if they occur. Also keep in mind that in order to be most effective, medication should be part of a treatment plan that includes intensive intervention and therapy.

HELPING YOUR CHILD AT HOME

The care you provide your child as a parent is just as important to your child's overall growth as is the care that any specialist provides. Your child knows you and trusts you to care for him or her. For this reason, your patient and consistent guidance is key to helping your child learn to manage his or her behavior. Your guidance also reinforces the care that your child gets from the specialists.

There are many ways you can help your child succeed at home, at school, and in social or community settings.

Promote positive behaviors Difficult behaviors are common in children with autism. Throwing a tantrum may be the only way your child knows to communicate needs, wants or feelings.

You can encourage positive behavior in your child by focusing on a few key steps (see also Chapter 16):

What's behind the tantrum? Look to see what's triggering your child's behavior. Maybe he or she is too tired to take on socializing. Or maybe plans have changed too suddenly for him or her. The answer to this question may provide inspiration as you look to problem-solve.

Ignore negative behaviors Ignore negative behaviors that don't cause self-injury or harm to others, especially behaviors such as whining or tantrums. Paying attention to a behavior — whether negative or positive — has the effect of reinforcing that behavior.

Praise positive behaviors Instead of continually trying to correct negative behaviors, shift your attention to positive behaviors. Model and explain to your child how to behave appropriately in different situations.

When your child shows positive behaviors, be quick to offer praise or a reward, such as a sticker or a favorite activity. Make a plan so that your child can earn privileges by engaging in desired behaviors.

Set consistent consequences Establish clear consequences for undesirable behaviors. Be consistent about sticking to the consequences, whether it be a loss of privileges or a timeout. With consistency and positive reinforcement, you can work toward helping your child improve his or her behavior.

Maintain a consistent schedule Your child will do best with a consistent schedule and routines. Many children with autism do not adapt well to changes. Challenging behaviors tend to happen more often when your child is out of his or her routine.

Teach social skills It may be hard for your child to use verbal and nonverbal communication skills. And it can be tough for your child to understand when other people communicate with him or her. Your child may not know how to act appropriately in different places. You can help your child learn how to interact with people.

There are four basic steps to use as you teach social skills:

1. Tell your child what to do and say.
2. Show your child what to do and say.
3. Practice at home, in school and in the community.
4. Reinforce the behavior. Praise your child when he or she does well.

It's a good idea to arrange play dates and interactions with other children. Show your child what to do with other children (see page 267). You likely will have to show it repeatedly. Be sure to have your child take turns in play and conversation. Teach him or her how to problem-solve when conflicts arise.

Tell "social stories," stories that give examples of what it's like to be in certain places or situations and how to act there. Examples include going to the store, sharing with other kids, choosing from a menu and going to the doctor or to school.

Encourage adequate sleep Many children with autism have sleep problems. Up to half of children with autism have trouble falling asleep, wake up during the night, wake up early, have nightmares or sleepwalk. Some simple things you can do to help your child sleep well are listed here.

- Have a set bedtime and wake time.
- Use a relaxing bedtime routine.
- Make your child's bedroom quiet and dark for sleep.
- Use the bed for sleep only, not for play or timeouts.
- Use a fan or play calming music in the bedroom to act as white noise.
- Avoid using electronic devices during the hour before bedtime. Being "unplugged" helps the brain calm down better than any electronic activity could.

When your child stays in bed as desired, be sure to reward him or her the next day. See Chapter 8 for more on sleep.

Offer a balanced diet Your child has the same nutritional needs as any other child. Yet it's common for children with autism to be picky eaters. It may be because they tend to process senses, such as smell or taste, differently than other kids do.

Often, children with autism show a strong preference for certain foods or eating patterns, which may result in weight loss or digestive problems, such as constipation. If your child has a low body mass index, make sure he or she is getting plenty of calcium and vitamin D for bone density. Talk to your child's medical provider if your child experiences digestive problems associated with his

BUILDING RESILIENCE AS A FAMILY

In the midst of days filled with caregiving, many families are pleasantly surprised to discover the ways in which their lives have been enriched through their experiences. These families note that over time they develop a greater sense of emotional strength, better communication, and increased levels of tolerance, empathy and patience. And when a problem or crisis does arise, they find they can address it head on with a sense of compassion, peace and focused energy.

Such a positive approach is possible because the family members have developed resilience, which enables them to bounce back, re-center and forge ahead, in spite of the challenges they face. These resilient families share many of the same values and priorities:

1. They make an effort to spend quality time together as a family.
2. They are able to balance the needs of the family member with autism with the needs of other family members.
3. They establish and maintain healthy routines in their everyday lives.
4. They hold shared values.
5. They find meaning in challenging circumstances.
6. They maintain flexible roles within the family structure.
7. Whenever possible, they take advantage of clinical support systems.
8. They communicate openly with each other.
9. They approach each challenge with a proactive mindset.

or her diet. Dietary modifications, such as a vitamin or fiber supplement, may be helpful. To help your child toward a balanced diet:

▶ Provide regular meals and snacks.

▶ Consider offering your child only water between snacks and meals.

▶ Create a consistent structure around mealtime: be calm; don't sit down until everything is on the table; limit other distractions; eat the same food together; allow enough time for dinner to flow at a leisurely pace.

▶ Have at least one food that your child likes at each meal.

▶ Offer new foods many times. It takes most kids a few times of trying the same "new" food before they get used to it or begin to like it.

Plan for safety Wandering off is a common tendency among children with autism, even as they grow older. Children wander off out of curiosity, for enjoyment or to escape an unpleasant situation. To keep your child safe:

▶ Fence your yard, add deadbolts to your doors, and install an alarm system on your home that alerts you when a door has been opened. Talk with your social worker or county assistant, as there may be grant money available for these renovations.

▶ Talk to neighbors about your child's wandering tendencies. If you feel comfortable doing so, provide them with your phone number or instructions on what to do if your child shows up at their home.

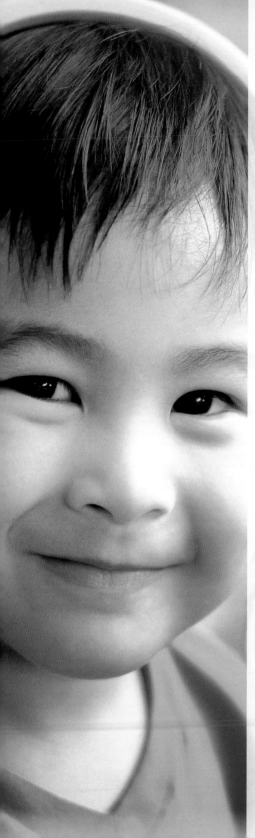

- Teach your child how to ask for or show you what he or she needs instead of wandering away.
- If it's a concept your child is able to understand, make sure your child is well-versed in how to stay safe around strangers.
- Have your child wear an ID bracelet that includes your name and phone number. GPS tracking systems may be useful as well, and they might be available through your local police department.

SELF-CARE

As a parent of a child with autism, you may find it all too easy to fall into a pattern of focusing on your child and forgetting to care for yourself. Hectic as life may be, it's important to try to take breaks from caregiving and make time for yourself.

Work to establish a regular routine that allows you to "recharge your batteries," even if it's just for a few minutes to sit and read your favorite magazine or do a quick exercise session.

If you have a partner, take turns getting out of the house to do something that you enjoy on your own. When possible, schedule times when you hire a sitter or have a family member watch the children while you and your partner spend quality time together.

If you have other children, set aside regular one-on-one time with each of your children as well. This reminds them that you care about them, value them as one of the family, and want to spend time with them.

With these strategies and resources close at hand, you will likely find that you are able to return to your caregiving duties with renewed energy, a more positive outlook, and more patience and empathy than you thought possible. Perhaps most importantly, the benefits of self-care tend to trickle down to other family members, improving their outlook and attitude as well. In this more positive home atmosphere, every family member has a better opportunity to thrive.

The importance of outside support

When stress becomes overwhelming, consistent, reliable support from extended family members can make a world of difference. In families where grandparents, aunts, uncles, mothers, fathers, brothers and sisters live nearby and are willing to help out, parents of the child with autism report feeling a greater sense of parenting satisfaction and improved family interactions.

In addition, lean into any professional support available to you, your child and your family. Families that take advantage of professional help report that they have a better sense of well-being and an improved understanding of autism and its symptoms. They also come away from discussions with therapists with an increased level of confidence in their own abilities as caregivers, greater resilience, and as a result, report that they experience less stress in the family.

Consider seeking out support groups for parents and families affected by autism spectrum disorder in your area. You may find that support group meetings become a touchstone in your life, a place where you can truly be yourself and know that group members will understand what you are going through. Fellow members may also be a source of emotional support, providing valuable insight into addressing challenging situations or ideas for coping with stress.

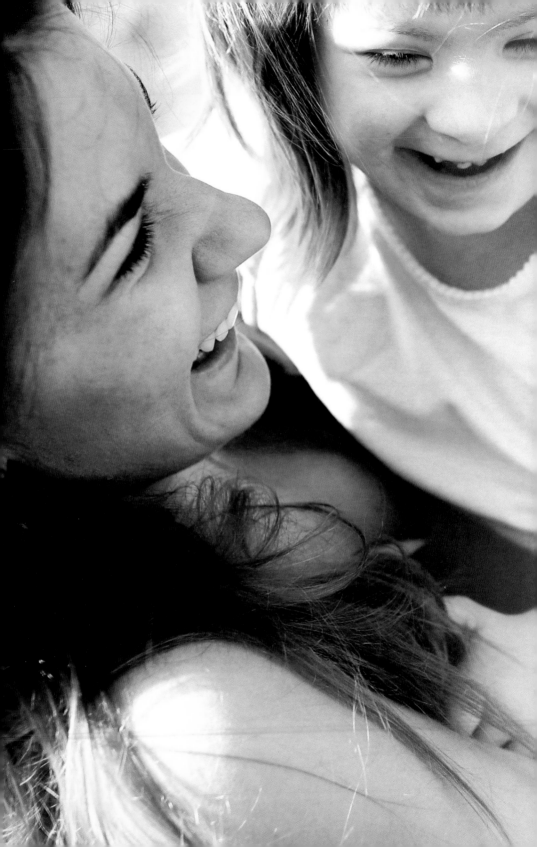

CHAPTER 24

Parenting complex needs

Parenting a child with complex health care needs due to a chronic illness, behavioral disorder or disability is similar in many ways to parenting an otherwise healthy child. Every child needs love, attention, supervision and a safe home. But a child with complex needs often requires more — more attention and supervision, more intense monitoring of basic needs and more time spent mastering the skills needed to meet your child's needs.

If it's been a while since your child's diagnosis, you've probably gotten through the initial adjustment and worked through some of the emotional upheaval that such a diagnosis often leads to. You've learned to manage treatment plans and the many appointments for follow-up care. You've become an expert in recogizing those small but sure signs that indicate when your child's symptoms are getting better and when they're getting worse. You know when it's time to call for help and you know what to do in an emergency.

Along with the added intensity of this kind of parenting, you also may have dis-covered added richness and unexpected joy in your family life. You may have seen your child achieve milestones you might not have thought possible.

As your child grows, you know that the challenges aren't going away, but neither are the rewards. With some planning, you'll be able to minimize the former and maximize the latter.

Along the way, make sure you don't let the condition or disability take over your child's life or your own. Focus on uncovering your child's many strengths and interests that aren't related to his or her medical condition. Enjoy being a family. Encourage independence. Plan for the future. Let your child know that you will be there, offering love and support, no matter what challenges he or she might face.

Although parenting a child with complex needs is a unique experience, many of the parenting principles found in this book apply equally to all parents. Feel free to explore other chapters and apply what works for you.

KEEPING YOUR CHILD SAFE

As your child gets into the preschool and school-age years, he or she likely is searching for more independence and mobility. Now is a good time to take a fresh look at your child's environment to make sure it's safe.

A helpful resource is your child's medical care team. Ask the team about what you can do to establish an appropriate environment as your child gets older — for when you're at home and away.

Preventing injuries and harm isn't that different for children with chronic conditions than it is for children without them. Each child is different, and the general recommendations to keep children safe should be set up to fit your child's skills and abilities. To help keep your child safe, know and learn about the unique concerns and dangers for your child. Keep in mind that your child's needs for safety may change over time.

With input from your child's medical providers, make a safety plan and share it with your child, your family, and other adults who spend time with your son or daughter. Consider the following factors when you make a safety plan:

Mobility Children who have limited ability to move or make decisions might not realize that something is unsafe, or they might have trouble getting away.

Carefully evaluate each place where your child spends time to make sure the environment is appropriate.

KNOW THE CONDITION

Every child is unique, even among those who have the same condition. Although your child will experience his or her particular condition in his or her own way, it helps to know as much as you can about the condition in general. How does life tend to progress? What are some of the challenges other parents in similar situations face? What are some of the rewards?

To gain this knowledge:

▶ *Find authoritative information.* Consider starting with an advocacy organization associated with your child's condition. For instance, the Cerebral Palsy Foundation's website provides videos, fact sheets, events and mobile applications.

▶ *Talk with professionals.* Your child's medical care team deals with a wide array of kids with the same condition as your child's. Team members understand what is typical for that condition and what isn't.

▶ *Talk with other families.* People living with a chronic illness or disability in the family are often dealing with the same issues you are. Chances are, they'll have insights and suggestions you won't gain anywhere else.

▶ *Trust yourself.* As you apply the knowledge you gain from other sources to your family, you'll gain experience on what works for your child and what doesn't. Remember that your child is unique, so a one-size-fits-all approach may not be ideal. Use your experience to tailor your approach to your child and family.

Check your child's clothing and toys. Are they suitable for his or her abilities, not just age and size? For example, clothing and toys meant for older children might have strings or attachments that aren't safe for a child who cannot easily untangle himself or herself. Toys for older children often have small parts that aren't safe for children who still put things in their mouths.

Safety equipment This varies depending upon your child's needs. Examples might include handrails and safety bars placed in key areas of the home to help a child who has difficulty moving around or is at risk of falling. Think outside the home, too. For example, you might obtain a life jacket specially fitted to help your child swim.

Communication Children who have problems communicating may need different ways to learn and retain rules about safety and danger. You might teach your child about safety using pretend play to rehearse safety drills and practice these on a regular basis.

You and your child may also need different ways to communicate immediate danger. For example, teaching your child to use a whistle, bell or alarm can alert others to danger. Tell adults who take care of your child about the ways you've agreed to communicate danger.

SETTING A ROUTINE THAT WORKS

A daily routine is the grease that makes many families run smoothly. Everyday routines provide the framework in which family members live out their values and connect emotionally over dinner, during

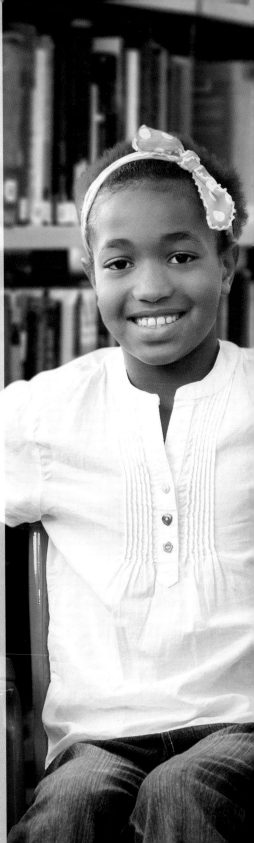

a shared television show or on rides home after school.

Regular routines also help children learn to take care of themselves and become independent. A predictable pattern to the day lets children know what to expect and when. It supplies them with ordinary tasks to accomplish and establishes the order in which things need to happen.

By mastering things such as getting dressed, doing homework and brushing teeth, children learn responsibility and gain confidence that they can navigate the world. A regular routine also helps kids develop healthy habits, such as washing hands and getting enough exercise and sleep.

When you first had your child, your daily routine probably centered on life within the family, such as nap times and feeding schedules. These days, your routine may be shifting more toward events outside the home — school, sports and play dates. If your child has a medical condition, this shift may be delayed a bit or occur in a different way than for other families.

Studies show it can be more difficult to establish firm routines for families who have children with complex needs, and there are a lot of reasons why. Sometimes it just takes longer to accomplish a task when there are limitations to contend with. Kids with disabilities or chronic illnesses tend to have more doctor appointments and therapy needs, which don't necessarily happen at the same time every day. And it's common for needs to change from day to day. But with a bit of planning and forethought, you can make the most of regular routines.

Having a regular routine will also help you as a parent. Routines can make daily decisions easier. For instance, if every Friday is leftover night, you don't have to expend mental energy figuring out what's for dinner. A "Taco Tuesday" can cut down on arguments over who gets to pick dinner that night. These little consistencies can help make you feel more in control when life gets busy. And they free up time and energy for other things.

The first thing to consider when developing a regular routine is what best suits your family. Would a more structured routine fit your family best, one where daily meals and fun activities are all planned out? Or does your family need a looser schedule that allows you to be more spontaneous?

Also keep in mind that a regular routine doesn't just mean your daily routine. It can include anything that you do in steady intervals, such as your weekly or even monthly routine. It's really anything that helps provide a safe and predictable landscape for your family. Whatever your routine type, aim to make it regular, predictable, well-planned and clear to all family members.

Set priorities To develop a successful routine, determine the goals you want to achieve that reflect your values. Maybe you place emphasis on having at least one meal together every day. Maybe you want to free up time so that you can do more fun activities together, such as a game or movie night. Or maybe you want to reduce screen time.

You might develop routines for yourself, each member of the family or the family as a whole, or any combination that makes sense to you. For instance, if you want to increase your child's independence, your child's routine might include:

▶ Picking up toys
▶ Getting cereal out for breakfast
▶ Doing homework after school

HELPING YOUR CHILD COPE WITH STRESS

The daily life of a child with complex needs can be just as stressful for the child as the parents. A child can get frustrated with his or her disorder, too, and resent that he or she isn't like most other kids.

Sometimes it can be difficult to recognize symptoms of stress in a child. It's not uncommon for children to try to adapt to stress by adopting a new behavior. Maybe they start to regularly complain about stomachaches. Or maybe they begin to lose focus when doing homework. Or they become upset more easily.

Start by talking with your child. Gently try to feel out what might be causing the increased stress. Maybe there's a problem at school or recent changes in routine. Also consider talking with your child's medical provider. He or she likely has experience with common stresses in children with your child's specific condition. The provider may help you come up with positive behavior alternatives to help your child adjust to stress — behaviors that ultimately increase your child's independence and resiliency.

To help you both unwind from time to time, find activities you both enjoy and can bond over. Maybe it could be spending an afternoon at the park or going for a long bike ride. These stress-free moments will not only help you relax but will also create memories you and your child will cherish.

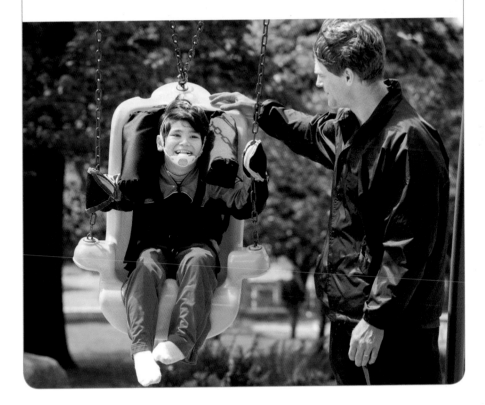

- Setting the table
- Doing dishes
- Getting ready for bed

It can be anything that you want your child to accomplish on a regular basis. Remember to also include activities your child enjoys, such as playing with friends or going for ice cream.

If you want to spend more time together as a family, your family routines might include:

- Dinner together
- Family fun nights
- One-on-one time with individual family members
- Planning the week ahead together
- Attending religious services
- Volunteering together

Talk to others If you are struggling with developing family routines or you just want to improve your routines, talking with others can help provide a fresh perspective.

Begin by talking with your family, including your child with complex needs. What are individual family members' daily obligations? How long do they expect regular tasks to take? How much free time do they need?

Use the feedback to tweak a routine to better meet everyone's needs. This will give your family members a sense of being on a team and a feeling that their input is valued.

Talk to people outside of your family who care for your child — child care providers, teachers, babysitters and grandparents. What do they expect to do for your child? What tasks should be taken care of before or after they spend time with your child?

Also talk to your child's medical care providers. They understand the specific needs of your child's condition. They may be able to give you ideas on how to build routines around those needs and build in opportunities for your child to learn and become independent.

Head off problems By now, you probably know the situations that are likely to create difficulty for your child. When planning your routine, try to minimize these situations.

For instance, if your child has attention issues, you've probably seen him or her struggle with getting ready in the morning. Picture yourself in his or her shoes. There's a timeline for getting dressed and

---

STAYING HEALTHY

When you have a child with a medical condition, taking care of the basics such as eating a balanced diet, participating in physical activities and getting enough sleep every night is especially important. It sets the foundation for better overall health and helps your child stay alert and focused. In addition, the principles for encouraging good behavior are the same for all children.

- For information on sleep, see Chapter 8.
- For information on fitness, see Chapter 12.
- For information on nutrition, see Chapter 13.
- For information on encouraging positive behavior, see Chapter 16.

eating breakfast; expected calm while eating; a parent's shifting attention as preparations for the day get underway; an imminent deadline of having to be out the door at a specific time; and the need for the child to do all of this when he or she might rather be sleeping.

Knowing the challenges your child is up against may help you create a plan that addresses problems before they occur. For instance, you might teach your child to do some tasks ahead of time, such as taking a shower or laying out clothes the night before, to ease the morning rush.

Make sleep a routine As kids get older and more independent, bedtime routines sometimes become less consistent. However, research shows that school-age children should be getting nine to 11 hours of sleep a night. Sleep is restorative. Getting enough sleep can improve alertness, concentration, behavior and the ability to cope with stressors, from doing homework to following treatment regimens. Try to establish a specific routine before bed to help your child wind down, and try to stick to the same bedtime every night, even on weekends and holidays.

Include downtime All kids need downtime, moments when they aren't expected to do something or act in a specific way. This can be especially true of kids with medical conditions. Giving them downtime to relax can help with overall behavior and help them learn to entertain themselves.

Don't forget to have fun. Many of the rewards of parenting come when you share time with your child, doing something you both enjoy, such as reading, watching a movie or cooking. Remember to set aside time for these moments.

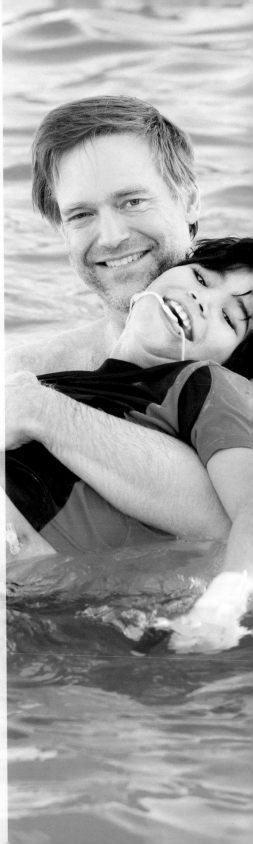

FOSTERING INDEPENDENCE

A long-term goal of parenting is to increase your child's independence. But how to increase independence while managing your child's condition can be tricky.

If you assign tasks that are too hard, you risk setting your child up for failure, which can result in feelings of frustration, anger, resentment and guilt for both child and parent. Repeated failures can be damaging to your child's self-esteem and create a sense of uselessness. Eventually your child may feel unable to accomplish anything on his or her own.

On the other hand, by not expecting your child to do anything at all or making tasks too easy, you risk sending the message that your child is incapable of being self-sufficient. You create a cycle of dependence that might be hard to break as your child gets older. As you develop tasks for your child, try to make sure that:

- Your child can do them
- The tasks are challenging enough that they increase your child's skills and independence

Finding the right balance is important in helping your child develop responsibility. It can be difficult to watch your child struggle. But it's in those moments, when a child overcomes a difficulty, that he or she gains the confidence to be independent. Here are some strategies that can help you encourage your child's self-confidence and independence.

Transfer knowledge In a way that's appropriate to your child's age and developmental level, help your child understand his or her condition and how it affects him or her physically, mentally and emotionally. Together, identify strengths your child has that he or she can use to offset weaknesses.

As your child grows and matures, you can relay more-complex details of the condition and incrementally transfer greater responsibility for managing the condition to your child. For example, you might set a goal that by the time your child is in the later elementary years, he or she will understand:

- The basics of his or her condition
- The importance of sleep, nutrition, fitness and germ control
- Key triggers that can make the condition worse
- The roles played by the people in his or her health care team
- The names of medications he or she takes and what they do
- How to perform daily treatment activities, such as setting up equipment or taking medication

Think about the future It's never too early to start thinking about your child's future. What do you hope your child might do after high school? Is he or she displaying any special interests or talents that might be helpful later in life? You certainly don't need to plan out every detail of your child's future, but asking these questions early will help you create opportunities to build toward specific independence goals.

Engage in life First-time experiences, such as the first day of school, can be a worrisome time for any parent and child. For parents of a child with complex health care needs, those worries may be much deeper as you wonder if your child will fit in with other children and how classmates will react to your child's condition. Try not to let your fears overcome your child's need to experience these moments on his or her own. For instance, if your child is terrified of getting on the school bus, offer to follow the bus in your car so that your child knows you'll be near, but refrain from just giving him or her a ride instead.

Be consistent Set rules with your child's particular needs and your goals in mind. For instance, a child with an intellectual disability may have different obligations than a neurotypical sibling. However, once you set the rules, make sure enforcement is consistent. This will help create a structure that gives your child a sense of stability and safety, which are important foundations for independence.

Consider creating rules and expectations together. That will help give your child a sense of responsibility for them. Add rewards, such as a favorite meal or a trip to the zoo, for good behavior or a job well done. Write everything out or create a chart showing what's expected of both of you.

Be flexible You can be consistent and flexible at the same time. The difference is knowing which of your child's behaviors are intentional and which are caused by your child's condition. This can be a

SUMMER CAMP

Parents of a kid with a chronic illness or disability often worry if summer camp is appropriate, and if so, if their child is ready.

It's perfectly fitting for your child to go to summer camp, regardless of his or her condition. Summer camp is an opportunity for your child to socialize and become more independent. After a year of school, of doing tasks he or she has to do, summer provides a chance to do things he or she wants to do and to have fun.

It's important to find a good match between camp and child. For some children, a mainstream summer camp is a great way to expand their horizons and get to know other kids. Other children may benefit from a more specialized summer camp. A quick internet search will reveal numerous camps all across the country focused on specific conditions, such as cerebral palsy, autism, spina bifida, asthma and others. Some camps accommodate a variety of conditions.

Another consideration is whether to attend a day camp or an overnight camp. If you select a camp for kids that share your child's condition, the camp will likely have a set of criteria that will help you decide whether staying overnight is appropriate. Read through the criteria carefully to make sure the camp is a good match.

If you're thinking about a mainstream camp, selecting day or overnight might be trickier. Is your child OK with routines and following directions? Also, how good are your child's social skills? Is he or she still struggling to make friends? If so, maybe select a camp that can strengthen those skills or talk to a counselor first.

You'll also want to consider your child's independence. Camp requires kids to do things on their own and be on their own. Does your child have experience being away from you? How did it go?

Summer camp is an opportunity for children to gain new experiences. Selecting the right camp for your child will help ensure those experiences are good ones.

challenge and may even change from day to day. For instance, a child with attention issues may be able to do homework one day but be overwhelmed the next. The goal is to understand the condition and know the difference between "I can't" and "I don't want to."

Avoid letting your child hide behind his or her condition or use it as an excuse for not meeting appropriate expectations. However, if you believe your child is truly struggling, take the time to consider the best approach forward and don't just automatically resort to corrective measures.

Acknowledge the struggle When your child has a task to do but says, "I can't," acknowledge his or her emotions and anxieties. Maybe share some of your own anxieties that you had as a child. This will let your child know that you understand and that you care about what he or she is going through.

But gently encourage your child forward. Maybe ask what he or she needs to successfully accomplish the task at hand. Helping your child work through obstacles and anxieties is an important step toward independence.

Allow for mistakes Everyone makes mistakes. Your child should be allowed to make them, too. If you see that your child is about to take a misstep, maybe with friends or in school, give your best advice, but allow him or her to make the final choice (as long as it's not a dangerous situation). By going through the decision process and experiencing the outcome, your child will gain self-awareness and learn individual responsibility.

Allow for discomfort It's likely your child has more than his or her share of uncomfortable moments. But making it

through these moments can help kids learn what they value and have confidence in their abilities to overcome difficulties. It creates resilience. Help your child see that he or she will still be OK and supported despite feeling miserable at times. For more information on developing resilience, see Chapter 17.

Allow free expression It can be tempting to speak for your child when he or she has a disability or chronic disorder. After all, you know him or her best. And sometimes kids with certain conditions can have a hard time expressing themselves, leading to awkward conversations with others, and even some embarrassing situations.

But by speaking for your child, you remove the opportunity for your child to make himself or herself heard and to improve his or her communications skills. You also signal that your child's thoughts and feelings aren't worth hearing.

Praise successes Always be on the lookout for ways to interact positively with your child. By praising behaviors you want to see in your child, you're more likely to see an increase in those behaviors. Also, by cheering your child's effort and persistence, you'll teach him or her that these are things that you value and appreciate.

Be patient Your child's road to independence won't always be smooth. Feelings of frustration are bound to occur. Be patient and try to model the behavior you'd like from him or her. If every frustration upsets you, your child will think this is how to act. But modeling patience in the face of difficulty is more likely to calm your child and allow your child to accomplish what's being asked of him or her.

HANDLING SLEEPOVERS

For many children, a sleepover is a rite of passage. It's like a mini-vacation away from a kid's usual routine of homework, early bedtimes and other responsibilities. During a sleepover, kids often develop deeper friendships over popcorn, video games and movies. It makes them feel like they're on their own, that they can navigate the world independently and advocate for themselves.

But a sleepover can be anxiety-inducing for parents, especially if their son or daughter has special health care needs. Will he be OK sleeping in a strange bed? Will she remember to use her inhaler?

It's important to know when your child is ready for a night away from home. Generally, if your child can sleep through the night without problems, be away from you for a few hours and do well socializing with others, he or she is probably ready for a sleepover. That doesn't mean the sleepover will go perfectly. But taking a few initial steps can help:

▶ *Give your child some sleepover experience.* Maybe stay in a hotel for a night or weekend. This will give your child a feel for what it's like to sleep in a strange bed and surroundings. You could also try letting your child stay overnight with a close relative.

▶ *For the first sleepover, pick a friend your child knows well.* If your child already has a close friend, he or she probably already knows your child's quirks and personality and is accepting of them.

▶ *Use the prospect of the sleepover to your advantage.* If a possible sleepover looms, tell your child that he or she needs to show for at least a week that he or she can get ready for bed — brushing teeth, getting pajamas on, getting into bed — independently.

▶ *Talk with the sleepover family.* If you have concerns about the sleepover, talk with the host family. The better the family understands your child, the more likely the sleepover will be a success.

▶ *Be prepared for a midnight trip.* Don't be surprised if you get a call in the middle of the night that your child needs to come home. And don't be discouraged — the first few sleepovers often fail for many children, not just those with complex needs.

CARING FOR YOUR OWN HEALTH

Caring for children with complex needs requires extra focus, extra coordination, and extra communication, planning and appointments. The financial burden can be heavy, as well.

All of that extra stress tends to result in higher levels of depression, greater feelings of isolation and poorer health than in parents whose children don't have complex health care needs. And the more care the child needs, the greater the stress levels.

But that's not the whole story. There are steps you can take to minimize these risks. With some critical thinking and careful planning, you can reduce health risks for both you and your family.

Identifying and managing stress
When parents are first told that their child has a chronic illness or disability, the resulting emotions can be overwhelming. Parents understand that their lives are changed forever and that the road ahead will be different than what they had planned. However, most parents go on to realize that, even with the additional strain and stress, their child brings them unexpected joy and pride.

Focus on the bright side Concentrating on the positives and drawing on your values, beliefs and goals creates a meaningful and enjoyable parenting experience. And having meaning in your daily life can increase your resilience to stress. For instance, caregivers who believe their caregiving role is positive overall report better health and less depression than caregivers who concentrate only on the negative aspects. Perhaps not surprisingly, many of the joys of raising a child remain the same despite the need for extra caregiving:

◗ The sharing of love
◗ Pleasure in providing care
◗ Opportunities to learn and grow
◗ A sense of accomplishment
◗ A strong family
◗ A strong sense of purpose
◗ Increased spirituality
◗ Higher confidence
◗ Larger social networks

Parents of children with complex needs also say their children give them greater personal strength. In one study, every participant said their child made them tougher and more confident. These parents say their child has changed their priorities and given them a greater appreciation of life. Experts say concentrating on the positives can help you adapt to the extra stresses of raising a child with complex health care needs.

Take care of yourself You, as the parent, are the core of your family. You are the one making the key decisions and dealing with all of the issues surrounding your child and his or her condition. You're the one who selects the appropriate child care, talks to your child's teachers, attends medical appointments, and sets and enforces goals for your child. On top of that, there are all of the other household duties such as paying the bills, cleaning the house, cooking meals, doing laundry and performing endless other duties.

That takes a lot of endurance. The bottom line is, you need to take care of yourself so that you can care for others. At times, all of the duties you need to perform will feel overwhelming. Taking a few small steps will ensure your body and mind are ready for them.

◗ ***Get regular exercise.*** Even a short walk around the block or a quick yoga session can help clear your mind and release stress from your body.

▶ *Eat a balanced diet.* It can be difficult to get regular meals amid the chaos of raising children, but studies show that good nutrition can have a strong effect on health and mood. Make regular meals at home together a priority for the whole family.

▶ *Get some rest.* When you're tired, it becomes more difficult to manage daily stress and unexpected situations — which are more common with children with complex needs. Getting enough sleep can make a big difference in your ability to manage stress.

▶ *Remember things you like.* Try to work in those things you enjoy. For instance, if you really like gardening or running, find opportunities to work it into your routine, even if it's only on occasion.

▶ *Get away.* Finding "me time" can be hard when you're caring for a child with complex needs. But it's during these times that you can clear your mind and think without being interrupted. Try to visit with friends to avoid becoming isolated. If necessary, ask someone close to you to watch the kids or find a caregiver who specializes in your child's condition.

Don't forget other family members It's important to make time to be with other members of your family, too.

You may not always be able to go out on a date night with your partner, but try to find time to connect, maybe over a cup of coffee or a favorite TV show after everyone else has gone to bed.

Talk to your other children about your child's condition. Encourage them to ask questions. Answer truthfully. Ask them about their fears or worries, and let them know how they can help their sister or brother, whether it's playing together or being a trusted friend.

DEALING WITH GUILT AND RESENTMENT

It's not unusual for a parent to feel guilty about a child's condition or disability. Some parents wonder if they somehow caused it to happen. Others feel guilty for wishing their child was different or that the child didn't have the condition at all.

Many parents fight the feelings of resentment that can accompany the loss of expectations about the future. Parenting is taking more time, energy and sacrifice than you ever imagined. In this context, it's only natural to have moments of resentment.

These feelings don't make you the worst parent in the world — they make you human. And it's how you deal with these moments that define your parenting skills.

Whatever the cause, it's important to realize that these emotions are normal. You're not alone in feeling this way. But it's also important to understand that dwelling on such feelings can be counterproductive, increasing stress and decreasing energy reserves.

Think about what may be causing these feelings of guilt or resentment. If people say or do things that induce guilt or make you feel bad about your situation, plan an appropriate response. Try to speak with others who know your child's condition well — it will help normalize what you're going through, which can help relieve some of your negative emotions. And realize that feelings of resentment can be a hint that you're overstressed and you need a break. Try to get away and unwind.

Other children in the family may sometimes feel upset about their sibling's condition and the extra attention he or she gets. And they may feel guilty for feeling upset. Those are normal feelings. However, each child needs individual time with you. If possible, on a regular basis, arrange for someone to care for your child with complex needs while you spend time with each of your other children.

Lean on your support network Take an honest look at the needs of your child, your family and yourself. Where do you need help? Perhaps the regular deluge of laundry is overwhelming. Or maybe the daily task of cooking dinner is a stressful chore for you. Then look over your support network and see where help is available. Maybe you have a sibling or friend who wouldn't mind helping in that specific area.

Remember that your support network extends beyond family and close friends. It can include caregivers, babysitters and others who provide your family with a regular service. It could also include social workers, teachers and therapists. All are familiar with your child's condition and may know of resources available in your area. Your child's medical team may include a case manager or service coordinator who can help access financial services and government programs in your community or county.

In addition, many support groups are organized specifically around a condition, such as epilepsy or Down syndrome. Connecting with families in similar situations can help you feel less isolated and give you a sense that what you're going through is normal. These parent-to-parent groups can provide a wealth of information — for example, the best child care for your child's condition, babysitter contacts, coping strategies for family members, transportation options in your area and more.

Studies show that the more social support a parent has, the more positive he or she is about the situation at hand.

Seek help when you need it All parenting is challenging. Parenting a child with a chronic condition can be especially so. If you feel like you need help, ask for it. There's no shame in admitting that what you're going through is difficult. Parents of children with complex needs are more susceptible to depression, anxiety, insomnia and chronic stress.

So if you're feeling persistently sad or overwhelmed with no relief in sight, seek professional assistance. Mental health experts can help you develop coping skills and build up resilience. They can diagnose depression and anxiety disorders and provide the help you need to manage them.

With the proper aid, you can increase your sense of well-being so that you can enjoy the experience of raising your child.

PART 7

Being a family

CHAPTER 25

Families of all kinds

During these middle years of childhood, family is central to your child. Not only does he or she receive the basics such as food and shelter at home but your child also looks to the family unit for security, acceptance and self-worth. In turn, you encircle your child with love and support, providing shared values, a sense of identity and a feeling of belonging.

The family can also serve as a microcosm of the world at large. It models how to build relationships, deal with conflict and handle a wide variety of situations. It is the rich soil that allows your child to grow and flourish.

Modern families take many forms. Although traditional two-parent families are still prevalent, a growing number of households are led by single parents, same-sex couples, grandparents or other combinations of adults. No matter what form it takes, at the heart of every functional family is an overarching spirit of unconditional love and acceptance and the belief that every family member is capable of achieving his or her full potential.

You can help maximize your child's success in life by intentionally strengthening your family and creating a warm, nurturing home environment that fits your particular circumstances. Through the years, you'll learn to meet your child's unique needs and adapt your parenting methods to suit his or her personality. As a result, family will continue to be a vital touchstone for your child as he or she grows in independence and self-reliance.

WHAT MAKES A FAMILY?

Although all children benefit from having a loving family, not all loving families need to look alike. In the past, the traditional family might have conjured up an image of a married couple, man and woman, and their children. Today's reality is more varied. For one thing, less than half of the children in the United States are living with biological parents who are in their first marriage.

Many families have gone through a separation or divorce, perhaps blending multiple families after a remarriage. Other families are led by a single mother or father raising a family solo or by a grandparent who has taken on the role of parent. More same-sex couples are stepping into the parenting role. Still other families grow through adoption or the foster care system.

All of these family structures can support and nurture a child. And while most of the work involved in parenting is the same regardless of who you are or how you came to be a parent, there are unique challenges and opportunities that can come with different circumstances. Following are some suggestions for making the most of various family formats.

CO-PARENTING

Co-parenting refers to parents who are raising a child together after a divorce or the breakup of a relationship. If this describes your situation, you and your child are in good company. It's estimated that about 40 percent of marriages in the United States end in divorce, affecting more than 1 million children each year.

It's not uncommon for the separation of two parents to bring up feelings of uncertainty, confusion, fear, sadness, loss and anger in all family members. These feelings are often strongest in the first year.

Even so, there's a lot you can do to smooth the way for yourself and your child. Together with your co-parent, you can support your child's well-being now and in the long term. Children are remarkably resilient and adaptable, and over time they'll adjust to their family's new normal. Co-parents can create an

atmosphere where a child can thrive by taking some of these steps.

Minimize conflict One of the best things you can do for your child is to strive for a positive working relationship with your co-parent. A high-conflict relationship between co-parents increases a child's risk of anxiety, depression and lower self-esteem. Children caught up in a high-conflict relationship between co-parents are also more likely to struggle in school and develop behavioral problems as teens.

To reduce tension with the other parent, try to accept that he or she is an important part of your child's life. Often, it helps to separate your personal feelings about your co-parent from who he or she is as a parent. When disagreements do arise, actively listen to the other parent and try to understand where he or she is coming from.

While certain events such as birthdays and holidays may continue to spark a sense of loss in your child, ongoing tensions between you and your co-parent are much more likely to cause your child distress.

Avoid undermining your co-parent Sometimes divorced parents avoid outright conflict only to express their negative feelings in less overt ways. Try not to be overly critical of your co-parent or get caught up in the blame game. Avoid speaking badly of the other parent to your child. These passive forms of hostility can be just as stressful to your child.

Focus on common goals Most co-parents, even if they have problems with each other, have one important thing in common: They want what's best for their child. When in doubt, try to view your co-parenting decisions through the lens of your child. Ask yourself what's best for your son or daughter. The answer may require you to set aside your own feelings about the other parent and make meaningful compromises.

Create a sense of security If you and your co-parent share custody, make sure that your child has everything he or she needs in both households. If your child's struggling with the switch between homes, suggest that he or she choose a favorite toy to carry from home to home. As much as possible try to maintain consistency in both households by abiding by similar rules and routines.

Seek help if needed If you and your co-parent are struggling to reach decisions about your child in a constructive, non-confrontational way, a family or divorce mediator may be worth considering. A mental health provider also may offer guidance and support if you or your child is struggling with anxiety or depression after a divorce, or you simply need a third party to talk to.

BLENDING FAMILIES

Even as divorce becomes more common, so does remarriage. An estimated 15 percent of American children belong to a blended family, which involves living with a stepparent and a parent.

Relationships in a blended family can be complicated, no doubt. Each family member must adjust to new roles and routines. This takes time and effort, but the payoff for your child can be great. By building and strengthening your blended family, you're opening up an expanding network of people who can care for and support your son or daughter.

Here are some ideas to help you create and maintain lasting bonds.

Form a shared philosophy For many couples in a blended family, a common source of tension is child rearing. That makes sense. You and your partner come to parenting with different experiences and expectations. Discuss your parenting strategies and styles on a regular basis, including the parenting roles each of you wants to take. Aim to find common ground and blend your approaches so that you can both feel respected and effective in the parental role.

Handle discipline with care If you're newly remarried, consider waiting a while to give your partner a disciplinary role with your children. This frees up your partner to focus on building a positive, close relationship with your child first. Once the child and stepparent have established a bond based on trust and affection, the stepparent can take more of a hand in enforcing family rules.

Spend alone time with your child If you're a biological parent in a blended family, schedule some one-on-one time with your child. This reassures your son or daughter that even if your family makeup has changed, your devotion to your child hasn't. If you're a stepparent, alone time with your stepchild can also be invaluable. Doing activities that you both enjoy will help strengthen your bond and open up lines of communication.

Honor the past but embrace the future It's not unusual for children in a blended family to want to hold on to the past. In contrast, a parent or stepparent may be more focused on building a future. Successful blended families balance these two needs. You can honor memories and traditions from your previous family by incorporating them into your current family's life. At the same time, it's important to establish new family traditions and experiences that are meaningful for everyone.

Focus on the little things As a stepparent, it might be tempting to try to win over a stepchild with a fancy new toy or an expensive vacation. While well-intentioned, these big gestures don't have the lasting impact that your steady, caring presence does. Helping with homework, playing catch in the backyard or listening when your stepchild has a bad day — these daily efforts are the glue that will bring you and your stepchild closer.

The same holds true for your family as a whole. Shared household activities such as chores or meals go a long way toward creating a cohesive family.

Be patient Often children under 10 adjust more easily to a new adult in their lives than do teenagers. Even so, it can take a couple of years — or even longer — for a new stepfamily to adjust to living together. Avoid pressuring your child or other family members to make new relationships work right away. Instead, encourage all family members to treat one another with decency and respect. If your child or another family member is struggling to adjust to your family situation, consider seeking the guidance of a mental health provider.

SINGLE PARENTING

Single-parent families are more common than ever — more than a quarter of the children in the United States live with a single parent, according to the U. S. Census Bureau. While most of these single parents are mothers, about a quarter of them are single dads.

Parenting without a partner brings special challenges. The responsibility for all aspects of day-to-day child rearing may fall squarely on your shoulders. Juggling work and child care can be financially difficult and socially isolating. But single parenting can also be rewarding, and it can result in an especially strong bond between you and your child. Many children growing up in single-parent families also learn to take on more responsibility at home and develop greater self-reliance.

Here are some suggestions to help you raise a healthy, happy child while tending to your own needs and happiness:

Seek and accept support One of the most important things you can do as a single parent is to maintain a strong support network. Practical and emotional support from others not only can help you handle your responsibilities but also boost your well-being. Your network might include trusted family members, friends, co-workers and support groups.

Find quality child care Staying home to raise a child is a luxury many single parents don't have. As a result, these parents find it crucial to enlist trustworthy child care while they're at work — both for the sake of the child's well-being and the parent's own peace of mind.

Look for a qualified caregiver who can provide age-appropriate activities in a safe and nurturing environment (see Chapter 9). Exercise your good judgment when asking a new friend or partner to watch your child. Anyone who cares for your child should be someone you know and trust and who has some experience with children.

Take care of yourself Single parenting is a constant juggling act that involves managing your career, finances, home responsibilities and child rearing. To help keep stress at bay, include physical activity in your daily routine, eat a healthy diet, and get plenty of sleep. Make sure you get some regular "me time" to replenish your energy and spirit. Consider arranging for a babysitter a few hours a week or month, if possible, or getting up early to enjoy a quiet cup of coffee each morning.

Prioritize family time Caring for a household single-handedly can put the squeeze on your time with your child, but doing special things together is important. Make quality time together a regular priority — even if it means having a messier house or not getting something else done that day.

Stay positive Make a conscious decision to focus on the positive and not dwell on the negative aspects of single parenthood. Try to keep your sense of humor when dealing with everyday challenges, and don't forget to have fun. If you're feeling down much of the time or find yourself stuck in a pattern of negative thinking, talk to your doctor or consult a counselor or psychologist.

GRANDPARENTING

When you raised your children and watched them grow up, you probably didn't count on being a parent again later in life. Yet here you are, stepping into the parenting role a second time around — and you're far from alone. It's estimated that about 10 percent of American children live with one or both grandparents, a number that has grown over time.

Many grandparents share the responsibility of child rearing with one or both parents, but it's not uncommon to be raising a grandchild on your own.

Raising a second family may not be what you anticipated, but it can be extremely rewarding. Many grandparents say they feel a renewed sense of purpose and appreciate having a second chance at parenting. They enjoy the deep bond they share with their grandchild and the opportunity to nurture a sense of security, identity and belonging.

As a grandparent, you're providing a safe, loving home in which your grandchild can thrive. You're also likely to face certain challenges along the way. To be a good caretaker while also taking care of yourself:

Acknowledge your grandchild's feelings Many grandchildren end up living with a grandparent due to difficult circumstances, such as a parent's death, divorce, substance abuse, mental illness or other difficulty. If that describes your situation, your grandchild may be struggling with feelings of insecurity, frustration, worry or grief. Let your grandchild know that it's OK to talk about these feelings. If your grandchild seems consistently anxious or depressed, seek the help of a mental health professional.

Provide a sense of security After playing a secondary role in your grandchild's life, it can be an adjustment for both of you when you become the primary authority figure. Do your best to set clear rules and expectations for your grandchild and enforce them in a consistent way. Establish predictable family routines, such as regular bedtimes and mealtimes. Doing these things will help to bring stability and security to your grandchild's life and order to your own.

Ask for support A strong support network is vital for any parent, but particularly for a grandparent raising a second family. Don't be afraid to reach out to trusted friends and family for help with babysitting, chores or other responsibilities. Join a support group for grandparents raising grandchildren. Look for additional support through your place of worship, your child's school, a local community center or government agencies.

Make your own health a priority With everything you have on your plate, you may think it would be selfish to put your own needs first. Nothing could be further from the truth. Taking care of yourself is of vital importance when it comes to caring for your family. Lean on your support network for help with child care so that you can go to doctors' appointments and tend to your health. Try to incorporate physical activity, healthy eating habits and relaxing downtime into your schedule. If you feel overwhelmed or overcome with feelings of guilt, disappointment or resentment, don't hesitate to talk with your health care provider or seek the guidance of a mental health professional.

Know your rights At some point, you may decide it's necessary to establish legal custody of your grandchild. A grandparent's rights vary from state to state, so consider meeting with a family law attorney who can help you navigate any legal issues.

Seek financial help It can be tough to make ends meet as a grandparent, especially if you are no longer working or had to give up a job to care for your family. You may qualify for help with housing, grocery or other bills, as well as clothing or school supplies. Reach out to your

MILITARY FAMILIES

Military families face unique challenges when it comes to juggling life's responsibilities. When a parent is deployed, it can put a strain on all family members, affecting the well-being of the child and the parent alike. The child misses the deployed parent. He or she may worry about the parent's safety and can face greater risks of mental health issues such as depression or anxiety. The parent on the homefront faces the added stress of holding down the fort without a partner. At the same time, the deployed parent may worry about maintaining a close relationship with his or her child and partner. There may be sadness, too, at missing out on important family events or childhood milestones.

The good news is that most families successfully manage the challenges of a parent's deployment. Here are some things you can do to help smooth the way:

▶ *Encourage honest communication.* Before and during a parent's departure, allow your child to express feelings and worries about the deployment. Answer questions as honestly as you can in an age-appropriate manner.

▶ *Seek support.* Lean on the support of family, friends and your spiritual community. Take advantage of programs for military parents and families if they're offered in your area. These programs often teach parenting skills or coping strategies to foster greater family resilience.

▶ *Stay connected.* Call, talk, text, video chat and email as often as possible. Take time to work though parenting concerns and other life issues as a couple. Stay in regular touch with your child to maintain a close bond. Some deployed parents make special videos for their children, such as reading a favorite bedtime story.

▶ *Take the re-entry slowly.* Although a parent's return to family life is cause for celebration, the adjustment for many families can be hard at first. As the returning parent, some of the challenges you may face are re-learning how to share parenting responsibilities with your partner, reconnecting with your child and adapting to the pace of life back home. Your child and partner will also be adjusting to your re-entry into their every-day lives. Be patient and give yourselves the time you need to create new routines.

grandchild's social worker, if one has been established, or check with your local government agencies such as social services, children and family services, child welfare or your local department of aging.

SAME-SEX PARENTING

Millions of children are being raised in the United States by at least one gay or lesbian parent. Often, the children are from previous heterosexual relationships, but many same-sex couples are conceiving or adopting children together.

Although same-sex parenting is becoming more common, you and your child may still face some challenges. One of them is a false assumption that same-sex couples aren't as equipped as heterosexual couples to raise a child. On the contrary, multiple studies show that children of same-sex couples fare just as well as children raised by opposite-sex couples. Research has also shown that a child's sexual orientation and gender identity aren't affected by the sexual orientation of his or her parents.

Even so, you may still worry. What if your child faces disapproval from other adults? What if he or she is teased by other children? You can't always control what happens away from home, but there's a lot you can do to support your child:

Be open The best way for your child to have a positive and confident outlook is for you to keep the lines of communication open within the family. Be matter-of-fact when discussing your family makeup and your sexual orientation while being mindful of what's age-appropriate. Be prepared to answer ques-

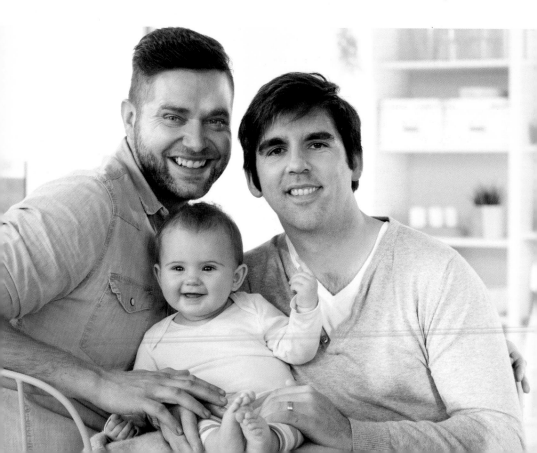

tions such as "Why don't I have a mom?" or "How was I born?" The more confident you are in your family structure, the more at peace your child will be.

Prepare your child At some point your child's likely to confront children or adults who don't understand or feel uncomfortable with your family's situation. This may range from expressions of genuine curiosity or confusion to deeply hurtful comments. Depending on your child's age, you may want to practice how to respond to these kinds of interactions with confidence. Reassure your child that you'll always be there if he or she needs help handling a challenging situation.

Find families like yours Read your child books showing different kinds of families. If possible, seek out other families led by same-sex couples, in addition to other kinds of families, so that your child knows that families can take many forms. If you don't know any such families in your community, consider joining or starting a support group. It can be reassuring for your child to spend time with other families that are similar to yours and connect with children in similar circumstances.

Share with your child's school The more your child's teachers know about your family, the better equipped they'll be to support your child at school. For example, you might want to explain that your child calls one parent Dad and the other Papa. You could also suggest books for the classroom that highlight different kinds of families, or donate some books yourself.

Know your rights If you and your partner are parenting a child together, it's important to understand the legal rights of the nonbiological or nonadoptive parent, even if you're legally married. Presumption of parenthood based on same-sex marriage varies from state to state. The American Academy of Pediatrics recommends that children be adopted by the second parent or co-parent in families headed by gay and lesbian couples. This provides the child the security and benefits of two legally recognized parents and preserves the co-parent's custodial rights. An attorney who specializes in family law can help you navigate the legal system.

Let your family be imperfect Many same-sex parents say they feel pressure to be a superfamily in order to prove that their family's valid. But no family's perfect. All families have squabbles, and all parents mess up. By accepting your family, warts and all, you're sending a powerful message to your child. You don't have to be perfect — or the same as everyone else — to be accepted and loved.

ADOPTIVE PARENTING

Whether your child joined your family through an international or a domestic adoption, as a baby or as an older child, he or she is at the center of your family's world. As with any parent, most of what your family needs to know about caring for a child is already in this book. At the same time, being the parent of an adopted child presents some unique opportunities and challenges.

Here are some ways your family can support your child in his or her journey through life.

Celebrate your family's story Many experts recommend that parents develop their own story of how their family was created and share it with their child regularly. Use the story to talk about your child's birth parents in an understanding way, explain why you chose adoption to build your family, and give your child a sense of personal history and belonging. Any details you can add to such a story about the joy of your first encounter will make it more delightful to your child.

Answer your child's questions honestly As you enter the middle childhood years, don't be surprised if your child starts asking more questions about his or her adoption story or birth family. Your son or daughter may also express some distress or sense of loss around being adopted. When talking about your child's background, be positive but factual. Resist the urge to embellish or add details that you don't know to be true. At the same time, don't feel the need to share all of the information with your child right away; there may be some details that are better saved until your child is mature enough to handle them.

Embrace your child's identity Many adoptive parents are raising a child with a different racial or ethnic identity from their own. Most experts recommend that families acknowledge and embrace these differences rather than ignore them. Incorporate your child's cultural background into family life by reading multicultural books, attending cultural festivals, exhibits or events, and eating traditional cultural dishes. Being sensitive to your child's identity may also mean talking about issues related to bias and discrimination in age-appropriate ways.

Seek out other families like yours Look to make connections with other families that have been touched by adoption — both the children and the parents will find this type of peer group helpful. Adopted children will get the added benefit of spending time with other children — and families — whose stories may more closely resemble their own.

Handle difficult remarks calmly Now and then, parents and children may be faced with ignorant or even hurtful remarks from others. A stranger may wonder how you and your child are related or who your child's "real" parents are. You don't have to answer every question, and you don't have to let everyone know you adopted your child. Instead, your response may be more for your child's benefit than to educate the person asking the question. Saying things such as "I'm his real parent" in a calm and assured way can help reassure your child.

Treat your adopted and biological children equally If your family includes both adopted and biological children, strive for fairness in how you treat them. It may be tempting to offer your adopted child special treatment or be looser with discipline, but this won't serve your child well in the long run. Keep in mind that equal treatment doesn't necessarily mean using the same approach with all your children. Each child will have different needs based on their individual strengths and weaknesses. What matters is that you accept your children for who they are and ensure that their needs are being met.

FOSTER PARENTING

As a foster parent you're a special kind of nurturer, devoting yourself to a vulnerable child who may only be in your life for a short while. It can be incredibly rewarding and life changing but also unimaginably hard at times. Many foster children have experienced abuse, neglect or both, and they're likely to have come from a household or community touched by poverty, violence, mental illness or substance abuse. This type of chronic stress during early childhood can have toxic effects on the developing mind and body, often leading to chronic developmental, behavioral, physical, emotional and educational problems.

Despite these negative early life experiences, your foster child is probably missing his or her birth family and struggling with the separation. He or she might act out or have built up a wall that can be difficult to break through. Although you might not be able to take away a child's pain, it's important to remember that you're providing something vital and irreplaceable: a safe, nurturing environment that shields a child from harm. That's no small thing.

To make the most of your time with your foster child, consider these tips.

Seek appropriate health care The American Academy of Pediatrics recommends that foster children have comprehensive medical, dental, developmental and mental health assessments within the first 30 days of being placed in a foster home. In addition, each child in foster care should have a medical file containing all relevant medical information that's been obtained so far.

Ultimately, your foster child's caseworker is responsible for these tasks, but it can be difficult to gather a child's medical history and determine who's legally responsible for making the child's health care decisions. If possible, work with your foster child's caseworker to find a pediatrician who can help you navigate your child's medical needs.

Support family connections The ultimate goal of the foster system is to reunite a child with his or her birth family. While you might have mixed feelings about the birth parents, it's important to honor their connection to your foster child. Be aware of your own biases or judgments and try to focus on your foster child's needs. Avoid speaking badly of birth family members, emphasizing instead their positive qualities. Offer support for your foster child before and after birth family visits or phone calls — encounters that can bring up mixed emotions in a foster child.

Help your child handle emotions Managing emotions is an important skill for any child to master. It can be especially difficult for a kid who's experienced stress or trauma. Teach your foster child words he or she can use to express feelings, and encourage open communication about thoughts and feelings — even if they're negative or upsetting. Act as a role model by responding to your foster child with warmth and consistency.

Let your kid be a kid Although painful experiences may have forced your foster child to grow up quickly, in the end he or she is still just a kid. Offer chances to do regular kid stuff, such as playing at a playground, pretending to be a superhero or working on a puzzle. Do activities together that you both enjoy, and provide opportunities for self-directed play. Give your foster child access to age-appropriate playthings such as books, play dough, art supplies, musical instruments or dress-up clothes.

Find support Being a foster parent can stretch you in ways you never imagined, which is why a supportive network is so invaluable. Reach out to friends or family members whom you can turn to for practical support, a listening ear or a much-needed pep talk. Connect with other foster families, whether in your community or online. They will know what you're going through and can offer specific encouragement and advice.

Accept your limitations One of the hardest parts of being a foster parent is not knowing how long your foster child will live with your family. It could be anywhere from a few days to over a year. Whatever time you have together, don't expect to solve every problem or turn the child's entire life around. Instead, set realistic expectations. Make a plan for what you'd like to accomplish and specific ways you hope to help your foster child. Then take things day by day, knowing you'll likely experience some incredible highs and lows along the way.

FAMILY MATTERS

Effective parenting doesn't depend so much on the exact makeup of the family but on the effort that goes into it. Children thrive on the warmth, respect and acceptance a family is uniquely positioned to provide. Along with this emotional nourishment, children are also absorbing how the members of a family treat one another.

Regardless of your particular circumstances, you can provide your child with the love and stability that your family is able to give. Warmth and affection, communication and togetherness, consistency and predictability, and limits and boundaries — these are the nourishing ingredients that can support a happy, healthy childhood.

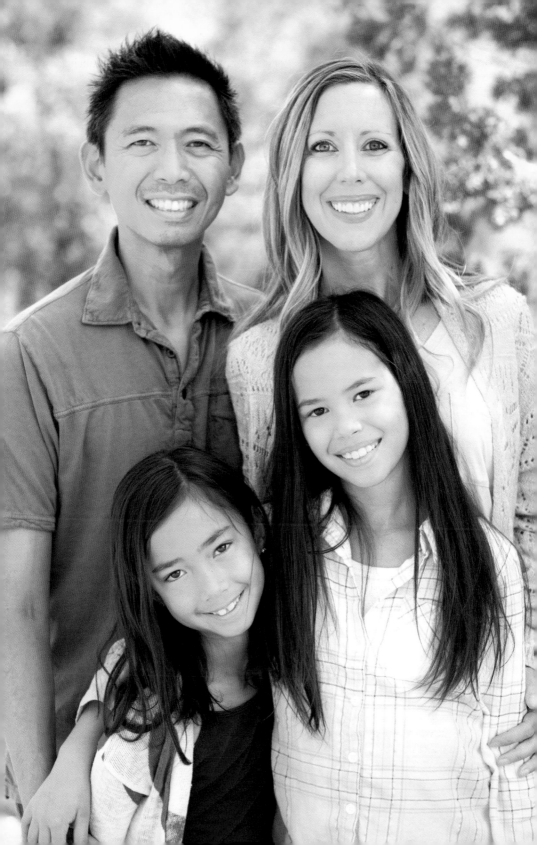

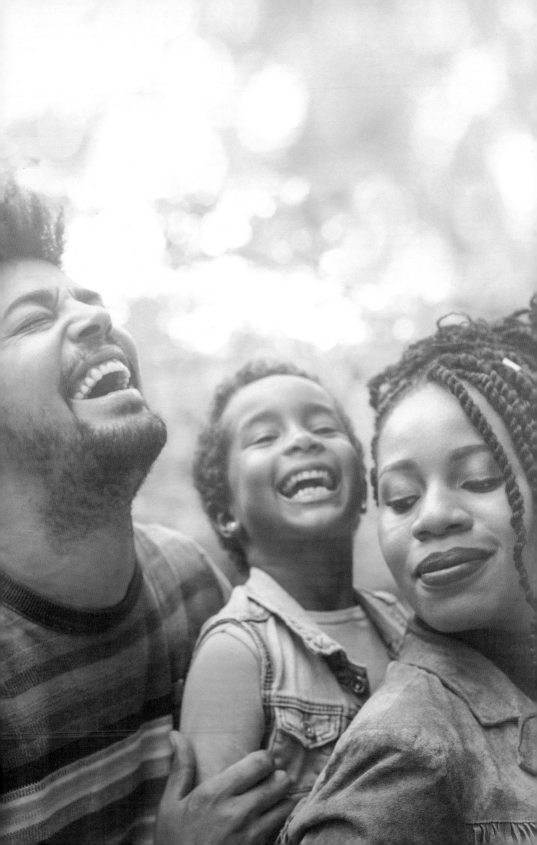

CHAPTER 26

Parenting together

Caring for a family can be a lot like managing a small business. You're in charge of making sure everyone's doing what they need to do, getting where they need to go, and receiving what they need to grow and flourish. It's a big job — one that takes coordination and cooperation with everyone involved. And in many families, there's not just one CEO, but two.

Parenting alongside another adult takes commitment, flexibility and mutual respect. Like any team, you may each play certain roles, yet these roles often overlap and shift depending on the needs of the moment. You won't always agree on every aspect of your child's life, but with open lines of communication, you can proactively work together to reach consensus and solve problems as they arise.

Parenting together means sharing the decisions and responsibilities of parenthood alongside its pleasures and joys. A solid parenting team strives for consistency in child rearing, mutual support and constructive problem-solving. The more that you and your parenting partner

can cooperate as a unit, the stronger your bond will be. The stronger your bond, the more effective you'll be as parents.

TAKING A CONSISTENT APPROACH

Whether your child's a young preschooler whose favorite word is "no!" or a school-aged kid who's constantly lobbying for extended freedom and privileges, you and your partner will be faced with countless decisions on a range of parenting issues.

Children do best when their parents are on the same page, sending a consistent message about their expectations and the consequences of misbehavior.

It helps if you work together to develop basic shared philosophies that guide you on how to handle a wide variety of parenting issues and challenges. That way, you'll be less likely to confuse your child with mixed messages and be better able to create clear and consistent expectations and limits.

Chances are, though, that you and your partner won't always agree on what those limits are and how to enforce them. In large part, that's because you've come from two different families that have passed down their own parenting strategies and beliefs — often from generations back.

Reflecting on your beliefs Many parents emulate their own parents in the way they raise their children — though some people make a point of doing the opposite of what their parents did.

It may be worthwhile to reflect on your own upbringing and how it's influenced your approach to parenting. What do you value about the way your parents raised you? Are there traditions you treasure and want to pass on? What do you hope to do differently? What beliefs and messages about parenting did you absorb from your childhood family?

Thinking through these kinds of questions will not only give you a clearer understanding of the kind of parent you are and want to be; it will allow you to communicate more openly and effectively with your partner about your parenting goals, hopes and concerns.

That kind of communication can go a long way toward understanding where both of you are coming from, increasing your ability to blend your parenting approaches and work off each other's strengths.

Some partners don't want to discuss their beliefs, hopes and worries because they're afraid that they'll reveal unbridgeable differences or start major conflicts. But confiding what you hope for as a parent and what you're concerned about strengthens the bond between you and your partner.

Blending your parenting styles
Another aspect of understanding yourself as a parent is identifying your basic approach toward or style of parenting.

Your core beliefs and attitudes about your role as a parent are played out in your parenting style, affecting how you interact with your child.

For example, do you tend to view yourself as an authority figure whose fundamental job is to raise your child with strict rules and high expectations? Do you enjoy showering your child with affection but feel less comfortable setting firm limits and enforcing rules? Or do you see yourself as a coach, guiding your child through the ups and down of life with an equal measure of structured limits and loving attention?

Some parents find that their styles are quite similar. They tend to agree on the big-picture issues, such as how to respond to misbehavior. But they may disagree at times on smaller things, such as whether it's OK to have a snack before bedtime.

It's not unusual, though, for parents to come at parenting with two different styles, which may lead to disagreements on everything from how many rules to impose to the types of consequences to adopt when rules are broken.

When you each take the time to identify your parenting style — and where it might have stemmed from — you may be better equipped to find common ground, as well as room for flexibility and compromise.

Talk to each other about your priorities when it comes to your child, as well as what you most hope to accomplish as parents. This can help you weave together your parenting philosophies and goals in a more cohesive way.

Keep in mind, though, that you don't necessarily have to go about parenting in

PARENTING STYLES

Some experts divide parenting styles into three or four overarching categories. While you may fit somewhere between one or more of the styles on the parenting spectrum, most parents tend to fall back on a particular style as their default.

Knowing the broad range of parenting styles and where you fall on the continuum can help you understand yourself and your partner better, allowing you to weave your styles together. Here's one way to think about different types of parenting.

Authoritarian Parents who adopt an authoritarian style often exert considerable control over their child and expect most rules to be obeyed without question. Because of this focus on maintaining clear authority, open communication and negotiation with the child is often less common. Parental expressions of warmth and nurturing may also take a backseat in favor of promoting strict expectations.

Permissive On the opposite end of the continuum is the permissive parenting style. These parents often express a lot of warmth and acceptance but are less likely to say no or set clear limits for their child. They're also less likely to exert control over their child, monitor his or her activities, or enforce consequences for misbehavior.

Authoritative Often considered the most effective form of parenting, the authoritative style falls somewhere in the middle of the other two parenting styles. Parents who are authoritative provide both warmth and limits, enforcing those limits in a caring way that takes into account the child's needs and feelings as well as the viewpoint and goals of the parent. Authoritative parents tend to balance firmness with flexibility and expectations with respect.

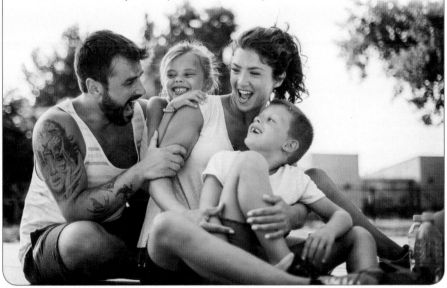

the exact same manner. For example, one of you may cuddle with your child when he or she gets hurt while the other is more likely to employ gentle humor or a playful distraction.

Different doesn't always mean better or worse. It can be useful to come at the same problem in two different ways. Complementary parenting styles can serve to enrich your child's perspective.

The goal is not to become carbon copies of each other but to strive for agreement on the big issues, such as rules, expectations and consequences.

WORKING TOGETHER

As your child grows, your parenting skills and philosophies are bound to evolve. Be sure to regularly discuss your goals with your partner or co-parent when it comes to child-raising so that you can remain on the same page.

It's especially important to agree on and observe the same rules and discipline guidelines. This reduces your child's confusion and need to test you.

Here are some ideas for how to keep your parenting goals and approaches in alignment so that you can work together to provide the love, attention, limits and routine your child needs.

Present a united front Send your child a consistent message by agreeing not to disagree about parenting decisions in front of him or her. Avoid contradicting each other in your child's presence when it comes to these matters.

Instead, try to make it a policy to work through major parenting decisions in private before presenting them to your child. Make it clear that those guidelines are coming from both of you.

You can always revisit your decisions again if one of you feels uncomfortable with the direction you've set for your child.

Back each other up Sometimes you or your partner or co-parent may end up making a parenting decision on the fly, before you've had a chance to talk it over. This can happen with small things, such as giving a reward for good behavior, or bigger issues, such as establishing a new policy around school performance.

Even if you disagree with the other parent's choice, try to maintain a united front by backing up the other parent in your child's presence. If you have strong feelings about the issue or are concerned about the long-term consequences, discuss those concerns privately. Later, you may choose to revise the previous decision in a way that you can both feel comfortable with. You can then present that decision to your child together.

Give yourselves time Your child accidentally smashes a lamp to smithereens while throwing a ball in the house, an activity that goes against a clear family rule. You want to impose an appropriate consequence, but you know your partner will probably also want to be part of the decision. What to do?

To show respect for your partner and avoid parenting disagreements later on, resist the urge to make an impulsive decision. Instead, consider telling your child that there will be a consequence for the behavior but that you need to talk to the other parent first. Once you've agreed on a course of action as parents, you can present it to your child together.

Avoid putting your partner in a tight spot Sometimes a parent's impulsive decision unfairly affects the other parent. One parent may impose a demanding punishment or make a big promise but won't be home to see that it's followed through.

That leaves the remaining parent with the dilemma of either carrying out a punishment or promise he or she may not be comfortable with, or going against the other parent's wishes.

To avoid this kind of situation, try not to make parenting choices that you won't be able to help put into action unless you and your partner or co-parent agree on it ahead of time.

Don't be divided and conquered
Your child comes to you after dinner asking if she can have a piece of last night's leftover apple pie. You say yes, but as you're handing her a plate, your spouse walks in saying that he'd already said no. Sound familiar? It's the classic divide and conquer method, one that many kids use to their benefit. It involves asking each parent for something separately until the child gets the desired result.

Instead of giving an answer right away, you can gently shut down this childhood strategy by saying something like "What did Dad say?" or "Let's check with Mom first." If you and your partner or co-parent get caught unwittingly contradicting each other, consider deferring to the first parent that your child approached. That way, you'll be sending the message that the divide and conquer method doesn't work.

Deal with problems as they arise
Sometimes when parents disagree about how to handle a parenting problem or dilemma they avoid it altogether, letting it go unresolved. In other cases, one parent will regularly defer to the other parent in the hopes of avoiding a conflict, leaving the other parent to handle most of the difficult issues.

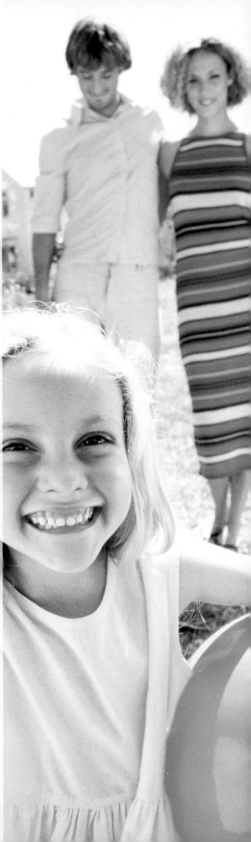

For the sake of your child, make a commitment to tackle problems head-on together. Two heads are usually better than one, and the compromise you reach will likely be more effective than what either one of you might have come up with on your own.

SUPPORTING EACH OTHER'S EFFORTS

Parenting can be a tough business, one that stretches you to the limit at times. While it's rewarding to see your hard work reflected in all the ways your child is maturing and thriving, you don't often get direct feedback on how you're doing. After all, no one's handing out evaluations or bonuses for a job well-done.

Most parents experience doubt sometimes, second-guessing their decisions or their effectiveness as caregivers. As a parenting team, you can boost each other's confidence and strengthen your ability to parent together by offering positive encouragement and responding to each other's needs.

When you support one another, you help to promote understanding, trust and connectedness. Those positive feelings often translate into fewer conflicts and better cooperation in child rearing and other areas of life.

Mutual support can also improve your confidence in your parenting skills, helping you to feel more effective when it comes to child-raising. That creates a positive snowball effect: When you feel better about your parenting abilities, you actually become a better parent. To support your partner or co-parent:

Focus on the positive Show your appreciation by taking the time to notice what you value in each other's approach

PARENTING AS A COUPLE

When you're a couple and also parents, it's important to nurture your couple relationship as well as your child. Research on married parents, for example, has shown that the quality of a spousal relationship not only affects the ability to parent successfully but also impacts the child's well-being. Negativity in a couple's relationship can expand to parenting and family interactions.

On the other hand, supportive, mutually satisfying couple relationships enhance the well-being of the whole family. Making a special effort to see yourself not just as a mother or father but as a partner is good for both of you — and your child.

Although time can seem like a scarce commodity, it's important for you and your partner to make time for each other and find ways to connect. If possible, set aside a regular time each week to be alone together without your child. Do something you enjoy or can laugh or talk about easily. Have a date night, go for a walk or just take a few minutes to sit together after your child has settled into bed.

to parenting. Perhaps your partner or co-parent uses humor with your child to great effect or has an amazing ability to soothe away worries. Let the other parent know how much you admire those qualities and express gratitude for all he or she does for your child.

Help each other evolve Of course no parent is flawless, and there may be times when it's useful to give or receive thoughtful suggestions. Nobody likes to be lectured, but if specific feedback is given in a gentle, caring way, you can strengthen each other as parents. By the same token, if you're on the receiving end of that kind of feedback, strive to listen with an open mind and with your child's best interests at heart.

Stand up for each other All children experience moments of resentment toward their parents. It's part of being a kid. If your child complains to you about the other parent, listen with empathy so that your child knows you care about his or her feelings, but avoid agreeing with or adding to your child's criticisms.

Depending on the situation, you may want to encourage your child to express those feelings to the other parent directly. That way, the two of them can work through any tensions together. If you feel your child has made some valid points, express them privately to the other parent in a supportive way.

Offer and ask for help All parents experience moments when they feel stretched a little too thin. Tell your partner what you need to feel supported, and do the same for him or her.

Ask for help in specific, concrete ways, such as giving your child a bath or help with a science fair project. If you notice that the other parent seems overburdened or worn down, offer to pitch in or take over a particular parenting job. For example, you might suggest that you help out with the evening's math homework so that your partner can have a few quiet minutes alone.

Switch things up Sometimes parents get stuck in certain roles, such as the disciplinarian, the problem solver or the homework helper. Don't be afraid to switch things up, giving each other a break from the routine and a chance to take on different roles in your child's life.

MODELING HEALTHY HABITS

To work together effectively as parents, one of the best things you can do is to maintain healthy interactions and habits in your adult relationship. A mutually respectful and caring partnership not only benefits the two of you but provides a sense of security and well-being for your child.

Your relationship also sets a powerful example. From the two of you, your child is learning how to treat others, handle differences and form deep bonds. When you and your partner support each other, tackle problems together and work through frustrations, you're giving your child lessons in building a healthy relationship.

Perhaps nothing challenges a relationship more than the inevitable disagreements you face as a couple. This may be over child-rearing decisions, household responsibilities, finances or any number of issues that come up on a daily basis.

Although it's unwise to hash out parenting disagreements in front of your child, kids may actually benefit from seeing their parents work through other kinds of differences in a constructive manner.

When you handle these differences calmly and respectfully, you're teaching your child invaluable conflict resolution skills, such as how to handle disagreement and negotiate compromise.

You're also modeling healthy ways of regulating strong emotions, such as stress, anger or frustration. What's more, you're showing that conflict isn't something to fear or avoid but is a normal part of any healthy relationship.

Healthy conflict can also help knit you and your partner more tightly together. When you know that you can work through your differences and still come out OK on the other side, you feel stronger and more secure in your relationship — and that allows for a greater sense of cooperation, trust and teamwork.

Here are some healthy problem-solving habits you and your partner can draw on when facing disagreements or conflicts.

Talk it out When facing a problem or disagreement, make time to discuss it together. Choose a time when you're both calm and able to listen with an open mind. Give each other turns to express your point of view. When your partner is speaking, try to truly focus on what he or she is saying instead of thinking about the points you want to make.

Stay focused Keep the conversation centered on the problem or issue at hand. Avoid pulling other topics or grievances into the mix, criticizing one another or assigning blame. Instead, focus on working together to resolve your differences and come up with a solution.

Stay engaged Facing conflict can sometimes be uncomfortable. It may be tempting to shut down the conversation and withdraw. Only by sticking it out will you be able to reach a satisfying compromise. If necessary, take a temporary break by saying that you need a chance to calm down and think. Then return to the conversation ready to engage.

Work toward understanding Make a genuine effort to put yourselves in each other's shoes. This can help you better understand your partner's perspective. It can also help you handle a conflict with greater sensitivity.

When you take the time to appreciate where your partner is coming from, you'll be more likely to find a way to incorporate each of your viewpoints into a compromise that satisfies you both. In many cases, joint problem-solving will yield a richer environment for your child to grow in.

Find balance There may be occasions where you realize that you simply aren't going to see eye to eye on an issue.

If it's something your partner feels a lot more strongly about, consider letting him or her take the lead in making the decision. He or she can do the same for you when something comes up that you have stronger feelings about.

This give and take allows for you to "agree to disagree" in a way that maintains a sense of balance and harmony.

A FIRM FOUNDATION

Your relationship with your partner or co-parent is a foundational aspect of your family. You make your foundation stronger by engaging each other with respect and mutual appreciation, supporting each other, and allowing each other to grow and develop as a parent.

By approaching parenting as a unified team, you create an optimal environment for your child to grow up in — a safe place where your child feels secure and wanted. You also set the tone for an affectionate, communicative family life. And you model what healthy adult relationships look like in a real-life setting — an important and lasting gift to any growing child.

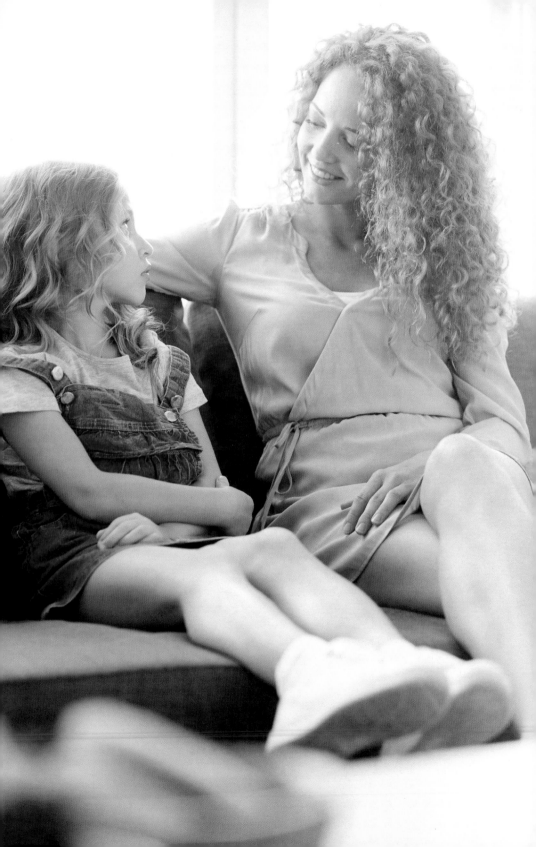

CHAPTER 27

Juggling act

A typical day as a parent can feel like one long sprint. It's a mad dash from the minute your feet hit the floor in the morning to the moment you sink into bed at night. Along with caring for your child, you may be juggling a job and relationships, not to mention trying to squeeze in some time for yourself.

The many roles you play in life can create a deep sense of meaning and fulfillment, but sometimes you may feel as if you're being pulled in too many directions. You wonder how you'll get it all done and still maintain some sort of balance. If only you could heap extra servings of time and energy onto your plate!

Take heart in knowing you're not alone. If you sometimes feel as if you're losing the battle for balance, it's not because you're inefficient or unmotivated. Many parents report feeling rushed in their day-to-day lives. They strive to do their best in all their roles but worry they're sometimes falling short.

Finding balance in daily life is a constant juggling act that takes organization, conscious choices and the willingness to ease up on yourself. While you may not keep all the balls perfectly in the air all the time, it's possible to manage and even thrive with the juggling routine. You can enjoy your many roles while making the most of these priceless years with your child.

JUGGLING WORK AND HOME

Being a parent in and of itself can seem like a full-time job. Add to that the fact that a majority of parents in the United States also engage in some type of paid employment and it's no wonder life can feel overly busy.

There's no wrong or right way to mix work with parenthood. The best arrangement is the one that works for you and your family.

For parents who work outside the home, achieving balance between their jobs and their family is the holy grail.

There's little doubt that being a parent can make work-life balance harder to achieve. Yet research has also shown that combining parenting with employment can positively affect your experience of both roles, making each area of life richer and more satisfying.

As a stay-at-home parent, taking care of your house and family requires time, effort and concentration. It is a job, though it may not be monetarily compensated. When you enjoy doing it and derive fulfillment from it, your passion will be passed along to your child.

When you are invested in what you do and draw pleasure and meaning from it, those good feelings can spill over into your family life and your interactions with your child.

There are times, though, when you may feel torn between your duties to your career, your home and your children. Generally, parents experience more stress from their work lives crossing over into family life, although some parents report that parenthood has impacted their career as well.

Despite the challenges of managing work, household and parenthood, there are things you can do to find more balance and draw greater enjoyment from all areas of life. Here are some big picture ideas to keep in mind.

Identify your core values Your values influence your goals at home and at work. The problem is that sometimes those values come into conflict with one another. You believe in being a superparent and a workplace hero. You prize keeping a spotless home and spending time with your child. It can be helpful to clarify for yourself what your most important values are. That will make it easier to prioritize your goals during this busy stage of life.

Embrace 'good enough' If you've always set high standards for yourself, this is the time to let go of perfectionism. Balance requires being good enough rather than perfect. Your home might not be as tidy as you'd like, and you might not have as much time to cook meals from scratch. Maybe you're not working as many hours as you did or you can't drop everything for a last-minute meeting. Strive to be your best without expecting the impossible.

Let go of guilt Sometimes, in the attempt to balance all your roles equally, you end up feeling as if you're letting everyone down. You may be especially worried that you're not devoting enough time to your child. That's when the guilt really sets in.

The truth is that compared to parents of previous generations, parents in the United States are spending more time on child care, not less — even if both parents are working. Research also shows that working moms spend nearly the same amount of time on educational and other beneficial activities with their children as their stay-at-home counterparts. Instead of worrying about what you're doing or not doing, focus on the positive aspects of your situation.

Redefine balance Balance doesn't necessarily have to be one thing that looks the same at all times. There may be periods when one area of life requires more attention or takes priority over the others. That's to be expected. If you notice that life's been off balance for too long, take some time to re-evaluate your priorities and make adjustments.

Get organized Make a daily to-do list. You might divide the list into tasks for work and tasks for home, or tasks for you and tasks for your partner. Identify what you need to do, what can wait — and what you can skip entirely. Organize household chores efficiently, such as running errands in batches or doing a load of laundry every day. Do what needs to be done and let the rest go.

Seek support Don't try to do everything yourself. Accept help from your partner, loved ones, friends and co-workers. Speak up if you're feeling guilty, sad or overwhelmed. If you can afford it, consider paying for weekly or biweekly housekeeping to have some extra time for your family or yourself.

SETTING LIMITS AT WORK

Because the number of hours in a day are limited, it's important to prioritize what goes into your schedule. If you're juggling full-time employment with parenting and housekeeping, one way to carve out more time for family, relationships and the activities you enjoy is to set some

limits on the job. Things you may be able to do to manage your work life include:

Make your job work for you The more flexibility and control you have over your hours, the less work-family conflict you're likely to experience. Ask your employer about flex hours, a compressed workweek, job sharing, telecommuting or other scheduling flexibility.

Not every work setting provides time to be a parent. But you might try offering compelling reasons why more flexibility could benefit your employer. The workforce is changing, and many employers acknowledge this. Consider working with other colleagues on a project or in your department to cultivate a work environment that offers a better balance of personal and work life — for parents and nonparents.

Provide key information Work with your colleagues, not against them. As much as possible, give your employer advance notice if a family obligation will affect your hours. Let your manager and your co-workers know so that you can get their support and be respectful of their needs, as well.

Manage your time Focus on being productive while at work, then learn how to put work down at the end of the day. Don't be afraid to respectfully say "no." If possible, cut or delegate tasks you don't enjoy or can't handle — or share your concerns and possible solutions with your employer. When you stop accepting tasks out of guilt or a false sense of obligation, you'll likely be more intentional at work and have more time for family and other activities that are meaningful to you.

Define your own boundaries Some parents find they achieve better balance when they draw clear lines between their different roles. They make a conscious decision to mentally separate work time from family time and strictly limit their use of work-related technology at home. Others may find it's less stressful to integrate work and family life more seamlessly, taking the occasional work call or completing some work tasks from home. Experiment with both options to figure out what feels best to you.

Keep your career options open Creating a sense of independence from a specific employer or career can give you the freedom to move between positions and companies, and possibly take some time off or consider starting your own business. Maintain your personal and professional networks and contacts, and build a strong reputation in your field.

WHEN YOU TRAVEL FOR WORK

Many jobs require some form of travel. While work travel can provide a break from the homefront, time away from home can also impact family life and routine. You can lessen the effect of work travel on your child by following some simple strategies.

- *Communicate.* Let your child know when you'll be traveling and for how long. If you have a preschooler, bring up your travel plans a week or a few days before you leave. Older children have a better understanding of time and may prefer to know about your travel plans further in advance.
- *Acknowledge negative feelings.* If your child expresses sadness or anger about your travel plans, don't dismiss those emotions. Listen, and offer understanding and comfort.
- *Don't prolong the goodbye.* Avoid dragging out your departure because of guilty feelings. On the other hand, don't try to sneak away without saying goodbye. Keep your goodbyes short and reassuring.
- *Stay connected.* Make video phone calls so that your child can see your face. Read to your child at night by phone or video chat. Share photos of your day. Send postcards that your child can collect.
- *Stick to routines.* Work with your partner and child care team to keep your child's schedule and routines as intact as possible while you're away.

SHARING THE LOAD AT HOME

Before becoming parents, you and your partner may have shared household tasks fairly equally. When a child enters the mix, traditional gender-associated patterns are more likely to assert themselves. If you're a stay-at-home parent, you're probably taking on an even greater share of parenting and household responsibilities.

Just as there's no one formula for mixing work and parenthood, there's no single way to share responsibilities on the home front. What matters is that you actively, deliberately and jointly work out a division of labor that distributes the stresses — and the rewards — of parenthood to the satisfaction of both of you.

Maybe sharing means one of you has chosen to put your energies into raising a family while the other focuses on career opportunities. Perhaps one parent has scaled back at work and shoulders more at home. Or maybe you've both decided to work fewer hours to carve out more time for child care.

It's not that you have to split all the responsibilities of life 50-50, but you want to come up with a plan that you can both embrace — one that allows you to work as a team in caring for your child and sharing decisions and tasks. Here are some tips to consider:

Communicate openly How much responsibility should you each take on at home? Make a list, and talk about what you can do, want to do and are good at. Structure the arrangement as an experiment, and tweak it as you go. Keep communicating about your expectations, what's working and what's not.

Recognize and acknowledge your different priorities — which may change over time. Sit down and discuss what matters most to each of you in terms of your child, your career, your free time and the chores. You and your partner aren't going to agree on everything — and probably won't find a perfect balance. Be willing to negotiate and compromise. When you're dividing up household chores, take into account your preferences and strengths and the most efficient use of your time.

Check your assumptions Sometimes what seems like a choice about how to divide up tasks is actually influenced by social or gender norms. For example, historically, mothers were often expected to be the primary caretakers for children, with fathers playing a secondary role.

Rather than feel bound by such gender roles, be flexible about how things get done. Couples who have less rigid expectations about their roles at home and as parents may experience less stress as individuals and more harmony in their relationship. What if your partner does chores and child care differently than you do? Agree that it's OK for both of you to have different ways of doing things, as long as you're providing consistency for your child.

Avoid keeping score You and your partner are on the same team — you don't need to keep score. Instead of taking an inventory of everything your partner is (or isn't) doing, trust that you're both committed to your family's success. Work together to solve problems, and avoid complaining about who has the short end of the stick. Pitting yourselves against each other shortchanges everyone.

Create systems to automate the tasks Devise systems around household chores that work for both of you: You do the laundry; your partner does the vacuuming and sweeping. Your partner cooks on weekends, and you handle the weekdays. You take turns putting your child to bed and giving baths. If you can afford it, think about hiring someone to help with the housework or yardwork. But be clear about whose responsibility it is to make those arrangements.

Have a plan for when your child gets sick Who cares for your child at home when a cold or stomach bug strikes? If both parents have work commitments, set up a Plan A, B and even C that you're both satisfied with. Perhaps you take turns staying home with a sick child. Maybe a friend, family member or neighbor is willing to pitch in when neither of you can get away from your job. Sick care for children may also be offered by some babysitting services, child care centers or hospitals in your area.

STAYING IN THE MOMENT

Have you ever found yourself on autopilot with your child? Perhaps you're playing a game of restaurant or superhero but your mind is a million miles away. You're too wrapped up in your own thoughts or worries to delight in your child's gap-toothed smile or marvel at the creativity unfolding before you. When you're stuck inside your head, you're less attentive to your child's emotions and needs. You're missing out on an opportunity to see the world through his or her eyes.

One way to combat this common parenthood pitfall is to practice mindful parenting. At its simplest, it involves staying focused on the present moment with your child, without any particular agenda for how your child will behave or what will unfold. Mindful parenting means bringing your full awareness to your child by actively listening and paying attention in a nonjudgmental, non-controlling way. It means bringing that same awareness and lack of judgment to yourself by noticing your own emotions and reactions to your child.

Research has begun to suggest that parents who practice mindful parenting may become more emotionally aware of their children, as well as more empathetic, accepting and compassionate toward their children and themselves. Mindful parenting may also have a positive effect on how parents interact with their children. For example, the practice of mindful parenting may increase positive parenting habits, such as showing affection and offering comfort or encouragement. By the same token, it may decrease less helpful parenting behaviors, such as yelling or being overly critical.

Learning how to stay in the moment with your child takes time and practice, but you may find it reduces stress and improves your relationship with your child. It's something you can incorporate into daily life, even during mundane tasks such as getting ready for school or helping your child prepare for bed. You can also bring a mindful awareness to one-on-one moments you and your child share together.

Here are some strategies you can use to incorporate mindfulness into your everyday parenting.

Bring your whole self When you choose to be mindful with your child, you're choosing to be present physically, intellectually and emotionally. If you find your mind wandering or if the day's stress starts creeping in, pause, take a breath and return your attention to what's happening right in front of you.

See your child Strive to see and appreciate your child for who he or she is rather than who you wish your child to be. Be aware of how your own unfulfilled needs, dreams or agendas may be interfering with your ability to accept your child in this moment.

Hear your child Whether you're having a conversation with your child, helping with schoolwork or just goofing around together, make an effort to pay attention to what your child is expressing. That includes both what your child is saying verbally and what he or she may be conveying through behavior and other nonverbal cues. The more aware you are

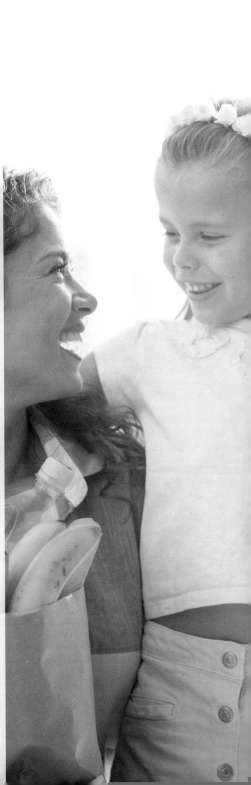

of your child's emotions, thoughts and perceptions, the more responsive you'll be to his or her needs.

Resist triggers Whether they realize it or not, kids have a way of pushing parents' buttons. When you're irritated by something your child is doing or saying, stop and notice how you're feeling or thinking. Don't judge yourself; just observe. What unconscious emotions might your child's behavior be triggering inside you? Before taking any action, consider the best way to respond to the situation.

Press the pause button You're folding a pile of laundry or cooking dinner when your child comes to you with a question or a story about his or her day. If you're able, stop what you're doing and make eye contact. Take a moment to fully listen and engage with your child before returning to your task.

Forgive yourself Even with your best efforts during moments of mindfulness, there will be times when you do get distracted, lose your patience or handle a parenting situation in a less than ideal way. Part of parenting mindfully is letting go of judgments of yourself. Strive to love yourself as unconditionally as you hope to love your child. In return, that love will flow back to your child.

STEPPING AWAY FROM SCREENS

If you're like many parents, there may be times when you're glued to your phone while playing with your child, pushing a swing at the playground or attending a little league game. Your child may complain that you're on your devices too much. He or she may even feel the need to compete for your attention by acting out. Part of the problem is that many parents feel pressure to answer texts or calls right away from friends, family and co-workers. And once the screen comes out, it's all too easy to get sucked in.

While your child doesn't need your undivided attention all the time, devices can come between the two of you too often. When you're staring at a screen, you're more distracted and less responsive to your child. Studies show that parents' screen time habits can interfere with or even reduce conversations and interactions with their children. On the other hand, when you put down your phone or tablet and focus on your child, you're sending the invaluable message that your child matters. This kind of attention is the precious commodity that helps a child to thrive.

Here are some suggestions that may help you better regulate your own media habits so that you can be more present in your child's life.

Be a good role model Studies show that children are heavily influenced by their parents' technology habits. When a parent's time on electronic devices increases, so does the child's. That's one more reason to limit the time you spend on your devices. You can also set a good example by putting your phone aside at mealtimes, when you're driving, and when you're directly engaging with your child and others.

Create device-free zones Consider setting up tech-free areas for the whole family. Perhaps devices are off-limits in the kitchen or at the dining room table. Maybe instead of pulling out the screens during short car rides, you engage in conversation or sing songs together.

EAT TOGETHER

Between soccer practice, ballet lessons and post-work errands, regular family meals may seem like a thing of the past. It's worth the effort, though, to try to make shared meals a priority in your family.

The kitchen table is a wonderful gathering place to connect as a family and build a sense of security and belonging for your child. Regular family meals can also benefit your child's overall well-being in other ways. Children who share meals with their family have been shown to eat a more balanced diet, have greater emotional health and take part in fewer risky behaviors. Eating together as a family may also reduce the risk of eating disorders and weight issues in children and teens.

For more on making the most of family meals, see Chapter 13.

Agree on tech-free times Establish times of the day when the entire family stays off devices. Mealtimes are a good choice. You might also set aside device-free time for an hour each evening and during certain periods during weekends.

Turn screen time into family time Watch age-appropriate shows and movies with your child or play some video games together. Talk about what you're watching or doing and ask questions. By interacting with your child during these enjoyable experiences, you're strengthening your bond.

CARING FOR YOURSELF

Many parents know in theory that they should make their own health and happiness a priority. In reality, though, it seems like there's always something (or someone) more important to attend to than yourself. With all of your responsibilities, you may feel that putting yourself first is indulgent at best and selfish at worst.

If that describes your thinking, think again. Nurturing yourself isn't just good for you. It's good for your child.

Consider the emergency instructions announced at the start of an airline flight: Put on your own oxygen mask before putting a mask on your child. Now apply that philosophy to your entire life as a parent. You need to make sure that you're functioning properly in order to properly care for your child.

When you consistently put yourself last, your emotional and physical resources get depleted. You become less capable of managing the stressors that come with parenting. Feeling some stress now and then can be good. It can motivate you to face a challenge or handle a

crisis. But when you're constantly under pressure, it can take a toll on your mental and physical health. Parental stress also impacts children, often leading kids to act out in negative ways, which causes even more family stress.

In some cases, neglecting your own needs may lead to mental health problems such as depression or anxiety. Poor mental health in parents not only can increase the likelihood of behavioral problems in children but also can increase children's risk of developing their own mental health issues.

On the other hand, when you continually replenish your reserves with self-care, you're ensuring that your own oxygen mask, so to speak, is securely in place. You're giving yourself what you need to nurture and support your child. You're also setting a powerful example for how to live life.

Children are more likely to engage in healthy behaviors such as eating well and being physically active when they see their parents engaging in these healthy habits. When your child sees you treating yourself well, he or she will learn the value of self-care. The bottom line is that when you're happier, your child will be happier.

Self-care involves prioritizing three fundamental elements of living: physical activity, diet and mental health. How much you move your body, what you feed yourself and how you tend to your emotional needs all contribute to your well-being. By tending to your needs in these areas, you'll have the energy, patience and resilience it takes to meet your child's needs.

Physical activity Regular physical activity is one of the cornerstones of self-care. Physical activity can help you control your weight, improve your bone health, and prevent or manage a wide range of health problems. Just as valuable, it can reduce stress, improve your mood and boost your overall energy.

Despite these undeniable benefits, parents tend to get less exercise — or stop exercising altogether — after they have children. Between child care, work and household tasks, many parents struggle to fit regular exercise into their routines. Parents also report feeling guilty about taking time away from their kids.

But by committing to your own physical fitness, you're shoring up your reserves as a parent and modeling healthy behavior for your child. As one parent says, "I just had to get over the guilt and the fear that people would judge me by making the choice to do what I needed to do for myself."

Aim for at least 150 minutes a week of moderate intensity exercise or 75 minutes a week of vigorous exercise. If that sounds daunting, know that some physical activity is better than none. Do what you enjoy — whatever gets you moving. Better yet, involve the whole family. Walk, bike, play basketball or go swimming. Mix it up!

If you're starting from a relatively low level of fitness, ease into increased activity to allow your overall fitness to improve over many months. If you're beginning a new exercise program, be sure to check with your doctor first to make sure it's safe for you.

A healthy diet Good nutrition is another key component to taking care of yourself. A healthy diet helps you control your weight and may lower your risk of certain health conditions such as heart disease and type 2 diabetes. A high-quality diet may also improve your mental health and emotional well-being. Plus, you'll be modeling healthy-eating habits for your child. These are all good reasons

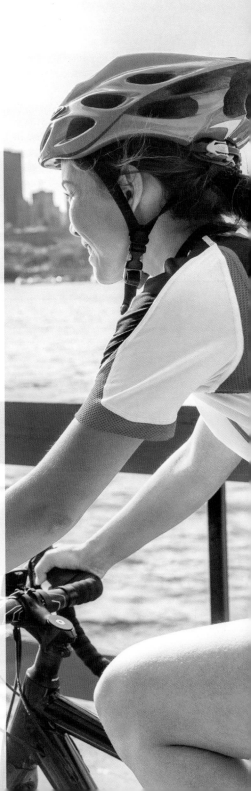

WHEN A PARENT STARTS DATING

If you're a single parent, part of taking care of yourself may include seeking a romantic partner and spending time with that person. While a new relationship can give you a fresh lease on life, it has the potential to create some anxiety in your child.

It's recommended that single parents avoid introducing their children to people they're casually dating. Instead, wait until a serious relationship has begun to develop. Prepare your child for the first encounter by sharing some details about your dating partner and what you like about him or her. Let your partner know about your child's personality and interests. You may even want to suggest some topics of conversation.

Keep the encounter casual and relatively brief, perhaps focused around an activity your child enjoys. Take things slowly, and give your child and your new partner a chance to warm up to each other. This will likely take time and a series of get-togethers.

Your child may feel threatened by your new relationship at first. Your child may express worry, sadness or even anger. Let him or her express these feelings, and help him or her work through those emotions. If you've gone through a divorce, your child may be hanging on to the idea that you and your ex-spouse will someday get back together. Offer reassurance that you and the other parent will continue to love your child the same as always, no matter what.

to make conscious choices about what — and how much — you eat.

Focus on fruits, vegetables and whole grains. Choose low-fat dairy and protein sources, and limit unhealthy fats and added sugars. Eat smaller portions and stay away from junk food. For more on healthy family nutrition, see Chapter 13.

Mental well-being Balancing parenthood with all your other responsibilities can leave you feeling stressed or emotionally drained at times. At the end of a long day, you may be facing a pile of dirty dishes in the sink, your child's bath time and an unfinished work project. Who wouldn't feel a little overwhelmed?

When you're low on your emotional reserves, you have less energy to draw on

for your child. That's why it's as important to invest as much in your mental health as you do in your physical health. When you tend to your emotional well-being, you're better able to cope with the stresses and challenges of parenting. You may still experience negative emotions such as worry or anger, but you can deal with those emotions in a productive way.

Getting regular exercise and eating a healthy diet are two key strategies you can adopt to protect your mental health. In addition, get enough sleep. A good night's sleep is essential for your mental and physical health. Most adults need at least seven hours of sleep a night.

Take time to relax and do things you enjoy. Although you may not have time for all the leisure activities you enjoyed before you had kids, you can still make room for fun. Try to schedule time each day to do something that gives you pleasure, whether it's reading, working out, taking part in a softball league, or quietly savoring a cup of coffee.

Seek out positive people in your life who can help you laugh and lift your spirits. Keep up with your friendships. For example, spend a night out with friends or call a friend just to talk. If you're feeling stressed, sad or frustrated, don't bottle it up. Lean on your social network for support and advice.

If you think you may be experiencing the symptoms of depression, anxiety or chronic stress, don't tough it out alone. Talk to your doctor or seek the guidance of a mental health professional.

ENJOYING PARENTHOOD

Parenthood is a grand adventure, one that challenges and inspires you in ways you may have never imagined. It can be downright terrifying at times, but it can also bring immense joy, opening you to a love and sense of purpose you didn't know was possible. There's nothing like seeing your child's unique personality take shape and celebrating his or her successes along the way.

Balancing that goodness with the demands of parenthood, a career and relationships can be tricky at times. But all of those joys and responsibilities add layers of meaning, purpose and richness to life.

As you continue down the parenthood path into the tween and teen years, remember that what your child will most likely remember in years to come isn't so much what you say or do at any particular moment, but more the person you are and the person you're working to become. If you strive to be your best self, you'll also be the best parent for your child. Trust that you know yourself, your child and your family best and that you have what it takes to navigate the ups and downs of being a parent.

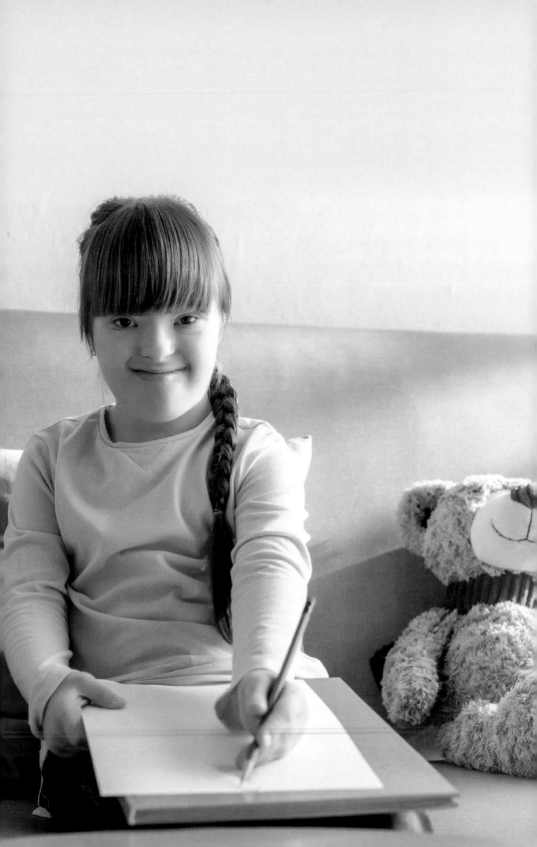

Understanding special education services

If your child is having difficulty with learning or development or has a condition, such as a learning disorder or intellectual disability, he or she may be able to get help at school through special education services. These services are mandated by the federal government under the Individuals with Disabilities Education Act (IDEA). This legislation provides for the free and appropriate public education of students who have certain qualifying disabilities. The law governs how states and public agencies provide these services, including early intervention, special education and related services.

You can start the process by sharing your concerns with your child's teacher and asking them to initiate individualized classroom-based interventions (pre-referral interventions) targeted to your child's school-based needs. Alternatively, you may request an evaluation from your school or school district for your child. If your child is found to be eligible for special education services, school staff will work with you to develop an individual-ized education program (IEP) for your child. An IEP is a written, detailed document outlining specialized instruction, related services and accommodations tailored to the individual student. If a student isn't eligible for an IEP, he or she may qualify for help under a Section 504 plan (see page 465).

For each state, school district and school there may be differences within each of these programs. Contact your local school district and, if necessary, your state Department of Education for detailed, current information about IEPs and Section 504 plans.

ELIGIBILITY

Eligibility for special education services is based on a student meeting criteria for specific disabilities. The national government defines the disabilities. But specific criteria for the disabilities vary by state.

Disabilities may include:

- Specific learning disability (SLD)
  - Oral expression
  - Listening comprehension
  - Written expression
  - Basic reading skill
  - Reading fluency skills
  - Reading comprehension
  - Mathematics calculation
  - Mathematics problem-solving
- Other health impairment (OHI)/other health disability (OHD), including Attention-Deficit/Hyperactivity Disorder (ADHD), Tourette's syndrome (TS), or a complex or long-standing (chronic) medical condition, such as epilepsy
- Visual impairment
- Hearing impairment
- Visual-hearing impairment
- Physical impairment (PI)
- Autism spectrum disorder (ASD)
- Emotional/behavioral disorder (EBD)
- Speech and language impairment (SLI)
- Developmental cognitive disability (DCD)
- Traumatic brain injury (TBI)
- Multiple disabilities, severely multiply impaired (SXI)

Using your state's guidelines, the evaluation team (which includes you) determines whether your child meets the criteria for one or more disability areas and whether he or she needs specialized instruction, related services or both. If your child does meet the criteria, an IEP will be developed by the team.

EVALUATION

Special education is designed for children who have one or more disabilities that interfere with their educational progress. Either school personnel or a parent may request an evaluation to see if a child is eligible for special education services.

Pre-referral interventions If a disability is suspected, a school may suggest initiating one or more pre-referral interventions, in accordance with state guidelines, prior to determining whether a evaluation for special education evaluation is indicated for your child. Pre-referral interventions may provide services that help your child in the mainstream classroom and provide valuable information for school staff to observe how your child responds to instructional or environmental adjustments. If you think your child's concern areas can be adequately addressed through one or more pre-referral interventions, a special education evaluation may not be necessary.

Requesting an evaluation If these interventions aren't meeting your child's needs, you can request a special education evaluation. Or the school staff may suggest moving forward with a comprehensive evaluation of your child if adequate progress isn't observed with the addition of classroom interventions. This evaluation can be started while the pre-referral interventions are being conducted.

When you make a request for an evaluation, the school will typically identify a team of staff members to work with you. With your help, the staff decides which areas your child needs to be evaluated in.

Keep in mind that you always have the right to have your child evaluated by specialists outside of the school district. Private evaluations are generally paid for by the parents. In many states, however, the school is only required to "consider" the recommendations of private evaluations.

SECTION 504 PLAN

If your child doesn't meet the criteria for an individualized education program (IEP) under special education services, another option is a Section 504 plan.

Section 504 is part of the federal Rehabilitation Act of 1973, which prohibits discrimination against people with disabilities. This law requires all schools to make reasonable accommodations within the classroom or other school environments for students with disabilities.

Either you or your child's school staff can request an evaluation for Section 504 plan services. To be eligible for services under a Section 504 plan, a child must have a documented physical or mental disability that significantly affects a body system. This disability must greatly impact at least one major life activity (function), such as walking, talking, hearing, seeing, reading, writing, doing math or learning in general.

The evaluation is conducted by school staff. With your permission, they may collect information from your child's health care providers, such as a doctor, psychologist or therapist to determine eligibility and how best to meet your child's needs.

If you choose, you may have your child evaluated by independent professionals at your own expense. The school district will review that information when you provide a copy to the staff.

Once a disability has been determined, and it's been decided that the student is eligible for services under Section 504, accommodations to help your child learn are considered. These accomodations are similar to those provided by an IEP (see page 468).

Make sure your child's plan is in writing, to aid follow-up and reassessments, if needed. Section 504 plans don't provide direct instructional services. Depending on your child's needs, these accommodations may be helpful enough for him or her to be successful in school. If the accommodations aren't sufficient, an IEP under special education services may be more appropriate.

If your child doesn't qualify for a Section 504 plan and you disagree with the evaluation, there are measures you can take, such as asking the evaluation team in writing to reconsider their decision, filing a grievance, or requesting additional information or testing.

HOW DO THE PLANS COMPARE?

The Section 504 plan and IEP are similar in terms of some of the services and accommodations they provide, but there are also key differences:

Section 504 Plan

Allows only for equal access to free appropriate public education, but there is no guarantee of "educational benefit."

Part of the Americans with Disabilities Act Amendments Act (ADAAA) of 2008.

A child receiving services through a Section 504 plan is not necessarily eligible for IEP services or IDEA protection.

The school system is not reimbursed for expenses related to the plan.

Some modifications and accommodations can be made for studies beyond high school. However, the student is expected to do all required course work at this level. Section 504 plans are also available if a worker has a disability that impairs a major life function — even if he or she still is able to perform the essential parts of the job.

Modifications and accommodations are provided within the typical classroom and school setting. Section 504 plans typically don't provide for direct teaching of skills.

Doesn't require that parents receive written notice about evaluations, meetings and changes to the plan.

Doesn't require monitoring of accommodations or keeping progress notes.

Doesn't require a meeting before changes can be made to the plan and no mandatory reviews.

Doesn't require that the school system and family agree before services are provided. Typically, both school and family work together to provide assistance for the child.

Individualized Education Program (IEP)

A child is entitled to an educational plan that is unique to the child. The child should receive educational benefit when she or he has an IEP.

Part of the Individuals with Disabilities Education Act (IDEA).

A child receiving special education services through an IEP is protected from discrimination under Section 504 of the Rehabilitation Act of 1973.

The school system is reimbursed for some expenses related to implementing an IEP.

Formal modifications and accommodations end once a child receives a high school diploma. Services at most colleges convert to a Section 504 plan.

IEPs provide specialized instruction for students, as well as modifications and accommodations in the classroom — to provide equal access.

Requires that parents receive written notice about evaluations, meetings and changes to the IEP.

Requires documentation of evaluation, placement decision, goals and progress notes.

Requires a meeting of the IEP team before changes can be made to the program.

Guarantees that parents have a right to an independent evaluation at the school's expense when there is disagreement about the evaluation. Identifies steps that may be taken to find a resolution to the problem if there is disagreement about a special education process or service.

As team members review your child's eligibility and needs, with your permission, they may look at records from your child's health care providers, such as your child's doctor, medical specialist, psychologist, or speech, physical or occupational therapist.

Using your state's guidelines, the evaluation team determines whether your child meets the criteria for one or more disability areas and whether he or she needs specialized instruction, related services or both.

Once the evaluation is complete, the team meets with you to share the results and discuss your child's eligibility for services. If your child meets the criteria for one or more disability areas, the next step is to develop an IEP within 30 days.

If you disagree with the results of the evaluation, you have the right to request independent testing outside of the school district at public expense. If the school refuses, there are processes set in place to resolve differences.

ESSENTIAL ELEMENTS

An IEP is a written document providing details of your child's education program. If you agree with the program as it's laid out, you sign it and your child should begin to receive services soon after. If you have concerns about any parts of the proposed services, you can work with the team to make changes before it's set in place.

If you aren't able to reach an agreement as an educational team through means such as mediation, conciliation or a neutrally facilitated IEP meeting, you can pursue additional measures, such as asking for a review of the evaluation, or requesting additional or independent testing. An IEP typically includes the following elements:

Goals and objectives "Goals" are what the team thinks your child should be able to learn or accomplish within the year of the IEP. "Objectives" are the steps that will lead to the accomplishment of those goals. The goals should be based on the needs identified in the evaluation.

Services These are the actions taken by school staff to help your child receive an education. In the services section of the program, there should be listed:
- Specific actions needed by staff to meet the IEP goals
- Amount of time needed this school year to meet the goals
- Expert skills needed to instruct the child so he or she can accomplish the IEP goals and make progress in the general curriculum

Accommodations These are changes needed to help a student learn. They give the student access to what other kids have. Accommodations are intended to meet the unique needs of a student. These accommodations might include:
- *Classroom accommodations.* These changes might include sitting close to the teacher, a contract that rewards desired behaviors, use of an FM system by the teacher to block out background noise or receiving copies of class notes.
- *Assignment accommodations.* Examples include extra time to complete homework, audio books or use of a keyboard to type notes.
- *Testing accommodations.* These accommodations might include taking tests in a quiet area, extra time to complete tests or use of aids such as a calculator or computer-based writing program.

Placement "Placement" is the appropriate location (setting) that will benefit the student. There are a few options for placement, ranging from the total-inclusion model to off-site placement. Some common examples are listed here. These options are typical but not required by law.

▶ *Inclusion model.* This model "includes"the child in the regular curriculum and classroom — for example, music, art, social studies, science — and activities — such as lunch, recess and field trips — as much as possible. For most children, the inclusion model is the most desirable opportunity. A classroom assistant or aide ("paraprofessional") may help integrate the student into the regular education setting. The specifics of this model can vary by school district, school and student.

▶ *Special education environment.* For part or most of the school day, a child may receive education in a classroom setting or "resource room" that can accommodate your child's needs. Examples include a smaller class size, increased one-on-one assistance and more-intensive instruction in certain core academics, such as reading.

▶ *Off-site environment.* Another option is the use of another school or a different setting that meets the child's needs. This option isn't needed often, but it must be available to meet the child's needs if necessary.

ONGOING REVIEW

Using the schedule recorded in the IEP, your child's progress toward meeting annual goals is reviewed by the school staff who provide services. Progress toward meeting the goals must be shared with you at least as often as the school shares progress (report cards) for children without disabilities. The IEP team must update the IEP goals annually.

By law, your child's needs must be re-evaluated every three years — to decide whether the child continues to be eligible for services and to update the child's needs. Re-evaluations may be done more often if a parent or teacher asks for it in writing or if other reasons make it necessary. For example, updates may be needed when your state's criteria change.

Making meals easier

Preparing meals at home doesn't have to eat up all of your time. With some advance planning, you can fit homecooked meals into your family's busy schedule.

In the pages ahead, you'll find a sample week's meal plan. You don't have to follow it step by step, but the suggestions listed will give you an idea of how one or two prep sessions in the kitchen can get you through the week. A few key recipes are provided. For other menu items, find easy recipes you like — say, for grilled chicken or roasted vegetables — in a cookbook or online.

Here are some key concepts for maximizing your time in the kitchen:

Schedule two prep days Set aside two times each week, including at least one weekend day, to do the majority of your food preparation. If you're chopping vegetables for one meal, chop all the vegetables you'll need for the next few days. Store them in clear containers so that you can easily find them when you need them. The same goes for meat or other proteins. If you're grilling or roasting chicken breasts, make a few extra. Use them in tacos or salads.

Make extra and freeze it Double recipes, so that you can eat half now and freeze half for later. This works well with many sauces and casseroles. It's also a good option for individual foods, such as pancakes and uncooked pita pizzas. Make the extras, and place them on a baking sheet in the freezer. Once they're fully frozen, wrap them in plastic wrap to use later.

Have a system Stick to a weekly theme. Taco Tuesday? Check. Meatless Monday? Yes. Kids generally like predictable traditions that they can look forward to. Involve your family in meal planning. They're more likely to eat what they've picked for the menu.

Use ingredients for multiple meals Intentionally plan for leftovers that you can use for quick meals later in the week. For example, extra flank steak on Sunday makes great tacos on Tuesday. A big batch of grains, such as brown rice or lentils, can be a side dish one night and topped with veggies as a main dish for another meal. Use your imagination — the sky's the limit!

SATURDAY MENU

Prep ahead
- Prep fruit and vegetables for the week. Try to keep the same 4 to 5 vegetables rotated through all the meals. Use frozen vegetables to cut down on prep time.
- Make muffins for Tuesday's breakfast (recipe on page 474).

Breakfast
- Whole-wheat blueberry pancakes*
- Fruit

Lunch
- Grilled cheese with whole-wheat bread and tomato slices

Snack
- Apples with cheese or nut butter

Dinner
- Grilled, broiled, sauteed or poached chicken breasts*†
- Brown rice* (follow package instructions)
- Steamed or roasted vegetables*†

Make extra chicken, rice and vegetables to use throughout the week.

*Good for multiple meals
†Use a favorite recipe

WHOLE-WHEAT BLUEBERRY PANCAKES
Makes 12 pancakes

Double this recipe and then freeze half the pancakes, separated by parchment paper. On a busy morning, just warm up frozen pancakes in the oven or toaster.

1⅓ cup white whole-wheat flour
2 teaspoons baking powder
1 tablespoon sugar
½ teaspoon cinnamon
1⅓ cup skim milk
1 egg, lightly beaten
1 tablespoon canola oil
1 cup fresh or frozen whole blueberries

1. In a large bowl, mix flour, baking powder, sugar and cinnamon together.
2. In another bowl, beat milk, egg and oil together. Add the liquid mixture to the flour mixture, and stir until the flour is moistened.
3. Add blueberries and stir gently.
4. Coat a griddle or skillet with cooking spray and heat to medium-high heat. Pour about ¼ cup of batter onto the hot griddle and cook until browned. Flip and brown the other side.

Per serving (2 pancakes):

Calories	158
Total fat	4 g
Saturated fat	1 g
Trans fat	0 g
Monounsaturated fat	2 g
Cholesterol	35 mg
Sodium	240 mg
Total carbohydrate	28 g
Dietary fiber	4 g
Sugars	7 g
Protein	6 g

SUNDAY MENU

Prep ahead
- Hard-boil eggs for snacks for the week.

Breakfast
- Veggie egg bake* (recipe on page 477; make extra and freeze for Thursday's lunch)
- Fruit

Lunch
- Chicken Caesar pita pockets‡

Stuff pita pockets with leftover chicken from Saturday's dinner and premade Caesar salad mix.

- Fruit

Snack
- Hard-boiled egg
- Fresh veggie sticks

Dinner
- Quick and easy chili*
  (make extra for Monday's lunch)
- Salad
- Cornmeal muffins

*Good for multiple meals
‡Use leftovers from previous meal

Per serving (about 1½ cups):

Calories	225
Total fat	11 g
Saturated fat	4 g
Trans fat	0 g
Monounsaturated fat	4 g
Cholesterol	39 mg
Sodium	260 mg
Total carbohydrate	24 g
Dietary fiber	8 g
Sugars	0 g
Protein	18 g

QUICK AND EASY CHILI
Serves 8

To make a vegetarian version, substitute a can of black beans or chickpeas for the ground beef.

1 pound extra-lean ground beef
½ cup chopped onion
2 large tomatoes (or 2 cups canned, unsalted tomatoes)
4 cups canned unsalted kidney beans, rinsed and drained
1 cup chopped celery
1½ tablespoons chili powder or to taste
Water, as desired
2 tablespoons cornmeal
Jalapeno peppers, seeded and chopped, as desired (not included in nutrition analysis)

1. In a soup pot, add the ground beef and onion. Over medium heat, saute until the meat is browned and the onion is translucent. Drain well.

2. Add the tomatoes, kidney beans, celery and chili powder to the ground beef mixture. Cover and cook for 10 minutes, stirring frequently. Uncover and add water to desired consistency. Stir in cornmeal. Cook at least 10 minutes more to allow the flavors to blend.

3. Ladle into warmed bowls, and garnish with jalapeno peppers, if desired. Serve immediately.

MONDAY MENU

Prep ahead
* Assemble the creamy cheesy macaroni so that it's ready to bake in the evening.

Breakfast
* Whole-grain cereal with fruit

Lunch
* Chili‡ (leftover from Sunday's dinner)
* Whole-wheat crackers

Snack
* Whole-wheat tortilla roll-up with banana and nut butter

Dinner
* Creamy cheesy macaroni* ······················
* Steamed broccoli

*Good for multiple meals
‡Use leftovers from previous meal

Per serving (1 cup):

Calories	300
Total fat	11 g
Saturated fat	5 g
Trans fat	0 g
Monounsaturated fat	4 g
Cholesterol	27 mg
Sodium	292 mg
Total carbohydrate	41 g
Dietary fiber	4 g
Sugars	0 g
Protein	18 g

CREAMY CHEESY MACARONI
Serves 10

Make an extra batch, wrap tightly with foil or plastic wrap, and freeze for another time.

1 package (14.5 ounces) whole-wheat elbow macaroni
1½ cups fat-free cottage cheese
2 tablespoons canola oil
½ cup flour
½ teaspoon ground black pepper
¼ teaspoon garlic powder
2 cups skim milk
2 cups reduced-fat sharp cheddar cheese, shredded
2 cups halved cherry tomatoes
Fresh parsley for garnish, optional

1. Cook macaroni according to package directions. Meanwhile, blend cottage cheese in a food processor or blender until smooth. Set aside.

2. In a large saucepan over medium heat, combine oil, flour, pepper and garlic powder. Stir until mixed. Gradually stir in the milk and bring to a boil. Cook for 2 minutes or until thickened and smooth. Add cottage cheese and cheddar cheese, stirring until melted.

3. Spray a 2-quart casserole dish with cooking spray. After the macaroni has been cooked and drained, place it in the prepared dish. Pour the cheese mixture over the macaroni and mix until blended. Bake at 350 F for about 30 minutes, or until heated through. Top with tomatoes just before serving.

TUESDAY MENU

Prep ahead
- Prep taco fillings*.

Breakfast
- Morning glory muffins* (made Saturday)
- Fruit

Lunch
- Barbecue chicken‡ salad

Shred cooked chicken from Saturday's dinner and toss with a small amount of barbecue sauce. Mound over a bed of greens and top with cherry tomatoes, corn and black beans.

Snack
- Vegetables and dip

Dinner
- Tacos†‡

Build your own tacos with a protein, vegetable and salsa in a tortilla shell. For example, combine baked fish sticks with shredded lettuce, guacamole and fresh salsa.

*Good for multiple meals
† Use a favorite recipe
‡Use leftovers from previous meal

Per serving (1 muffin):

Calories	180
Total fat	8 g
Saturated fat	1 g
Trans fat	Trace
Monounsaturated fat:	2 g
Cholesterol	31 mg
Sodium	156 mg
Total carbohydrate	26 g
Dietary fiber	2 g
Sugars	14 g
Protein	3 g

MORNING GLORY MUFFINS
Serves 18

Freeze the muffins you won't eat, and pull them out of the freezer as needed. Freezing the muffins keeps them fresher longer. Warm the muffins slightly before serving. For variety, try shredded zucchini in place of the chopped apples.

1 cup all-purpose (plain) flour
1 cup whole-wheat flour
¾ cup sugar
2 teaspoons baking soda
2 teaspoons ground cinnamon
3 eggs
½ cup vegetable oil
½ cup unsweetened applesauce
2 teaspoons vanilla extract
2 cups chopped apples (unpeeled)
½ cup raisins
¾ cup grated carrots
2 tablespoons chopped pecans

1. Heat the oven to 350 F. Line a muffin pan with paper or foil liners.

2. In a large bowl, combine the flours, sugar, baking soda and cinnamon. Whisk to blend evenly. In a separate bowl, add the eggs, oil, applesauce and vanilla. Stir in the apples, raisins and carrots. Add the egg mixture to the flour mixture and blend just until moistened and slightly lumpy.

3. Spoon the batter into muffin cups, filling each about ⅔ full. Sprinkle with chopped pecans and bake until springy to the touch, about 35 minutes. Let cool for 5 minutes, then transfer the muffins to a wire rack and let cool completely.

WEDNESDAY MENU

Prep ahead
• Remove the veggie egg bake from the freezer for Thursday's lunch.

Breakfast
• Scrambled eggs with veggies
• Whole-wheat toast

Lunch
• Black bean and cheese quesadilla[†‡]

Warm a large tortilla in a skillet and top with black beans and cheese. When cheese is melted, fold tortilla in half and slip onto a plate. Dip in salsa.

Snack
• Hummus with fresh veggie sticks

Dinner
• Fried rice[‡]

Use leftover rice from Saturday's dinner.

• Fresh-cut fruit, such as oranges or pineapple

[†] Use a favorite recipe
[‡] Use leftovers from previous meal

Per serving (about 1 cup):

Calories	279
Total fat	16 g
Saturated fat	3 g
Trans fat	Trace
Monounsaturated fat	7 g
Cholesterol	47 mg
Sodium	116 mg
Total carbohydrate	31 g
Dietary fiber	4 mg
Sugars	0 g
Protein	6 g

FRIED RICE
Serves 4

Rice that's been cooked and refrigerated overnight (or longer — up to 3 days) makes better fried rice because the rice tends to clump together.

2 cups cooked brown rice
3 tablespoons peanut oil (or vegetable oil)
4 green onions with tops, chopped
2 carrots, finely chopped
½ cup finely chopped green bell pepper
½ cup frozen peas
1 egg
2 tablespoons low-sodium soy sauce
1 tablespoon sesame oil
¼ cup chopped parsley

1. In a large heavy skillet or wok, heat the oil over medium-high heat. Add cooked rice and saute until lightly golden. Add green onions, carrots, green pepper and peas. Stir-fry until vegetables are tender-crisp, about 5 minutes.

2. Hollow out a circle in the center of the skillet by pushing the vegetables and rice to the sides. Break the egg into the hollow and cook, lightly scrambling the egg as it cooks. Stir the scrambled egg into the rice mixture. Sprinkle with soy sauce, sesame oil and chopped parsley.

3. Serve immediately.

THURSDAY MENU

Prep ahead
* Start the pizza dough for Friday, if making it from scratch.

Breakfast
* Morning glory muffins‡

Lunch
* Veggie egg bake‡
* Fruit

Snack
* Cheese stick with crackers or handful of nuts

Dinner
* Pasta with sausage,* bell peppers and onions†

  Cook sausage (reserve extra for Friday night's pizza). Add sliced bell peppers and onions. Cook until vegetables soften. Toss with cooked pasta and a small amount of pasta cooking water.

*Good for multiple meals
† Use a favorite recipe
‡ Use leftovers from previous meal

FRIDAY MENU

Prep ahead
* Assemble the pizza so that it's ready to bake in the evening.

Breakfast
* Whole-wheat blueberry pancakes‡

Lunch
* Hard-boiled egg and avocado on toast, or nut butter and banana sandwich
* Sliced veggies

Snack
* Yogurt cup with fruit

Dinner
* Whole-wheat pizza with sausage‡ and broccoli

  Use a ready-made pizza crust or pita bread or make your own favorite dough. Top with pizza sauce, reserved sausage from Thursday's dinner, lightly steamed broccoli and shredded mozzarella. Bake until crust is crisp.

‡Use leftovers from previous meal

VEGGIE EGG BAKE
Serves 6

Double this recipe, and split it between two pans to have extra for freezing (or use a muffin pan for individual servings). You could also prepare this casserole the night before and refrigerate. The next morning, let the casserole stand at room temperature while oven heats and then bake as directed.

1 cup frozen chopped spinach, thawed
6 large eggs
1 cup skim milk
1 teaspoon dry mustard
1 teaspoon dried rosemary or 1 tablespoon minced fresh rosemary
½ teaspoon salt-free herb-and-spice blend
¼ teaspoon ground black pepper
6 slices whole-grain bread, crusts removed and cut into 1-inch cubes
¼ cup chopped onion
½ cup diced red pepper
4 ounces thinly sliced reduced-fat Swiss cheese

1. Heat oven to 375 F. Coat a 7-by-11-inch glass baking dish or a 2-quart casserole with cooking spray.
2. Place the spinach in a strainer and press with the back of a spatula to remove excess liquid. Set aside.
3. In a medium bowl, whisk together eggs and milk. Add dry mustard, rosemary, spice blend and pepper; whisk to combine.
4. Toss spinach, bread, onion and red pepper in a large bowl. Add egg mixture and toss to coat.
5. Transfer to prepared baking dish and push down to compact. Cover with foil. Bake for 30 minutes or until the eggs have set.
6. Uncover and top with cheese. Continue baking for an additional 15 minutes or until the top is lightly browned.
7. Transfer to a wire rack and cool for 10 minutes before serving.

Per serving (a 3½-by-3½-inch piece):

Calories	258
Total fat	10 g
Saturated fat	4 g
Trans fat	0 g
Monounsaturated fat	2 g
Cholesterol	137 mg
Sodium	465 mg
Total carbohydrate	25 g
Dietary fiber	3 g
Sugars	0 g
Protein	17 g

PAIN RELIEVER DOSAGE BY WEIGHT

Acetaminophen (Tylenol, others)

Dosage

Weight	Infant or children's oral suspension 160 mg per 5 mL	Children's chewable tablet 80 mg	Junior strength chewable tablet 160 mg	Adult tablet 325 mg	Adult extra strength tablet 500 mg
6 to 11 lbs.	1.25 mL (40 mg)	–	–	–	–
12 to 17 lbs.	2.5 mL (80 mg)	–	–	–	–
18 to 23 lbs.	3.75 mL (120 mg)	–	–	–	–
24 to 35 lbs.	5 mL (160 mg)	2 tablets (160 mg)	1 tablet (160 mg)	–	–
36 to 47 lbs.	7.5 mL (240 mg)	3 tablets (240 mg)	1½ tablets (240 mg)	–	–
48 to 59 lbs.	10 mL (320 mg)	4 tablets (320 mg)	2 tablets (320 mg)	1 tablet (325 mg)	–
60 to 71 lbs.	12.5 mL (400 mg)	5 tablets (400 mg)	2½ tablets (400 mg)	1 tablet (325 mg)	–
72 to 95 lbs.	15 mL (480 mg)	6 tablets (480 mg)	3 tablets (480 mg)	1½ tablets (487.5 mg)	1 tablet (500 mg)
96 to 146 lbs.	–	–	4 tablets (640 mg)	2 tablets (650 mg)	1 tablet (500 mg)

Source: Mayo Clinic

Use only the enclosed medication dispenser that comes with the product. (Kitchen teaspoons are not accurate measures for medication.)

Dose may be given every 4 hours. Do not use the medication more than 5 times in 24 hours.

The following abbreviations are used on this dosage chart: • Milligram (mg) • Milliliter (mL) • Pounds (lbs.)

Not applicable: –. This form of medication should not be given to a child of this weight.

Ibuprofen (Advil, Motrin, others)

Weight	Infant drops or oral suspension 50 mg per 1.25 mL	Children's oral suspension 100 mg per 5 mL	Children's chewable tablet 50 mg	Junior strength caplet or chewable tablet 100 mg	Adult tablet 200 mg
			Dosage		
12 to 17 lbs.	1.25 mL (50 mg)	–	–	–	–
18 to 23 lbs.	1.875 mL (75 mg)	–	–	–	–
24 to 35 lbs.	–	5 mL (100 mg)	2 tablets (100 mg)	1 tablets (100 mg)	–
36 to 47 lbs.		7.5 mL (150 mg)	3 tablets (150 mg)	1½ tablets (150 mg)	–
48 to 59 lbs.	–	10 mL (200 mg)	4 tablets (200 mg)	2 tablets (200 mg)	1 tablet (200 mg)
60 to 71 lbs.	–	12.5 mL (250 mg)	5 tablets (250 mg)	2½ tablets (250 mg)	1 tablet (200 mg)
72 to 95 lbs.	–	15 mL (300 mg)	6 tablets (300 mg)	3 tablets (300 mg)	1½ tablets (300 mg)
Greater than 95 lbs.	–	20 mL (400 mg)	8 tablets (400 mg)	4 tablets (400 mg)	2 tablets (400 mg)

Source: Mayo Clinic.

For a child who is younger than 6 months old, ask your child's medical provider before giving ibuprofen.

If giving less than 100 mg, use infant drops.

Use only the enclosed medication dispenser that comes with the product. (Kitchen teaspoons are not accurate measures for medication.)

Dose may be given every 6 to 8 hours. Do not use the medication more than 4 times in 24 hours.

The following abbreviations are used on this dosage chart: • Milligram (mg) • Milliliter (mL) • Pounds (lbs.)

Not applicable: –. This form of medication should not be given to a child of this weight.

Additional resources

AMERICAN ACADEMY OF PEDIATRICS
www.aap.org
Find the latest news and research, helpful tips, and more.

AMERICAN RED CROSS
www.redcross.org
Register for a class on pediatric first aid and CPR near you.

CENTER FOR PARENT INFORMATION AND RESOURCES
www.parentcenterhub.org
Explore information for parents of children with disabilities. Use the search tool to find your local parent center.

CENTERS FOR DISEASE CONTROL AND PREVENTION
www.cdc.gov
Learn about vaccines, healthy travel, food safety, common illnesses, and more.

CHILD MIND INSTITUTE
www.childmind.org
Find information on the child brain, associated disorders and mental health.

CHOOSEMYPLATE.GOV — CHILDREN
www.choosemyplate.gov/children
Explore interactive resources on balanced nutrition, different food groups and picky eaters, and find kid-friendly recipes.

COMMON SENSE MEDIA
www.commonsensemedia.org
Get age-appropriate reviews and ratings on movies, books and more.

CONNECTSAFELY
www.connectsafely.org
Get the latest parent-directed information on social media apps, online safety and cyberbullying.

FAMILIES EMPOWERED AND SUPPORTING TREATMENT OF EATING DISORDERS (F.E.A.S.T.)
www.feast-ed.org
Connect with a coalition of parents that advocates for research and education on eating disorders and provides a network of support to families affected by the disorders.

HEALTHYCHILDREN.ORG FROM THE AMERICAN ACADEMY OF PEDIATRICS
www.healthychildren.org
Find expert information on children's nutrition, safety, behavior and wellness, geared especially toward parents.

MAYO CLINIC
www.MayoClinic.org
Visit Mayo Clinic's online health information portal, which includes a range of articles related to children's health.

NATIONAL EATING DISORDERS ASSOCIATION
www.nationaleatingdisorders.org
Learn about eating disorders; find support for getting started on the road to recovery.

NATIONAL HIGHWAY TRAFFIC SAFETY ADMINISTRATION — CAR SEATS
www.nhtsa.gov/equipment/car-seats-and-booster-seats
Use the interactive guide to find the right car seat or booster seat for your child; get tips for installation.

NATIONAL INSTITUTE OF MENTAL HEALTH
www.nimh.nih.gov
Get the basics and more on a variety of behavioral and mental health conditions that affect children.

PACER CENTER
www.pacer.org
Find information, workshops and other resources on education for children with disabilities or complex health care needs.

PACER'S NATIONAL BULLYING PREVENTION CENTER
www.pacer.org/bullying
Find out what parents need to know about bullying, and learn what adults and children can do to address and prevent bullying.

POISON HELP
www.poisonhelp.org
Get online help for a possible poisoning. Call 800-222-1222 in the U.S. to talk to someone directly.

Index

O

obesity
avoid "diets" and, 220
avoid teasing and, 221
avoid weight talk and, 220–221
BMI measurement and, 228
causes of, 227
childhood epidemic, 229
determining, 228–229
eating at home and, 230
eating better together and, 230–233
family lifestyle choices and, 227
5-2-1-0 method and, 232
managing resistance and, 234–235
overview, 227
physical activity and, 233–234
preventing, 219–225
problem, not ignoring, 235
sweet drinks and, 231
technology and, 64
OCD (obsessive-compulsive disorder)
behaviors, 289
defined, 289–290
diagnosing, 290
exposure and response prevention
therapy and, 290
medications, 290
parenting a child with, 290–293
tics, 291
treating, 290
See also mental health concerns
ODD (oppositional defiant disorder)
ADHD and, 374
consistency in approach to, 300
defined, 299
finding help for, 299–300
symptoms of, 299
treatment for, 300
**off-site environment, special education
services,** 469
omega-3 fatty acids, 212
organization
time management and, 63
in work and home balance, 450–451
OSA (obstructive sleep apnea), 125
outside time, 234
overdosing medicine, 304
"overscheduling," 29

P

parasomnias
confusional arousals, 122–123
defined, 122
nightmares, 124–125
sleep talking, 124
sleepwalking, 123–124
See also sleep and nighttime issues
parent-coach relationship, 194–195
parenthood, enjoying, 461
parenting
adoptive, 433–434
appreciating child and, 19
child with OCD (obsessive-compulsive
disorder), 290–293
complex needs, 408–423
co-parenting, 426–427
enjoying, 19
foster, 434–435
grandparenting, 429–432
helicopter, 256
humor and, 21
key points in, 19–21
mindful, 454–456
same-sex, 432–433
self-care and, 19–21
single, 428–429
time for reflection and, 19
trusting instincts and, 19
parenting together
agreed course of action and, 442
avoiding tight spots and, 442–443
backing each other up, 442
beliefs, 440
blending styles and, 440–442
characteristics of, 439
communication, 440
consistency and, 439–442
couple relationship and, 445
dealing with problems as they arise
and, 443–444
helping each other evolve and, 445
modeling healthy habits and, 446–447
offer and ask for help and, 445–446
positive focus, 444–445
priorities, 440
relationship as foundation, 447
standing up for each other and, 445
styles, 441
supporting each other, 444–446

IMAGE CREDITS

The individuals pictured are models, and the photos are used for illustrative purposes only. There is no correlation between the individuals portrayed and the subjects being discussed.

Cover, spine and page 477 photographs by Bill Tyler. Illustrations on pages 168, 169, 173, 176 and 177 by John Karapelou. All photographs and illustrations are copyright of MFMER, except for the following: